Moreton Morrell Site

D1586749

Feline
Medicine

A Practical Guide for Veterinary
Nurses and Technicians

Moreton Morrell Site

For Elsevier:

Commissioning Editor: Mary Seager
Development Editor: Rebecca Nelemans
Project Manager: Caroline Horton
Designer: Andy Chapman
Illustration Manager: Bruce Hogarth

Feline Medicine

A Practical Guide for Veterinary Nurses and Technicians

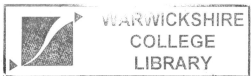

Edited by

Martha Cannon BA VetMB DSAM(Fel)
RCVS Specialist in Feline Medicine

Myra Forster-van Hijfte DVM CertVR CertSAM DipECVIM
MRCVS
European and RCVS Specialist in Small Animal Medicine

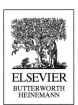

ELSEVIER
BUTTERWORTH
HEINEMANN

Elsevier Butterworth Heinemann

Edinburgh   London   New York   Oxford   Philadelphia   St Louis   Sydney   Toronto   2006

ELSEVIER
BUTTERWORTH
HEINEMANN

First published 2006

ISBN 0 7506 8827 0

British Library Cataloguing in Publication Data
A catalogue record for this book is available from the British Library

Library of Congress Cataloging in Publication Data
A catalog record for this book is available from the Library of Congress

Printed in China

Working together to grow
libraries in developing countries

www.elsevier.com | www.bookaid.org | www.sabre.org

ELSEVIER   BOOK AID International   Sabre Foundation

The Publisher's policy is to use **paper manufactured from sustainable forests**

CONTENTS

CONTRIBUTORS

Graham Bilbrough MA VetMB CertVA MRCVS

Rachel Burbidge PHC VN

Martha Cannon BA VetMB DSAM(Fel) MRCVS

Julie Cory DipAVN(Medical) VN

Myra Forster-van Hijfte DVM CertVR CertSAM DipECVIM MRCVS

Rebecca Giles C&G CertSAN VN

Susan Howarth DipAVN(Surgical) DipAVN(Medical) VN

Annette Litster BVSc PhD FACVSc(Feline Medicine)

Paul Manning MA VetMB MSc(VetGP) MRCVS

Valerie Pollard DipAVN(Surgical) VN

Jacquie Rand BVSc DVSc DipACVIM

Perdi Welsh BSc(Hons) DipAVN(Surgical) CertED VN

PREFACE

"The smallest feline is a masterpiece."

Leonardo da Vinci

As specialists in feline veterinary care we have long been aware of the unique value of working with competent, caring nurses who really understand cats and their needs. Veterinary nurses are at the heart of every small animal veterinary practice: they are key providers of patient care, and form a vital link between pets, vets and owners. A good veterinary nurse is an immensely valuable member of any veterinary practice team, and as the nursing profession continues to develop and expand, their role becomes ever more significant.

Cats are wonderful creatures, but they can be challenging to work with and they are different to other pet animal species in so many ways. The aim of this book is to provide a practical guide to all aspects of feline veterinary nursing and to encourage nurses to give cats the individual care and consideration that they deserve. It has been written by authors who have a depth of practical experience either as veterinary nurses or as veterinary surgeons, all of whom understand the pressures and challenges of modern veterinary practice.

We hope that all veterinary nurses, from the newest student to the most experienced feline nurse will find something new and interesting in this book, and that as well as offering a wealth of tips on cat care, cat handling and common nursing procedures it will also be a rapid reference source to help to answer those difficult telephone enquiries that crop up so often in day to day veterinary work. If this book helps to explain why cats are so special, and helps to make working with them safer and more enjoyable, then we will have achieved our aim.

Martha Cannon
Myra Forster-van Hijfte

CHAPTER 1

FELINE BEHAVIOUR

Julie Cory, DipAVN(Medical) VN

An understanding of feline behaviour and of the cat's social structure is important when handling or owning a cat. A knowledge of normal feline behaviour helps us appreciate what issues are relevant to a cat, understand how behavioural problems may arise and decide what can be done to modify the animal's behaviour.

1.1   SOCIAL BEHAVIOUR

Feline social behaviour is very different from that of other domestic animals. Dogs, sheep, cattle, etc. live in large groups and have a hierarchical system in place to determine who makes the decisions. Dogs are known for being territorial, but often they are more attached to their owners or to other dogs, than to the physical place that they live in. In contrast the cats that we keep as pets have evolved from the 'small' wild cats. They are solitary hunters of small prey so they do not require the help of others and do not need to remain in groups for survival – hence no dominance hierarchy and no underlying motivation to stay in a particular area or with particular individuals. It is not unusual for a cat to move next door if the conditions at home are not favourable.

The domestication process in cats has evolved more gradually than for other species, involving an association between people and cats rather than a domination of cats by people. From a management point of view, this means that cats are more independent and self-sufficient than other domestic animals. As the saying goes 'a dog will hear your command and rush to obey, a cat will hear the command and get back to you!'

Social groups

Cats work on a system of mutual tolerance and will accept company, but will not go looking for it. This has lead to the common belief that they are a solitary species, disdaining all company. This is a generalisation, and while some cats will spend large amounts of time alone, others can be very affectionate to their owners and other cats in the household. Feral cats may live in large communities, often sharing duties such as raising the kittens or spending time mutually grooming each other (allogrooming). Cooperation between these cats requires certain key factors to be in place, and while there is no sharing of resources as can be seen in truly social animals like the dog, there is little fighting over the resources either.

Feral groups of cats occur in areas where food is plentiful, often supplemented by humans. Food is acquired on a 'first come, first served' basis and access to it is not determined by rank, so there must be adequate supplies if everyone in the community is to eat. Access to space and shelter work along the same principles, with favourite areas being occupied rather than defended. If the cat is not in the resting area, another cat can sleep there without causing offence – providing other areas of seclusion and safety are available.

These key resources of space and food may be lacking in a home environment that is closely controlled by humans, leading to disharmony between cats in the household. Cats are frequently acquired because of physical appearance (e.g. breed, coat length or colour) or are acquired as strays, without due consideration being given to their personalities, and to whether there is adequate space for the newcomer. This frequently causes problems with the existing cat(s) in the household as the newcomer establishes itself within the territory.

The population dynamics of large feral cat communities are also interesting when compared with those of the home environment in which pet cats are expected to live. Most feral communities consist of related female cats, with a resident tom (or two, depending on the number of females present). From a management and behavioural point of view keeping groups of female cats within a household may be preferable to keeping groups of males. Similarly, cats raised together from a young age may be more tolerant of each other than older cats that are introduced to the group later in life.

As we have seen cats are often more attached to their territory than to their owners. The home ranges of owned female cats generally cover their house and garden, and may extend into neighbouring gardens if there are no resident females there. This home area will be claimed by marking the periphery with faecal deposits. A male's home range can be three times the size of a female territory and overlaps several female home ranges. The exact size will depend on the number of females, whether it is the breeding season and whether the male is neutered or not. With the increasing incidence of neutering, the home range of an entire tom can be very considerable in order for him to find an un-neutered female.

It is now known that a cat's personality characteristics are largely inherited from the father. It appears that confident, bold fathers produce confident, bold kittens regardless of their mother's personality. The majority of friendly, affectionate males are homed and neutered, whereas entire males tend to be the less social, more aggressive cats that do not settle into a pet cat home. Could this be leading to an 'evolutionary' change in the personality of mixed breed kittens? If so, educating these kittens during their critical socialisation period (see below) may become more important than ever.

The socialisation period

The early weeks of a kitten's life are a critical period in its behavioural development. It is a period during which a sense of what is normal and what is potentially dangerous becomes established, which will help to orientate the adult animal in a human-centred world. During this vital window of time, known as the 'socialisation period', the kitten learns to cope with living with other animals. Exploration, play and interaction with mother and litter mates prepares the kitten for social encounters with other cats and develops behaviour patterns for maintaining social bonds with its own species and with any non-feline species such as humans and dogs that the kitten is in contact with. This early socialisation to humans may be an important factor in the acceptance of human affection later in life, and in developing tolerance of our primate displays of social attachment – hugging, stroking and so on.

The socialisation period starts a little earlier in kittens than in dogs, but is equally important in establishing normal parameters for the things that the cat will share its life with. This critical period of development starts at around 2 weeks of age when the kitten's ears and eyes open and it starts to discover an exciting world. Young kittens are notorious for getting into mischief involving curtains, furniture, people's legs, dogs, and so on; their thirst to explore, investigate and try new things is unquenchable, and this helps to build a picture of their world, as well as to develop strength and coordination. This is a period of reduced fear, but it is not completely absent so that very frightening encounters will be remembered and avoided for the duration of the cat's life.

The timing of the end of the socialisation period is less clear, but from around 8 weeks of age, or perhaps a little later, the kitten enters a new stage of development marked by a more cautious approach to life and to new experiences, with a degree of restraint being shown before a new cat, dog or person is approached and investigated. This new suspicion of novelty can extend to food items, with different textures or tastes being refused in preference to more familiar items.

Ensuring that young kittens are raised in a complex, interesting environment, and that they are handled by a wide range of people, and exposed to other cats and to dogs, will go a long way towards ensuring that the kitten grows up to be a friendly, confident and 'well-adjusted' pet. This is made more challenging in cats than in dogs, because kittens often remain with their breeder until after the socialisation period has finished, so the responsibility for socialisation falls on the owner of the kitten's mother, rather than on the kitten's new owner.

Owners should be advised to question breeders on their socialisation programme for kittens, while hand-reared kittens should also be gently exposed to a variety of situations so that novelty is seen as good and does not induce fear.

Applying social behaviour to pet cats

By understanding the normal social structure of cats we can look at the environments we place them in, and suggest ways of reducing stress and improving their quality of life in our care.

Cats live in a three-dimensional world, and as solitary animals that rely on their physical strength to hunt for food they need to look after themselves, and look out for potential danger at all times. This may help to explain why they feel more secure in a raised area where they are out of harm's way and can see trouble approaching. At home we can utilise the space within quite a small area by providing shelves, cupboards, climbing frames, and so on. This not only allows the cat to escape unwanted attention, but allows several sleeping areas if there are multiple cats in the household. By providing several raised areas each cat can choose where they want to sleep at any one time, and this reduces conflict over occupied places. Similarly, other resources such as litter trays and feed bowls need to be numerous, to avoid the need for two cats to use the same 'station' at the same time as another cat, which increases the potential for conflict.

Movement between different resource sites, especially sleeping areas, can improve the relationship between cats in the household, or between cats and their owners, through the sharing of communal scent. Familiar scents on resting places such as cat beds, sofas or human beds help cats to develop a sense of group identity that more gregarious species achieve through body language, allogrooming and social play. The feline system of shared scent is more subtle, but no less meaningful in providing a sense of familiarity and therefore security.

BOX 1.1   KEY POINTS

- Cat society does not involve a hierarchy so they are more self-sufficient and independent.
- Cats do not require the help of others, so social groups are tolerated rather than actively sought.
- Ample resources are required for numbers of cats to live together harmoniously.

1.2   FELINE COMMUNICATION

To understand feline behaviour, we need to appreciate the different ways in which cats communicate with each other and with humans. The signs are often there, but are less conspicuous than in some species and are easily missed. The owner's account of the cat's behaviour at home, or careful observations over a period of time will be required to determine what is going on in the cat's mind.

Body language

Cats are not a gregarious social species and their body language and vocalisations are more subtle than dogs. They are less forthcoming with their intentions and their communication repertoire is smaller, particularly with regard to the 'come closer' signals, so understanding feline communication can be quite challenging. Nevertheless, since vision is the human's primary sense, we find this method of communication the easiest to interpret and can become fairly good at identifying the messages being portrayed.

The most familiar type of communication in cats is the 'stay away' set of signals, involving raised hackles, arched back, flattened ears and accompanying hissing or growling (see Fig. 1.1). This set of gestures is generally very obvious and effective.

Dogs have several different facial expressions, body postures and gestures that encourage others to interact, fuss or play with them. Cats have far fewer 'come closer' gestures, although that is not to say that they are absent. Some postures have developed to communicate with humans, such as the 'tail up' signal seen when greeting owners or familiar people. The cat's tail is held vertical with a slight kink at the tip (see Fig. 1.2), often gently quivering, similar to a spraying posture but much more relaxed – and without producing any urine. Used in combination with vocalisations such as chirruping or meowing, and scent marking such as rubbing, this is a clear message of ownership, familiarity and social bonding.

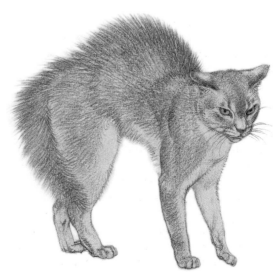

Figure 1.1 'Stay away' signals – with raised hackles, arched back, flattened ears and accompanying hissing or growling.

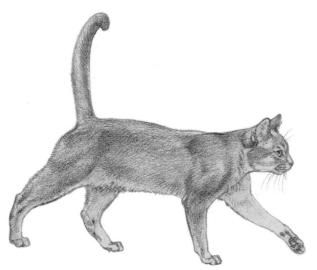

Figure 1.2 When greeting familiar people the cat's tail is held vertical with a slight kink at the tip.

Tail wagging in cats is often seen as a sign of displeasure, but a gentle, relaxed wave can indicate contentment. It may be helpful to compare tail wagging in cats to foot tapping in people. A gentle tap can indicate contentment, whereas stamping and agitated tapping often conveys annoyance. A relaxed gentle swaying can escalate to a rigid, purposeful swish of the tail if the cat becomes more agitated.

Eye contact is another area of body language in which the difference between relaxation and aggression can be subtle. A fleeting glance combined with relaxed facial muscles is acceptable to cats, whereas tense facial muscles and a prolonged stare from other cats or humans can be very intimidating and threatening.

The combination of ear position and height of body can be used to communicate a perceived level of threat. The lower the body to the ground and the flatter the ears, the more intimidated the cat feels. Ears that are folded back as well as flat suggest a frightened cat (see Fig. 1.3), while ears that are flat and pointed away from the head suggest an annoyed cat without as much fear (see Fig. 1.4). Again, there are important differences between dogs and cats here. In a dog, a lowered body posture indicates fear and submission. In a cat, it simply allows the cat to roll over and release

Figure 1.3 A frightened cat, with ears that are folded back as well as flat.

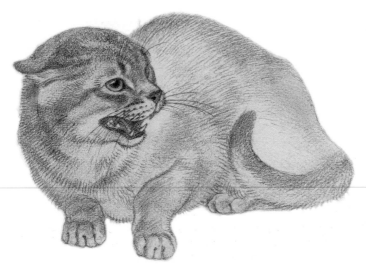

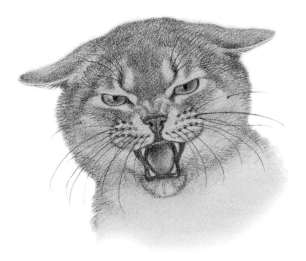

Figure 1.4 Ears held flat and pointed away from the head suggest an angry, but frightened cat.

all its weapons, i.e. its teeth and claws. Raised body postures in cats, such as an arched back, are often adopted in response to surprise or insecurity and maintain the option of running away.

Communicating by marking

Humans are very poor at communicating by scent. Strong smelling aromas such as coffee or freshly baked bread can elicit certain feelings of wellbeing or evoke associations with previous memories, however, this ability is very crude compared with a cat's sense of smell. As previously described, shared scents and the smell of familiar cats can communicate friendship and acceptance. Cats have a number of sebaceous scent glands in their skin, especially around the head, the base of the tail, and the feet. These can be used to deposit scent markings by rubbing the side of the face or the chin on objects, other cats, and even human companions. Scratching floors, walls and trees will release scent from the glands in the feet to perform a similar function.

Urine and faeces are also deposited at particular sites to communicate territory or ownership. Urine spraying within the house can be a sign of territorial marking in adolescent, entire male cats, but can also indicate insecurity and a need to identify a core home area. 'Middening' is the deposition of faeces in prominent places, again as a means of establishing ownership of territory.

All of these forms of scent marking will generally be used to mark objects in busy pathways within the house or garden so the scent will be encountered by as many other cats as possible. Strange cats will investigate these markers, and the chemical messages contained may elicit the 'Flehmen' response (see Fig. 1.5) where the cat's top lip is raised to reveal its upper incisors, and air is taken into the vomeronasal gland (or 'Jacobsen's organ') for analysis. This is particularly common during the breeding season when males identify the reproductive status of the females.

Vocal communication

Vocalisations can be very informative in cats. Many individuals are 'chatty' and regularly chirp conversationally with their owners and some breeds, e.g. Siamese and Oriental breeds, are characteristically more 'talkative' than others. Talkative chirrups, mews and meows are often used for greeting and social bonding interactions with owners, but are rarely used between cats.

Purring is commonly believed to be a sign of contentment, but it may be more appropriate to consider it as a care-soliciting and care-giving message. Purring is usually heard when the cat is relaxed, with or without company, but more commonly occurs when the cat is interacting with humans or other cats. Having said that, cats also often purr in stressful situations or when in pain, and this may be an 'I'm a kitten, please look after me' vocalisation, reminiscent of the purring, suckling kitten.

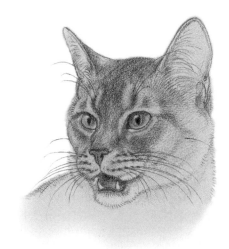

Figure 1.5 The Flehmen response: the cat's top lip is raised to reveal its upper incisors, allowing air to be taken into the vomeronasal gland for analysis.

More dramatic vocalisations occur when the cat is stressed or angry and wishes the other party to go away. As previously mentioned, these 'stay away' signals are more obvious than the relatively subtle 'come closer' signals, and they serve to reduce the likelihood of a physical encounter. Growling, hissing and spitting are used in combination with body language to communicate the animal's displeasure and will rise in volume in response to the cat's increasing agitation. As with aggressive behavioural patterns in dogs, aggressive displays by cats are designed to prevent conflict and the risk of injury. Only when these signals are ignored will the cat engage in actual biting and scratching.

BOX 1.2   KEY POINTS

- Signs of stress or discomfort in cats are more subtle than those of other species.
- Scent can be used to declare territory or ownership.
- Vocalisations can be used for social bonding as well as a defence strategy.
- Body language can be subtle, using combinations of multiple signals rather than discrete signs.

Mixed messages: when human to cat communication goes wrong

Social structure and communication signals are very different between humans and cats, and sometimes this can cause problems. Humans instinctively respond as humans, whereas cats will interpret the response from a feline perspective.

For example it is often believed that cats are attracted to people that don't like them, and this may be taken to mean that cats are perverse, and enjoy making people uncomfortable. In fact this apparent contradictory behaviour may arise as a result of differences in the way that humans and cats use eye contact. As humans, eye contact is an important way to identify others that we are interested in, so people who wish to interact with a cat are likely to try to maintain eye contact with it – which to a cat is very threatening. People who don't like cats tend to ignore them, and avoid eye contact, which the cat finds reassuring. This is an interesting theory, but a recent study into maintaining eye contact in cats suggests it may not actually be the case.

There has also recently been increased interest in the problem of obesity in our pet cats (see p. 48) and it may be that, in addition to other factors such as palatability of food and method of feeding, a misinterpretation of communication signals may contribute to the problem. Eating is a social occasion for humans, with the sharing of food symbolising friendship and social acceptance. For cats, eating is a purely functional activity; however they can learn that eating enables social interactions with their humans. When a cat approaches its owner it is generally engaging in a social bonding behaviour involving rubbing, scent marking and vocalisation. The owner often interprets this as asking for food and will offer a food treat. The cat is designed to eat little and often and will frequently accept this offering, reinforcing the owner's perception that the cat is begging for food. Mixed messages such as these can lead to confusion and conflict in the human/feline relationship.

1.3   FELINE BEHAVIOUR AND THE HOSPITALISED CAT

By appreciating the subtleties of feline communication and behaviour, we can gain an insight into a cat's state of mind either when living with it, or when nursing it. Many aspects of feline nursing rely on accurately interpreting changes in behaviour and differentiating what is normal and what is significant. Recognising the signs of stress can prompt changes in accommodation or handling that can reduce stress, leading to an increase in appetite or a speedier recovery from illness or surgery. Correctly identifying signs of pain is essential for an appropriate pain management programme, and this is an area where nursing care and time spent with the patient can make a world of difference.

Social behaviour and hospitalised cats

Cats present a unique challenge when introduced to a hospital environment. A major concern is that cats are very bonded to their own territory, leading to increased stress levels simply as a result of being in a strange environment. Hospitalised cats feel vulnerable, and often show it by hiding in their litter trays or under their bedding. Constraints of size and the facilities available make it difficult to get round this problem within the practice environment. However, there are often small changes that can be made which can provide a more acceptable area for the cat, e.g. by providing more appropriate hiding places, or by removing stressful distractions such as a barking dog or the presence of another cat directly opposite and within visual contact.

For long-stay patients, a raised shelf within the kennel may be advantageous, especially for separating sleeping areas, food bowls and litter trays. In more standard kennels, the use of cardboard boxes that can be disposed off when the patient goes home, or 'igloo' type beds that can be washed and disinfected, can provide the cat with a safe and defendable sleeping place. The provision of a toy or blanket carrying the owner's scent, or that of cats from home, can supply some familiarity and security. The use of feline facial pheromones may also provide calming signals in an inherently stressful environment.

Identifying abnormal behaviour patterns in hospitalised patients can prove challenging. For cats, sitting at the back of a cage, disdaining to interact with their carer may be normal behaviour for a solitary species, however it also means that it is not always obvious that a hospitalised cat is distressed, or in pain. Only by spending time with the individual and getting to know their responses can a full understanding of their condition be reached. Subtle changes in piloerection, muscle tone and facial expressions may be the only clue that the patient is in a lot of pain and that analgesia is required.

Our own body language will also make a major contribution to how relaxed or agitated our feline patients are quiet, relaxed, gentle movements are much preferable to tense, jerking movements when handling cats. Avoiding sustained eye contact by looking over the cat's head or at its chest can be less intimidating while still allowing close monitoring of the patient. A relaxed stare with intermittent slow blinking can be used to indicate a lack of threat. This imitates the communication used between cats themselves: when two cats meet they may circle one another for long periods before one slowly walks away. The conclusion to the encounter is often heralded by one of the cats slowly blinking in surrender. Cats appear to accept the same gesture in humans, and use it as a cue to relax after an intimidating encounter, such as someone reaching into their kennel to touch them, or to remove soiled bedding or used dishes.

BOX 1.3   KEY POINTS

- Feline nursing requires good observational skills and an ability to read the cat's language.
- Cats suffer from more stress as a result of feeling vulnerable in strange environments.
- Cats will pick up on our body language, and become more agitated or more calm depending on how they are handled.

1.4   COMMON FELINE BEHAVIOUR PROBLEMS AND THEIR TREATMENT

Feline behavioural problems are an increasingly important aspect of feline veterinary care. They appear to have become more common in recent years, and this may be for a number of reasons. Behavioural therapy for a number of species has been well publicised, with television programmes regularly featuring an animal behaviourist. Cat owners are better informed about the availability of behavioural advice, and are becoming more inclined to seek advice on their cats' problems. Secondly, the relationship between cats and their owners has changed over recent years, with cats becoming more integral to family life and less independent. They therefore spend more time indoors, so that behaviours such as scratching and aggression are more noticeable. Restriction to indoor living, highly palatable and readily available foods, and owners who work all day may cause frustrations in cats that lead to inappropriate behavioural displays. Finally, a major cause of perceived behavioural 'problems' is the owner's perception of what their cat should and should not be doing, with normal feline behaviours sometimes causing distress to their owners.

In general the range of behavioural problems encountered in a domestic species will depend on the level of control exerted over them by their owners and their lifestyle. Behavioural problems now recognised in dogs are many and diverse, while cat behavioural problems currently seem less varied, although this profile may change over the coming years. It must also be remembered that the behavioural problems for which owners seek advice from a veterinary clinic or animal behaviourist probably do not represent the whole picture of behavioural problems in the species. Certainly in dogs many issues are ignored by owners, or are not talked about owing to an owner's perception that they are 'minor' problems, or due to embarrassment. This is probably also the case with cats, and it is likely that elimination problems are more common in the general population but that many owners are reluctant to talk about this for fear of ridicule, and because they are prepared to live with the problem.

The most common behavioural problems currently seen in cats involve aggression towards either humans or other cats, and elimination problems. These will be discussed further with a look at possible causes and approaches for managing the problem using solutions that hopefully suit both the owner and the cat. Less common problems such as scratching furniture, fabric eating and over-grooming will also be discussed.

When considering any behavioural problems it is important to remember that they often have complex causes involving the lives of the cat, other cats in the same house, the owners and other people the cat encounters. It is essential that these complex problems are approached in the right way, in order to reach an accurate diagnosis and formulate a management programme suitable for all concerned. This is especially important when there are elements of stress, fear or aggression. 'First do no harm' is equally applicable to behavioural management as to veterinary medicine, and it may be better to refer the owner to a more knowledgeable or experienced source of advice.

Problems of aggression

Aggression covers many behavioural patterns, and it should be analysed objectively without projecting human emotions onto the animal's behaviour. Obtaining an accurate case history coupled with careful observations of the behaviour will be needed to ensure the correct diagnosis is made and that the reason for the aggression is correctly identified. The world of feline behavioural therapy is currently less litigious than canine behavioural therapy, but even so, when aggression to people is involved the treatment programme needs to be safe for all concerned and must always avoid the risk of owners getting bitten or scratched.

Cats live in a mutual tolerance society rather than a dominance hierarchy (see p. 1), so aggression is generally less motivated by possession or status but often involves insecurity and/or fear. Given the option, most cats will retreat rather than attack, however this is not always the case and is not always an option, which can cause problems in a hospital setting where escape is not possible. Aggression over resources such as food or resting areas can occur if the cat feels vulnerable or if there are not enough resting areas for all the cats in the household.

Aggression towards people

Displays of aggression to people can often be easily explained, for example an injured cat in a hospital cage is likely to show aggression towards its carers due to stress, fear, pain and a feeling of vulnerability. This type of aggression is understood and easily forgiven, whereas cats that attack their owners when being stroked can cause much more distress, fear and anger. The management of aggressive cats within a hospital environment is covered elsewhere, with advice on kennelling, reducing stress and handling techniques (see pp. 55, 65).

The treatment of aggression at home can be more challenging, especially as it can be difficult for the clinician to observe the behaviour and get accurate descriptions of body language and feline interactions from the owner. The increase in popularity of recording cameras can help enormously here, allowing the owner to video aggressive encounters, which will enable you to observe the behavioural displays first hand. An accurate case history will always be required with questions asked about the animal's history, including where the cat was obtained, and at what age, how long the behaviour has shown, when the behaviour occurs and who is present during the attacks etc. The taking of a thorough behavioural case history is beyond the scope of this book, and anyone who intends to become more involved in behavioural work will need to read more widely (see p. 15) and undertake further training in the subject.

There are several types of aggression that can be directed at owners, or at strangers entering the cat's territory:

- Fear aggression.
- Predatory aggression.
- Close contact aggression.
- Territorial aggression.

FEAR AGGRESSION
Probably the most easily understood form of aggression is when it is motivated by fear. Rescued cats may be more highly represented in this type of

aggression, due to the inherent insecurities of a new home and new owners. The upheaval of being rehomed may cause significant stress in a territory-based species. A history of abuse or maltreatment is not always the cause of fear aggression in rescue cats, although these cases do genuinely exist and should be considered. The socialisation period is as important in cats as it is in dogs, for the development of social attachment and the acceptance of other species. Stray and rescue cats may have had poor socialisation with humans during this sensitive period, and will consequently be more distrusting of people, even familiar people, than well-socialised kittens. In addition physical pain, for instance because of road traffic accidents, cat fights and arthritis, should be ruled out as a cause of fear and aggression by a veterinary health check.

Recognising fear aggression often involves examining the general behaviour of the cat. Body language and facial expressions seem similar in all cases of aggression, whatever the underlying motivation. By investigating the full behaviour of the cat more specific signs can often be seen. The fear-aggressive cat will often spend its time away from the main business of the house, such as in a little used room, under a duvet, or on top of a wardrobe. It may accept attention from familiar people, but will rarely initiate social contact and will often slink away at the first opportunity. Owners can often tell that their cat is uncomfortable with fussing and that attacks occur if they persist in stroking or picking up the cat. Such behaviour may be directed at unfamiliar people, with the cat happy and relaxed around the family but disappearing whenever anyone comes to visit. If aggression is concentrated on one member of the family or a particular visitor it is tempting to believe that the person must have abused, attacked or otherwise frightened the animal intentionally. This is not always the case, and human males particularly can cause fear just because they are larger, have deeper voices and are more deliberate in their actions than females.

When treating fear aggression, owner education is paramount to prevent injury and also to appreciate the extent of the problem. Often explaining to an owner that this particular cat does not like social company can be all that is required, allowing the owner to appreciate that it is not essential to constantly pick the cat up and hug it, and that this will always provoke defensive actions in this particular cat. Describing the body language shown by the cat and explaining to the owner that this is defensive communication can prevent owners from invading the cat's personal space and provoking aggressive attacks.

Treating the underlying fear felt by the cat is a lot more difficult to achieve, with cats being more difficult to bribe than dogs. The bottom line is that cats do not need social companions. Dogs have an evolutionary motivation to seek social bonds, cats do not. Forcing the issue of social attachment is likely to reinforce that cat's distrust of humans rather than cause acceptance of the attention. Building the cat's trust needs to be done slowly, with the first steps involving approaching the cat, using minimal eye contact, then retreating without any physical contact at all. If the cat likes certain food types such as cheese or ham, these can be used to reward the cat whenever people approach. Progression may involve approaching the cat, giving a quick stroke around the ears then leaving again, all the while being sensitive to the cat's stress and tolerance levels.

Creating a less threatening environment for the cat can also help to calm stress levels and increase the cat's tolerance of attention from the owner or visitors. Providing plenty of 'bolt-holes', where the cat can feel safe within the house can leave the cat feeling less vulnerable. Allowing the cat to maintain height with raised platforms for sleeping areas, or allowing access to cupboards and wardrobes can increase the cat's feeling of security. Hidden areas such as cardboard boxes, igloo-type beds or open drawers can allow the cat to relax in an easily defendable area. Pheromone therapy may be useful in a quiet area of the house such as a spare bedroom to provide a sanctuary away from the main thoroughfare of the home.

Many owners will feel that it may be helpful to get another cat to calm the fearful one, but this is not usually a good idea. It may occasionally help the cat settle and become more confident, however, it is more likely that the two cats will hate each other and that the presence of the newcomer will increase the stress levels within the house. Cats have low motivation to form social bonds with other cats just as they do with humans, so the introduction of a new cat into the household should be done carefully and not as a solution to a problem.

PREDATORY AGGRESSION

This form of aggression towards humans is particularly common in young cats and kittens. Cats will practice their hunting skills on any available object such as toys, pieces of paper, pens or moving targets such as hands and feet. This type of behaviour is often encouraged, especially by children, whose running around and squealing adds to the excitement of the game. Ambush techniques from behind the stairs or furniture are often practised, with the cat hiding until the appropriate moment, rushing out for the attack then running away again. For the cat, this is a good game and important for future life skills, however, for the owner it can cause serious problems with deep scratches and bites being common.

Generally kittens grow out of this behaviour, and focus their attention on outside prey rather than their owners. Cats kept within a highly controlled environment, such as indoor cats, can continue this behavioural pattern as an outlet for hunting behaviours. Owners should be encouraged to play with their cats in a more acceptable manner, such as chasing balls or dangling toys and to avoid handling the cat in ways that might encourage hunting behaviour, such as stroking its belly or rapidly wiggling their fingers or toes. When kittens have a tendency to bite and scratch, it is important to convince the owner to keep still and not snatch the hand away, which will encourage the cat to continue the game. 'Playing dead' will soon diminish the cat's interest in inappropriate games, while actively rewarding the cat by spending increased time playing with chasing toys allows the instinct to be expressed appropriately.

CLOSE CONTACT AGGRESSION

With this form of aggression the cat actively seeks attention then attacks for no apparent reason, and this can be particularly disturbing for owners. Clues as to why this behaviour is displayed in cats lie in their social structure. These cats like the attention of their owners and feel the need to maintain social bonds with close contact, such as sitting on a lap or close to the owner. The owner will interpret this as permission to stroke and fuss the cat, but after a while the cat attacks the hands of the owner sometimes quite viciously. It is believed that the cat feels an internal conflict between wanting to maintain social cohesion, but at the same time feeling threatened by such prolonged social contact. Because they are an essentially solitary species, cats do not have the communication tools available to them to modify social interaction and tend to change from a happily purring cat to a growling aggressive cat very quickly.

This lack of warning signals from the cat, and the apparent sudden rejection of the owner, makes this type of aggression very upsetting. Again, educating the owner about normal cat behaviour and explaining to them that their cat does like them, but is evo-

lutionarily ill-equipped to deal with overt displays of attention, can often reassure the owner greatly. Restricting the attention to a couple of strokes or a quick tickle behind the ear, and allowing the cat freedom to jump off the lap at anytime can often prevent this type of aggression. Often the best social relationships cats have are with people that generally ignore them because of their busy lifestyles.

TERRITORIAL AGGRESSION

Territorial aggression is sometimes seen in cats, with occasional stories of them attacking the postman! This behaviour may be attributed to the defence of a territory or home range, by male and female cats, in an area that is short of viable territories. It may also be seen in fearful animals, who feel threatened by strange people. The latter can be managed by the principles discussed above for fear aggression, whereas territorial aggression can be much harder to deal with, because it is not usually possible to significantly expand the amount of territory available.

BOX 1.4 KEY POINTS

- Aggression occurs in many forms and it is essential to identify the root cause of the behaviour.
- Controlling fear aggression often requires promotion of a sense of security for the cat.
- Predatory aggression is common in young cats learning hunting skills.
- Social aggression often stems from the cat's inability to communicate effectively during close social contact.

Aggression towards other cats

Aggression shown between cats is often a result of the factors already discussed, such as fear or lack of resources. Cats can have personality clashes just as people can, and this should be considered before bringing a new cat into an existing community. As with fear aggression to people, fear aggression to cats can be heightened in rescue cats; however this is less common than defensive aggression following bullying or an attack.

AGGRESSION OUTSIDE THE HOME

Aggression shown to cats outside the home can occur for a number of reasons, but is usually a combination of sexual aggression and territorial aggression. Increased aggression is likely to be seen during the breeding season as males fight for females, and the females fight off advances from the males. The general noise of yowling cats on a summer night can be the sounds of mating, as well as fighting! Testosterone-fuelled behaviour can occasionally be seen in neutered toms, particularly if they have been neutered later in life and have learnt the rewards of behaving aggressively. Territory disputes and the desire to control a neighbourhood can persist after the male has been castrated, although early castration often prevents such problems.

A dictatorship can occur in cat communities, with one individual bullying other members of the community – both male and female. Aggression can be seen in both parties but it is not unusual for the aggressor to appear passive while the victim shows all the aggressive postures and vocalisations.

Managing aggression outside the home is notoriously difficult, largely because of lack of control over the other cat(s) involved. Other owners that do not want to neuter their cat, or do not admit that there is a problem, can make it difficult for the owner who has sought your advice to resolve the problem. Often the only way to reduce the fear in the victim is to manage the situation at home. Magnetic cat flaps can help prevent other cats entering the house, so the victim has a safe haven. Alternatively, restricting the victim's access to outside may need to be considered; while this may seem more like punishment than help, it will at least stop the bullying and reduce the stress suffered by the victim.

AGGRESSION WITHIN THE HOUSEHOLD

Aggression between cats within a household is a common problem, which may manifest in a number of ways.

Fear aggression shown by cats within the same household is easier to deal with than when an external cat is involved, but it does take commitment from the owners and an understanding that some cats just don't like each other and will never be friends. The availability of resources is the first area to consider. Conflict may occur over food stations, sleeping areas or even attention received from the owner and there should be plenty of all these resources for each cat, such as a number of feeding areas and litter trays. The positioning of these resources must also be considered:

- Are they in acceptable places for the cat?
- Are they all placed together in a small area or are they in too busy an area?

- Does a cat have difficulty accessing them as a result of medical conditions such as arthritis?

Even if all these conditions are satisfactory, aggression can still occur with one cat denying access for the others.

Silent aggression is a behavioural pattern seen in cats where resources are restricted, or a favoured resource such as a sleeping place or litter tray, is occupied. The owner complains about the defensive aggression displayed by the victim cat, as this is the one showing all the classical signs of aggression – vocalisations, flattened ears, lowered body posture, and so on. The other cat often looks quite relaxed and 'all very innocent'. The aggressor exploits the essentially non-confrontational nature of cats, positioning itself between the victim and the resource. By simply occupying this area, the aggressor cat can restrict the victim's access to a resource, or its chance of fleeing. Victim cats can be cornered on bookshelves or under furniture, but the owner may interpret the close proximity of the two cats as a social bonding signal. The body postures of the two cats will give clues, as well as the behaviour displayed by the victim at other times – actively avoiding going into the same room as the aggressor, or leaving as the other cat approaches.

Owners are often concerned about aggression seen in cats that ambush, scratch, pounce and roll on each other, with or without vocalisations. This is often play behaviour and hunting practice, displayed by cats that are socially coherent. If each cat spends an equal time being victim and aggressor, there is usually no problem, however should one cat dominate this play session the owner may need to intervene. As with silent aggression, the aggressor should be discouraged with a raised tone of voice or sustained eye contact. It is, however, paramount that the correct cat is reprimanded, and these treatment programmes should not be entered into if you are unsure as to which cat is causing the problem.

The dynamics of a cat's social structure should also be considered, with a group of males being more likely to bicker and fight than a group of females, although groups of males can in some cases live together happily. Prevention is obviously better than cure, with owners being advised against keeping large groups of male cats, but often you are faced with a pre-existing situation and an owner who is unwilling to part with the cats they have. The availability of resources is often the key to success here, with cats being allowed their own space within different rooms if necessary. Placing newly met cats together in a small area and expecting them to learn to get on quickly is destined for failure. Feline relationships take time to develop and are based on a non-threatening environment.

BOX 1.5   KEY POINTS

- Aggression towards a cat outside the home can be difficult to resolve.
- Fear aggression between cats is generally due to bullying by a particular aggressor.
- Ample resources will be required within multi-cat households.
- Female groups are generally more harmonious than male groups.

Elimination problems

Inappropriate toileting in cats is the second most common behavioural problem seen in practice after aggression, because it is something many owners find difficult to live with. Embarrassment from the owner is an important factor in these problems, and they should be dealt with sympathetically because there is a widespread assumption that all cats are habitually clean.

Cats may eliminate in the house for a number of reasons, and these should be investigated fully before attributing the problem to a particular cause. Of particular concern is the cat that has previously used the litter tray but has recently stopped, indicating a behavioural or medical problem rather than lack of training.

Inappropriate urination

Bladder disease is a very common cause of inappropriate urination problems in cats and should always be eliminated as a cause by a veterinary health check before pursuing a behavioural treatment plan. All behavioural modification plans will fail unless any underlying medical condition such as cystitis, diabetes mellitus or renal disease is treated appropriately, quite apart from the possibility of the medical condition becoming worse without prompt veterinary care.

The first step in investigating a urination problem is to differentiate between emptying of the bladder and territorial marking or spraying. Observing the posture of the cat while voiding urine (if possible), the location of the urine and the volume of the urine

passed will enable the observer to differentiate between the two (see p. 13).

When managing any inappropriate urination problem it is also important to remove any scent of urination from the inappropriate areas, as animals are attracted to communal toileting areas by the smell of urine or its component ammonia. Disinfectants such as bleach contain ammonia and can encourage the cat to return to that site, so any accidents should be cleaned with a biological washing solution – after checking this will not discolour any carpets or rugs!

INAPPROPRIATE EMPTYING OF THE BLADDER

Normal urination occurs with the cat squatting (see Fig. 1.6), although this may be less obvious if the cat has any hind-limb pain. Urine will usually be found on horizontal objects such as carpets, beds, mats, and so on, and relatively large volumes of urine will be passed, unless the cat is suffering from lower urinary tract disease (see p. 147).

Behavioural reasons for a sudden onset of inappropriate bladder emptying can involve a change in the environment of the cat, particularly changes involving the litter tray. Silent aggression and lack of resources have already been identified as potential causes of problems; lack of access to the litter tray or a tray that has been used by other cats can result in the cat toileting elsewhere. A change in the litter substrate is a common reason for cats to disdain the litter box, and the owners should be asked whether they have changed litter

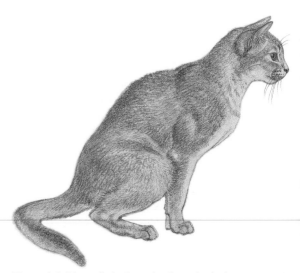

Figure 1.6 When eliminating urine the cat adopts a squatting posture.

brand recently or changed the amount of litter provided. The position of the litter tray should be assessed to establish whether the tray is positioned too close to food and water sources, in a busy area of the house, too close to an external door or within the presence of a dog, which may prevent the cat feeling sufficiently secure when using the box. Adult cats with medical conditions and young cats may have difficulties holding their urine for a long period of time. If the litter tray is positioned downstairs, they may not have enough time to get to it from an upstairs room, and litter trays upstairs and downstairs may need to be provided.

Despite popular opinion, some kittens do not learn to use a litter tray, or fail to learn that inappropriate surfaces such as carpets are not acceptable areas to toilet. In these cases basic house-training needs to begin with the cat being restricted to a small area containing a litter tray with the cat's preferred type of litter. The cat can be allowed free access to the house under supervision after toileting, but should be returned to the indoor kennel or playpen after a short while. The cat will soon learn to use the preferred litter, although there may be lapses if the cat is stressed or the litter tray is not clean. When encouraging cats to toilet outside, earth or turf can be used in the tray.

URINE SPRAYING AND TERRITORY MARKING

Spraying can be differentiated from urination by the standing posture adopted during voiding (see Fig. 1.7), the marking of vertical objects (from which

the urine may then drain onto a horizontal surface), and the small volume of urine passed on each occasion. Spraying will often be targeted onto areas of prominence such as doorways, sofas or beds.

The two main reasons for spraying are stress and hormones. Entire male cats will often spray to declare their territory to other cats, and this is not usually a problem when it occurs outside. Spraying within the house can occur if territories are crowded or the cat is kept entirely indoors. Neutering entire toms usually resolves the problem, although it may persist for a while in older cats. Cleaning the area with a biological washing solution so the enzymes break down the ammonia is equally important, so the cat is not tempted to over-mark the same areas.

Spraying urine is also used to proclaim territory, and can be used by a cat who feels its security and safe area are under threat. Stress caused by moving house, the introduction of a new cat/dog/baby, a feline dictator in the neighbourhood, a silent aggressor in the house or other cats entering the home can all trigger spraying in neutered males and female cats. Again, management of the cat's environment is the key to resolving the problem, with an assessment of hiding and resting places, the presence of aggression towards the cat, and the general stress levels within the home. Busy households can be stressful for sensitive cats with no way of escaping the hustle and bustle of family life. Providing hiding areas in quiet places, restricting the access of any dogs to the cat's preferred resting areas, providing a magnetic cat flap to prevent strange cats entering the house and providing extra help through pheromones may reduce the stress levels sufficiently to resolve the spraying, and improve the cat's welfare.

Inappropriate defaecation

The deposition of normal faeces in inappropriate places ('middening') can have a similar root cause to urination problems, and with similar solutions. Medical conditions such as diarrhoea and faecal incontinence should be ruled out before proceeding.

Restricted access to a litter tray, or a litter tray that is full, is probably the main cause of inappropriate defaecation. Sometimes owners overlook the obvious, with normally outside toileting cats being restricted to indoors for some reason but not being offered a litter tray. Trays that are too close to feeding stations or external doors can prove unacceptable to the cat, whereas a quieter, more secluded site is preferable to the cat.

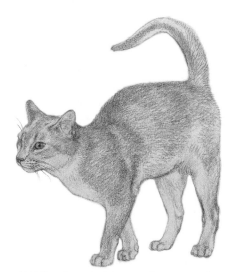

Figure 1.7 When 'spraying' the cat adopts a standing posture and directs the urine onto a vertical surface.

Faeces can be deposited in times of stress, with the defaecation occurring in areas the cat wishes to proclaim as theirs, such as bedrooms or resting areas. This can be distressing to the owner, particularly if the faeces are deposited in the bed. As with spraying, the environment should be assessed, dogs or children restricted from the cat's resting area and multiple hiding places offered, particularly at a height.

BOX 1.6   KEY POINTS

- Inappropriate elimination may take the form of urination, spraying or defaecation.
- Medical causes should always be ruled out before commencing behavioural modification.
- High stress levels are a common cause and steps should be taken to reduce these.
- Neutering may help to prevent spraying, but spraying does not always have a hormonal cause.
- Cleaning up accidents should be done with a biological washing solution to break down the ammonia content of urine or disinfectants.

Other behavioural problems

Cats can develop many strange and bizarre habits that can cause concern to their owners. Aggression and elimination problems are by far the most common complaints, but occasionally other behavioural patterns can occur, involving either abnormal behaviour or normal behaviour displayed inappropriately. With any abnormal behaviour pattern, medical causes should be excluded such as dietary imbalances, neurological diseases or endocrinological disorders, and a full veterinary health check is essential.

Scratching behaviour

Cats use many ways to communicate ownership of territory, and this often involves scents that humans cannot appreciate. Urine and faeces have been described earlier; the rubbing of cheeks and chin along people and furniture is often tolerated well by owners but scratching around the house can cause problems. The scent glands on the feet leave an impression of the cat, as well as the visual marker of torn sofa, carpet, wallpaper, or curtains. Again, when this behaviour is displayed outside it rarely causes complaint, but even cats that have access to the outdoors will often scratch inside the house. Some cats will choose vertical markers, while others prefer horizontal surfaces, and texture is also important, with certain fabrics and weaves being particularly attractive. This is a natural behaviour being shown by the cat, rarely indicating stress or fear, but it can be intolerable for the owner.

The key to resolving this problem is to provide more acceptable targets for the behaviour. Marking is often performed in conspicuous places, or in areas of much activity such as hallways or living rooms. Providing commercial scratching posts and activity centres in these areas can encourage the use of acceptable marking sites rather than expensive furnishings. The positioning of these posts should be carefully considered, with their placement as close to the site of destruction as possible, and they must reflect the cats preferred texture and position – vertical or horizontal. If caught in the act the cat can also be discouraged from using the furniture with tone of voice and eye contact. Alternatively, applying unacceptable textures, such as foil or sticky plastic, can restrict the damage when the cat is unsupervised. Denying unsupervised access to that room may be a more practical solution, depending on the geography of the house.

Over-grooming and self-mutilation

This problem involves abnormally obsessive grooming behaviour, carried to the point of self-mutilation. Affected cats will initially over-groom themselves and pull out the hair from favoured sites ('barbering') but will often then progress to licking and damaging the skin once the hair has been removed. Fortunately, the vast majority of cats that present to a veterinary practice because of over-grooming have a treatable medical cause such as ectoparasites, allergies, or lower urinary tract disease. These conditions can usually be successfully managed provided that veterinary advice is sought promptly.

Where there are true behavioural causes overgrooming is often associated with obsessive, compulsive behaviours requiring pharmacological management, and careful consideration should be given to referral to a behavioural specialist. Simple first aid measures such as applying aversive creams and ointments, fitting buster collars or active discouragement by the owner rarely succeed, with the cat turning attention to another area of the body or becoming more secretive in its grooming habits. Referral to a behaviourist who can determine the cause of the obsessive behaviour is generally advisable in these cases.

Pica

Pica, the ingestion of inappropriate and even potentially harmful substances, is another distressing behaviour problem that is occasionally encountered in cats. Cats often become attracted to strange substances such as sticky tape or wood, but rarely ingest these so the behaviour does not cause any problems. Other cases of strange appetite, such as wool eating in Oriental breeds, can be more dangerous and intestinal obstructions are commonly associated with this behaviour. As with inappropriate elimination and over-grooming, it is important to exclude medical causes, in this case possible hormonal imbalances and nutritional deficiencies. Where there is a behavioural cause there is often an obsessive component, and again referral may be the most appropriate route.

Further reading

Beaver BV 1980 Feline behaviour: a guide for veterinarians. WB Saunders, Philadelphia.

Bradshaw JWS 2002 The behaviour of the domestic cat. CABI Publishing, Wallingford.

Fogle B 1991 The cat's mind. Pelham Books, London.

Horwitz D, Mills D, Heath S (eds) 2002 BSAVA Manual of canine and feline behavioural medicine. BSAVA, Cheltenham.

Overall K 1997 Clinical behavioural medicine for small animals. Mosby, St Louis.

Turner DC, Bateson P (eds) 2000 The domestic cat: the biology of its behaviour, 2nd edn. Cambridge University Press, Cambridge.

PREVENTATIVE HEALTH CARE

CHAPTER **2**

Rachel Burbidge, PHC VN

Helping our clients to maintain their pets in good health is becoming an increasingly important aspect of modern day veterinary practice. Veterinary nurses have a valuable role to play in this, through client education and advice on all aspects of preventative health care, and by promoting the services their practice can offer.

2.1 ENDOPARASITES

Endoparasites are internal parasites that live within the host animal's body. The most common feline endoparasites are the intestinal worms, but there are also types of parasites which can inhabit the lungs and even the heart and blood vessels.

Infection with endoparasites can affect the health of the individual cat, and in some cases there are also implications for human health. Testing for worm infections involves faecal analysis (see p. 102), but this is relatively expensive and time consuming. Broad spectrum antihelmintics are safe, effective and inexpensive, so regular worming of all adult cats and kittens (see p. 20) is a more practical approach than routine faecal screening to identify infected cats.

Nematodes

The nematodes, or roundworms, are cylindrical worms that taper at one or both ends (see Fig. 2.1). They are white or pale cream in colour and may have a translucent look due to the presence of a colourless cuticle. Within the host animal's body they feed on mucosal fluid and cell debris.

There a large number of nematodes that can infect cats (see Table 2.1) but they all share a similar life-cycle. The adult female worm lives inside a suitable host animal and produces eggs, which are passed out via the host's faeces. A larva develops inside the egg casing and can remain within the eggshell for long periods before emerging. As the larva matures it will moult (shed its cuticle) four times, and these larval stages are desig-

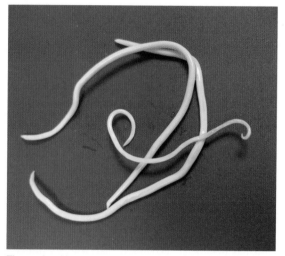

Figure 2.1 Nematodes are pale, cylindrical worms that taper at one or both ends.

nated L1 to L5. The L5 stage is an immature adult stage. Only L2 larvae can establish an infection in a new host, and this is known as the infective stage. Some nematodes have a **direct** life-cycle, in which all stages of maturation and multiplication occur in one host species, while others have a more complex **indirect** life-cycle involving 'intermediate' or 'paratenic' host species. An intermediate host is one that is required by the parasite to support one or more of the stages in its development from egg to adult, while a paratenic host is an 'optional' host that can carry the parasite but does not contribute to its maturation.

Table 2.1 Nematodes of the cat	
Ascarids	*Toxocara cati*
	Toxascaris leonina
Hookworms	*Uncinaria stenocephala*
	Ancylostoma tubaeforme
Lungworm	*Aelurostrongylus abstrusus*
Heartworm	*Dirofilaria immitis*

Ascarids

TOXOCARA CATI

This ascarid lives in the small intestines of the cat. In most cases infection is asymptomatic, but heavy infections in kittens can cause stunting and a pot-bellied appearance. Occasionally kittens will pass worms in vomit or faeces.

Kittens and adult cats can be infected by ingesting infective eggs (e.g. when grooming fur that is contaminated with faeces) or by consuming a paratenic host e.g. a rodent or bird. Lactating queens can also pass the infection to their kittens through their milk (L3 larval stage) but larvae cannot pass across the placenta to infect kittens in utero.

Once an infective egg is swallowed the L2 larva hatches from the egg and burrows through the intestinal wall into the host's blood stream. It is then carried to the liver, to the right side of the heart and finally to the lungs. Here it moults to the L3 stage, which is then coughed up and swallowed, returning to the intestines to finish its moults before becoming an adult. The time taken from ingestion of the egg to maturation into an adult female passing new eggs (the 'pre-patent period') is approximately 7 to 8 weeks.

It has now been recognised that *Toxocara cati* is a potential hazard to human health. The L2 stage can infect humans and can lead to tissue damage due to larval migration (ocular and visceral migrans). This is of special concern in young children, so it is important to make owners aware of the importance of cleaning up cat faeces in the garden and covering children's sand-pits so that they don't get used as litter trays. It takes about 1 month for the toxocara egg to mature to the L2 (infective) stage but after that time the encysted L2 stage can remain infective for many months.

TOXASCARIS LEONINA

This roundworm can infect both cats and dogs. It seems that large worm burdens of this species are fairly well tolerated and do not normally cause clinical signs.

This worm has a simple, direct life-cycle. Infection is by ingestion of infective eggs, or by eating an infected intermediate host such as a mouse or rabbit. After ingestion larval development takes place in the small intestine, and there is no migration to other body tissues. The pre-patent period is 11 weeks.

Toxascaris leonina cannot cross the placenta to cause pre-natal infection nor is it passed on via the mother's milk, so infection is usually seen first in adolescent animals.

Toxascaris leonina can infect man but has not been shown to cause disease.

Hookworms

Hookworms are so called because of their hook-shaped head. They attach themselves to the host's intestinal wall by their mouthparts causing damage to the intestinal lining, and they then feed on the damaged tissue.

These worms are not very common in cats in the UK, but there are two genera worth a brief mention:

UNCINARIA STENOCEPHALA

Uncinaria is most commonly found in dogs kept in a kennel type of environment with access to grassed runs. Cats are unlikely to become infected unless allowed access to these areas. Infection is by ingestion of infective eggs or can occur directly, by larvae burrowing through the skin. Signs of infection are undetectable unless there is a very heavy burden, in which case diarrhoea and loss of condition may occur.

ANCYLOSTOMA TUBAEFORME

A. tubaeforme is not found in the UK but it is endemic in more southern parts of Europe where the warmer climate supports its life-cycle. This intestinal hookworm feeds on the blood of the host cat and can cause weakness and inappetence due to anaemia. The introduction of the PETs travel scheme has now introduced the possibility of seeing cats with this worm in the UK and VNs should be aware of this.

A. tubaeforme is not recognised as a major zoonotic risk but it has been suggested that if humans are infected, the migrating larvae can cause damage.

Lungworm

AELUROSTRONGYLUS ABSTRUSUS

These are black, thread-like worms that live within lung tissue. Infected cats may show no signs, or may develop a cough. The cough is usually mild and self-limiting unless there is an exceptionally heavy burden.

Aelurostrongylus has a complex life-cycle involving three different host species. Cats are the **definitive** host, i.e. the host in which mature adults produce infective eggs. The adult lungworms produce larvae that are coughed up and swallowed by the infected cat; these are then passed out in the cat's faeces. The L1 are then ingested by slugs and snails, which act as an intermediate host for the larva to moult to L2 and L3. Frogs, birds and rodents are potential paratenic hosts, which may eat an infected slug or snail, and may then themselves be caught and eaten by cats. The L3 larva then burrows through the intestine wall to the blood stream and is carried to the lungs where it completes its maturation into adulthood.

Heartworm
DIROFILARIA IMMITIS
This worm does not occur in the UK but again with the PETs travel scheme veterinary personnel should be aware of cats returning to this country from endemic areas. *Dirofilaria* are common in southern Europe, especially around the Mediterranean. Mosquitoes are the intermediate host, and the maturing larvae are passed on via the insect's bite. Adult worms cause coughing, dyspnoea, vomiting, lethargy, weight loss and inappetence. Cats are less susceptible to heartworm infection than dogs, but if they do become infected it can be devastating, and there is a risk of sudden death. Preventative measures are recommended for all cats travelling to areas in which *Dirofilaria* is endemic.

Cestodes

Cestodes, or tapeworms, are flat and ribbon-like in appearance. They consist of a scolex (head) and proglottids (segments) (see Fig. 2.2). New segments grow sequentially from the lower part of the scolex to produce the worm. The proglottids farthest from the head are the largest, most mature segments, and contain the eggs. These terminal segments are called gravid segments. Tapeworms have an indirect life-cycle, which requires involvement of an intermediate host.

At maturity the gravid segments break away from the main worm, but maintain viability and are able to

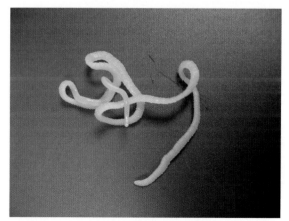

Figure 2.2 Cestodes are flat ribbon-like worms consisting of a head (scolex) and multiple proglottids (segments).

move independently. They are either passed in the host's faeces or they make their own way out of the anus. These small, creamy white segments can often be seen moving over an animal's coat especially around the anal area. This is the most common way in which tapeworm infections are identified since infection with these worms is rarely associated with clinical signs of disease. Once out of the body the gravid segments dry up, and look like 'grains of rice', and may be seen sticking to the cat's coat or on bedding.

To complete the life-cycle the segments must be ingested by a species-specific intermediate host. The embryo within the proglottid then develops into a metacestode. Metacestodes are sac-like structures containing a head or heads of new tapeworms (metacestodes vary in size and structure depending on the type of tapeworm). Once ingested by the final host the metacestode releases the scolex, which then attaches itself to the intestinal wall by hooks and suckers and begins to produce new segments.

The three types of tapeworm that can infect cats are *Dipylidium caninum*, *Taenia taeniaeformis* and *Echinococcus multilocularis*. Only *D. caninum* and *T. taeniaformis* are currently found in the UK.

DIPYLIDIUM CANINUM
Flea larvae and immature adults are the intermediate hosts for this tapeworm. The flea larva ingests the tapeworm egg, which has been shed into the environment. As the flea matures the larva develops into a metacestode and the cat then swallows the flea while grooming itself. The metacestode is released into the cat's intestines and a new tapeworm develops. The pre-patent period is 3 weeks. Heavy worm burdens can cause loss of condition but in most cases the cat will appear to be unaffected. Regular flea control can help prevent infection with *D. caninum.*

TAENIA TAENIAEFORMIS
Rats and mice are the intermediate host for *T. taeniaeformis,* and the life-cycle is completed when the infected rodent is caught and eaten by a cat. The pre-patent period is 7 weeks and again infection rarely causes clinical signs but owners may see the gravid segments around the anus. Since owners are unable to control hunting, regular worming of cats that are allowed access to the outside is important.

ECHINOCOCCUS MULTILOCULARIS
Although this tapeworm is not found in the UK it is worth a mention as it is present throughout the rest of Europe,

from Poland in the north to parts of France in the South. It is a highly zoonotic parasite that can cause very serious disease in humans. In order to prevent its spread to this country cats must be treated with an effective cestocidal wormer before entering the UK. Small rodents are the intermediate host, so only cats that are allowed outside to hunt are at risk. The pre-patent period is 28 days; monthly worming with a cestocidal is advised for cats that visit areas in which *E. multilocularis* is endemic.

Recommended worming treatment regimes

What to use
There is a wide range of antihelmintic treatments that are available to pet owners. The spectrum of activity and pharmacy classification of the drugs most commonly used in the UK are shown in Table 2.2.

When to worm
KITTENS

In very young kittens the main concern is the nematode *Toxocara cati* which can be passed on via the mother's milk. Kittens should be wormed at 2, 5, 8 and 12 weeks using an antihelmintic that is effective against nematodes.

Juvenile cats should be wormed again at 6 months of age and then every 3 months, as for adult cats.

ADULT CATS

The current recommendation is to worm adult cats every 3 months with an antihelmintic that is effective against both nematodes and cestodes. The lifestyle of the cat should also be taken into account when advising on a worming regime. As previously discussed the pre-patent period for *D. canium* and *T. taeniaeformis* are 3 and 7 weeks respectively, so a cat that has fleas or goes out hunting may need worming more frequently.

PREGNANT CATS

Care should be taken when worming pregnant cats as the majority of worming products are not licensed for this use. The worming requirement here is mainly for roundworms and an anthelmintic containing fenbendazole is currently the wormer of choice. It is recommended to worm the queen once, at around the time of birth and then at the same time as the kittens.

2.2   ECTOPARASITES

Ectoparasites are organisms that live and feed on the surface of another animal. In the cat the most common ectoparasites are either insects e.g. fleas and lice, or acarids, e.g. ticks and mites.

Fleas

The flea is a brown, wingless insect, with a flattened profile (see Fig. 2.3) which allows it to move freely through the host animal's coat. It has specialised mouthparts for piercing skin and sucking blood. Flea saliva contains an anti-coagulant, and when the flea bites its host it injects saliva into the puncture site to prevent the host's blood from clotting, so that the flea can take in a full meal of blood. It is the flea's saliva that can trigger a powerful

Table 2.2 Currently available anthelmintic treatments			
Active ingredient	Trade name	Classification	Range of activity
Fenbendazole	Panacur, Granofen, Zerofen	NFA-VPS GSL	N: 1,2,3,4,5 C: 2
Imidacloprid/moxidectin	Advocate	POM-V	N: 1,4,6 (also fleas, ear mites)
Milbemycin/praziquantel	Milbemax	POM-V	N: 1,4,6 C: 1,2,3
Piperazine	Endorid	AVM-GSL	N: 1,2,3
Praziquantel	Droncit	AVM-GSL	C: 1,2,3
Praziquantel/emodepside	Profendor	POM-V	N: 1,2,4 C: 1,2,3
Pyrantel/praziquantel	Drontal cat	NFA-VPS	N: 1,2,5 C: 1,2,3
Selamectin	Stronghold	POM-V	N: 1,4,6 (also fleas, ear mites)

Nematodes: N1, *T. cati*; N2, *T. leonina*; N3, *U. stenocephala*; N4, *A. tubaeformae*; N5, *A. abstrusus*; N6, *D. immitis*.
Cestodes: C1, *D. canium*; C2, *T. taeniaeformis*; C3, *E. multilocularis*.
N.B. Before recommending any drug, always check the current data sheet for its suitability for the individual cat.

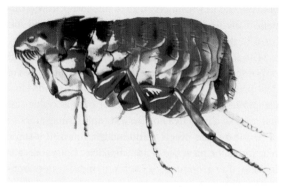

Figure 2.3 The adult flea is a brown, wingless insect, with a flattened profile. Reproduced with permission from Bayer Animal Health Division.

allergic reaction in the host animal, causing severe itching and hair loss in affected animals.

There are a number of flea species that may be found in companion animals, but studies have shown that in over 90% of cases it is *Ctenocephalides felis* (the 'cat flea') that is found on cats and dogs.

Life-cycle

Adult fleas are permanent parasites that stay on the same animal throughout their life, however the eggs that they lay do not remain on the host animal. They are shed from the fur into the environment, where they hatch into larvae which themselves remain in the environment as

they mature into juvenile fleas, before seeking out a new host animal to complete their life-cycle (see Fig. 2.4).

ADULT FLEAS

Adult fleas only represent 5% of the total flea population, and therefore only account for 5% of the flea problem within a household. The female flea finds a host, and then mates with a male flea; she then consumes a blood meal to provide the energy to produce and lay her eggs, between 24 and 48 hours later.

FLEA EGGS

A female flea can lay an average of 20 to 30 eggs per day, and flea eggs account for around half of the total flea population within a house. Flea eggs are creamy-white smooth oval structures that are barely visible to the naked eye. The eggs do not adhere to the host animal's coat, so the majority of them will be groomed off the coat by the cat and the rest will drop off into the environment, where they will eventually hatch. The length of time before the eggs start to hatch can be anything from a few days to a week depending on the environmental conditions.

FLEA LARVAE

Once it is ready to hatch, the larva inside the egg uses an 'egg tooth' to break through the shell. Larvae have the appearance of small maggots; they have three larval stages, and as they mature they change colour from

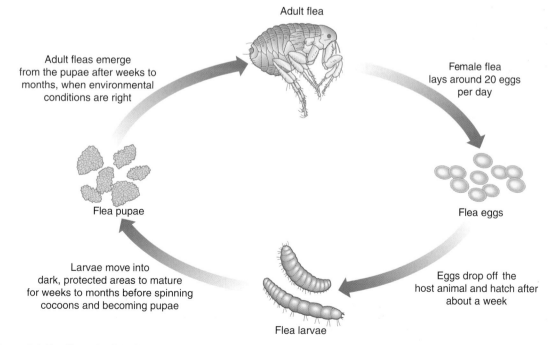

Adult flea

Adult fleas emerge from the pupae after weeks to months, when environmental conditions are right

Female flea lays around 20 eggs per day

Flea pupae

Flea eggs

Larvae move into dark, protected areas to mature for weeks to months before spinning cocoons and becoming pupae

Eggs drop off the host animal and hatch after about a week

Flea larvae

Figure 2.4 The life-cycle of the flea.

yellowish white, through reddish brown to opaque white. The development between these larval stages can take anywhere between a few days to a few months. The larval stages account for around one third of the total household flea population. They feed on organic debris, e.g. flea faeces and dead skin cells, and it is the larval stages that may ingest tapeworm eggs if they encounter them, allowing fleas to act as an intermediate tapeworm host (see p. 19). Flea larvae are mobile, and are sensitive to light. They tend to move into darker areas, in deeper layers of carpets and underneath items of furniture.

THE PUPAE

Approximately 2 weeks after the last larval moult has occurred the larva spins itself a cocoon and becomes a pupa. This stage of the flea life-cycle accounts for about one tenth of the total flea population, and is the most difficult to destroy due to its thick protective cocoon. The outside of the cocoon is sticky, allowing the pupa to adhere tightly to soft furnishings and it also quickly becomes covered in debris which acts as camouflage.

The adult flea develops within the cocoon, and these 'pre-emerged' adults can survive for considerable periods within the cocoon. They are sensitive to vibration, warmth, humidity and carbon dioxide and will not emerge until the environmental conditions are right, and until they sense an external stimulus from a suitable host, indicating a ready food source for the adult flea.

The total length of time the life-cycle takes to complete therefore depends on the environmental temperature and humidity. Temperatures below 3°C and above 33°C are lethal to flea development and the winter climate in the UK is such that the flea will almost never survive or complete its life-cycle outside. However the combination of centrally heated homes, pets with free access to the home and abundant fitted carpets and soft furnishings means that the flea problem is now an all year round problem and is not confined to the spring and summer as in years gone by.

Recognising a flea infestation

FLEA BITES

Once fleas become established in a household they may cause itching and irritation to the pets within the household, and may also bite the people living in the house. A human being is not a suitable host for a cat flea to live on, but newly emerged cat fleas may jump onto and bite a human if they cannot find a more suitable host. Most people react mildly to flea bites, developing a small, itchy pink spot at the site of the bite. Flea bites most commonly occur around the ankles and lower legs because the newly emerged fleas are living in the carpets. If the flea infestation extends to bedding and soft furnishings bites may occur anywhere on the body.

The severity of the clinical signs that a cat develops in response to a flea problem will depend on the number of fleas present on the cat, and the ability of the individual cat to tolerate that particular number of fleas. Some cats can tolerate a high flea burden with only a small amount of pruritus while others will develop a marked allergic reaction to the presence of just a few fleas. Common signs include over-grooming, scratching, miliary dermatitis and alopecia. In cases of severe infestation, especially in young kittens or geriatric cats, anaemia can develop.

IDENTIFYING THE PRESENCE OF FLEAS

It is not always easy to find adult fleas themselves because they are highly mobile, fast moving creatures. If live fleas are seen, then it is likely that the cat has a heavy flea burden. If live fleas themselves cannot be seen it is worth looking more carefully for evidence of their presence. After feeding on a meal of blood the flea passes faeces (flea dirt), which contains dried blood. Flea faeces can be recognised as small black flecks in the coat. A flea comb is an effective tool for finding flea dirt, and the 'wet paper test' (see Box 2.1) is also a valuable means of proving the presence of fleas to a sceptical owner.

Flea allergic dermatitis

Some cats have a hypersensitivity to antigens in flea saliva, and develop flea allergic dermatitis (FAD) if they are bitten by fleas.

Clinical signs of FAD include:

- Pruritus.
- Over-grooming.
- Miliary dermatitis.
- Symmetrical alopecia of the lumbar region, hindquarters and abdomen.

BOX 2.1   THE 'WET PAPER TEST' FOR IDENTIFYING THE PRESENCE OF FLEAS

- Take a sheet of white paper and wet it under a tap.
- Hold the wet paper under the cat, while you rub its coat up and down, allowing any debris from the fur to fall onto the white paper.
- Flakes of dead skin and specks of grit will remain unchanged when they touch the wet paper, but flea dirt is composed of dried blood and will dissolve, leaving a small reddish brown streak on the paper.

FAD is a common cause of over-grooming and symmetrical alopecia. Cats commonly use their barbed tongues to 'scratch' itchy skin, and one effect of the over-grooming is to break hairs off at their base. In many of these cases fleas are never seen, because the hypersensitive cat is constantly grooming itself and swallowing the fleas, so it can sometimes be hard to convince the owner that fleas are the root of the problem.

Treatment and control of fleas

There are many different types of flea treatment available to owners, from sprays to spot-ons, tablets to injections, and the range of products available can become confusing to clients.

Treating a flea infestation involves three important aspects:

- Killing the fleas on the pet(s) in the household.
- Killing the immature life-stages within the environment.
- Preventing re-infestation.

KILLING ADULT FLEAS

Treatments that kill adult fleas on the cat are commonly referred to as 'adulticides'. There is a wide range of available products, in a number of different formulations (see Table 2.3).

Adulticides that contain organophosphates have now been largely superseded by newer drugs which are both safer and more effective, although they are also more expensive. Some drugs (e.g. the permethrins) that are safe for use on dogs are highly toxic to cats, so it is essential owners understand the differences between these products, and that they only use products that are licensed for use in cats. Most of the newer flea adulticides are safe to use in kittens, but it is important to check the relevant data sheet before recommending a product for use in kittens or pregnant cats.

For prevention of infestation adulticides should be used all year round, as centrally heated homes provide an environment that allows fleas to multiply all year round.

KILLING IMMATURE LIFE-STAGES IN THE ENVIRONMENT

Adult fleas account for only 5% of the total flea population within a household, so in order to control a flea problem it is essential to address the environmental life stages as well as the adult fleas. There are two ways to approach this.

A household spray (see Table 2.3) containing a long acting insecticide can be used to spray all carpets and soft furnishings. When using a household

Table 2.3 Currently available flea treatments		
Active ingredients	Formulation	Product name
Adulticides		
Fipronil	Spray, Spot on	Frontline
Imidacloprid	Spot on	Advantage, Advocate
Nitenpyram	Tablets	Capstar
Diazinon	Collar	Preventef
Selemectin	Spot on	Stronghold
Insect growth regulators		
Pyriproxyfen	Spot on	Cyclio, Fleeguard
s-methoprene	Collar	Freedom Cat Collar
Lufenuron	Suspension, injection	Program
Combined adulticide and IGR		
s-methoprene + fipronil	Spot on	Frontline Combo
Environmental control		
s-methoprene + permethrin	Household spray	Acclaim
Pyriproxyfen + permethrin	Household spray	Indorex

spray it is important to spray all areas that may contain flea larvae and pupae. Flea larvae are mobile and tend to move away from the light and away from areas that are walked over frequently, so it is important to spray the edges of the room, and under heavy items of furniture. The spray will kill all larval stages, but the pupae, within their protective cocoons, are not affected until they hatch into newly emerged adults, which are then susceptible to the residual insecticide.

Vacuum cleaning prior to spraying increases the effectiveness of the treatment. Thorough vacuuming will remove 20% of larvae and 30 to 60% of eggs from carpets. It will also remove organic debris and flea faeces, which are a food source for the larvae. The action of the vacuum cleaner improves penetration of the spray by aerating the carpet. The vibrations created by the vacuum cleaner will stimulate the pupae to hatch out.

Boiling a kettle in the room with the windows closed will also help to increase the air to the right humidity to encourage emergence of new fleas from the pupae.

Insect growth regulators (IGRs) can be used to interfere with the development of the immature stages of the life-cycle. These products (see Table 2.3) are applied to the cat, and are a valuable source of environmental control.

Ear mites

Ear mites (*Otodectes cynotis*) are oval in shape with four pairs of legs (see Fig. 2.5). They can infect many species including cats and dogs.

Life-cycle
The ear mite has a simple, direct life-cycle, involving four stages from egg, via larva and nymph to adult. All four life-stages take place on the host animal. Adult ear mites feed on the tissues lining the host animal's ear canal and the female lays her eggs in the horizontal ear canal. The larvae hatch out and mature into adults within 14 to 21 days. Transmission between animals is by direct contact.

Clinical signs
Signs that suggest the presence of ear mites include head shaking, scratching at the ears and the presence of a brown waxy exudate in the external ear canal. Affected cats also exhibit a hind-limb scratch reflex when their ears are rubbed.

Treatment
Ear mites can be treated using topical aural acaricides (ear drops) or using a parenteral treatment. As ear mites are spread by contact all cats and dogs in the house should be treated.

TOPICAL TREATMENT
After the ears have been cleaned and inspected for damage to the ear canal and eardrum a topical aural acaricide can be applied in the form of ear drops. Treatment needs to be continued for long enough to treat two generations of adult mites. This can be done by treating both ears for seven days, then stopping for seven days to allow new mites to hatch out, then treating both ears for a further seven days.

Topical treatment should not be used in cats with a perforated tympanic membrane (ear drum).

PARENTERAL TREATMENT
Selamectin (Stronghold Spot-On) and imidacloprid (Advocate Spot-On) are licensed for the treatment of *Otodectes cynotis* in cats. These presentations are ideal for those owners unable to apply ear drops, or for use in cats with damaged ear drums.

Ivermectin has also been found to be very effective against ear mites in cats. It is not licensed for use in cats but it appears to be well tolerated, and may be considered if none of the licensed products are appropriate for use in an individual cat.

Ticks

There are many species of tick worldwide and they have a significant role in the spread of a number of diseases. The most common type in the UK is the 'ixodid' or hard tick. *Ixodes ricinus* (sheep tick) is the most prevalent, closely followed by *Ixodes hexagonus* (hedgehog tick). The adult female is light grey in colour and can increase up to 200 times in size when engorged with blood (see Fig. 2.6).

Life-cycle
Ticks have a life-cycle that involves four stages of development (from egg, via larva and nymph to the adult form) and three different host animals, which may be of different species (see Fig. 2.7).

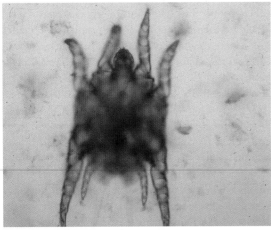

Figure 2.5 An ear mite (*Otodectes cynotis*). Reproduced with permission from Leo Animal Health.

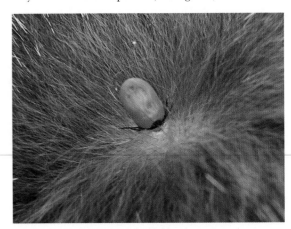

Figure 2.6 A tick engorged with blood.

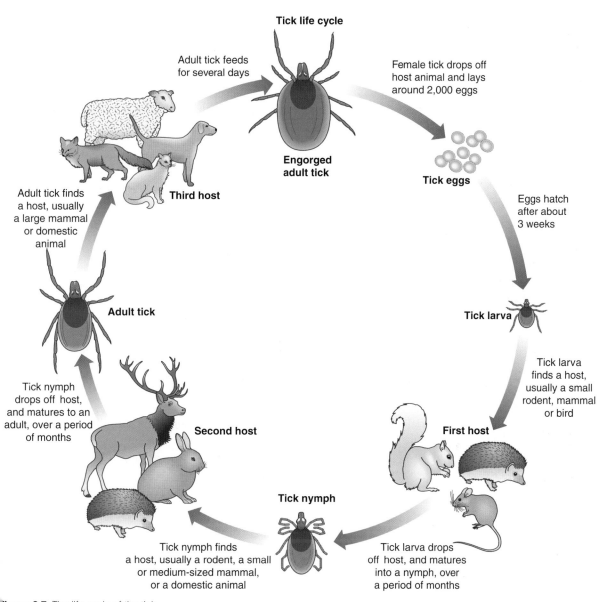

Tick life cycle

Adult tick feeds
for several days

**Engorged
adult tick**

Female tick drops off
host animal and lays
around 2,000 eggs

Tick eggs

Eggs hatch
after about
3 weeks

Adult tick finds
a host, usually
a large mammal
or domestic
animal

Third host

Tick larva

Tick larva
finds a host,
usually a small
rodent, mammal
or bird

Adult tick

Tick nymph
drops off host,
and matures to an
adult, over a period
of months

Second host

First host

Tick nymph

Tick nymph finds
a host, usually a rodent, a small
or medium-sized mammal,
or a domestic animal

Tick larva drops
off host, and matures
into a nymph, over
a period of months

Figure 2.7 The life-cycle of the tick.

The life-cycle can take up to 3 years to complete. The larvae, nymphs and adults attach themselves to a host animal for a few days each year to feed before dropping to the ground to moult to the next stage. The adult female, after engorging with blood, will drop to the ground to lay her eggs and then die. Ticks prefer warmth and humidity to complete their life-cycle, which accounts for their seasonal emergence in spring and autumn.

Clinical signs

The adult tick may be seen on the cat (see Fig. 2.6), or a local skin reaction to a tick bite may be seen. Ticks will usually attach themselves in areas where the hair coat is thinner i.e. ears, face, feet and abdomen. When distended with blood the tick's body can become dark-brown or black and owners sometimes confuse them with small skin tumours.

Treatment and control

Ticks can be manually removed, but care must be taken not to leave their head and mouthparts embedded in the skin as this can result in the formation of an abscess. Manual removal is possible either using a proprietary tick removal device (e.g. an O' Tom Hook™) or by first loosening the tick's hold by covering it with cotton wool soaked in a suitable acaricide (e.g. Fipronil). It is important to educate clients of the danger of leaving the mouthparts behind when removing a tick.

Cats that frequently pick up ticks can be partially protected using a suitable licensed product (e.g. fipronil) on a regular basis. This will not prevent ticks from attaching but should kill them within 48 hours, minimising the risk of tick-borne disease, e.g. Lyme disease.

Mites

Neotrombicula autumnalis

Harvest mites (or berry bugs) are seen as bright red pinhead dots with three pairs of legs. They are usually found in the interdigital spaces, around the eyes or on the ears. They may cause local irritation. Diagnosis is by direct observation but can be confirmed if necessary by microscopic examination of a tape strip (see p. 104). Topical treatment with a flea adulticide is usually effective in eliminating the mites.

Cheyletiella blakei

These mites cause excess scaling of the skin and are just large enough to be visible to the naked eye, hence their colloquial name 'walking dandruff'. *C. blakei* are usually only found on cats, especially younger cats, but they can also infest humans. Diagnosis is by direct examination of the coat with a magnifying glass or by taking samples using adhesive tape (see p. 104).

Notoedres cati

This is a mange mite (similar to *Sarcoptes* in dogs), which is particular to cats. It is a burrowing mite, and is highly infectious and also zoonotic, but fortunately this mite is quite rare in the UK. Clinical signs are moderate to severe itching leading to alopecia, with yellow crusty lesions usually on the ears, face and neck. Diagnosis is based on identification of the mites in skin scrapings.

Demodex cati

This cigar-shaped mite can be found in low numbers in the hair follicles of healthy cats. They only cause a problem if present in very high numbers, which is rare in the UK, but may occur in young animals causing a local form of demodectic mange, or in older immunosuppressed cats resulting in the very rare generalised form of infection. Clinical signs are red, itchy skin with alopecia, progressing to thickening of the skin and development of pustules in extreme cases.

2.3   VACCINATION

In recent years the subject of vaccinations, for companion animals and for humans, has become a much-debated subject. The widespread use of vaccination has certainly reduced the frequency and severity of some cat diseases and if routine use of vaccinations were to cease, we would be likely to see an upsurge in feline infectious disease, some with a possibly fatal outcome.

However, concerns have been raised as to whether vaccines are being given more frequently than necessary. Adverse reactions can occur following vaccination (see Table 2.4) but they are uncommon and in most cases are not life threatening. In general, if an individual cat is at risk of catching a particular infectious disease the benefit of vaccinating against that disease is likely to be far greater than the very small chance of an adverse reaction. However this is a complex area: the number of diseases that can be vaccinated against continues to grow, as does our understanding of the duration of immunity provided by vaccination and the potential adverse effects of vaccination.

Currently available feline vaccinations

Vaccine types

There are two principle types of vaccine that are currently available for use in companion animals:

Killed (or inactivated) vaccines contain dead organisms, which when injected into the body will stimulate a mild, local reaction. In order to amplify this reaction into a full immunoprotective response it is usually necessary to incorporate an 'adjuvant' which helps to stimulate a strong immune response to the killed organisms.

Modified live vaccines contain antigen in the form of living pathogens that have been modified ('attenuated') so that they will not cause significant disease. These attenuated pathogens retain the ability to multiply in the body and so are able to stimulate a full immune response without the need for an adjuvant.

Modified live vaccines have the advantage that they provide rapid immunity without incorporating an adjuvant. However in some circumstances the attenuated organisms may still cause mild signs of disease. For this reason killed (inactivated) vaccines are often recommended for use in pregnant queens and those cats that are immunosuppressed due to concurrent disease, or drug treatment.

Table 2.4 Possible adverse effects of feline vaccines

Adverse effect	Comment
Local inflammation	Some cats may develop local inflammation and irritation at the site of vaccination. These local reactions can be uncomfortable but should resolve within 6 weeks. It may be appropriate to use a different type vaccine when the next booster is due.
'Off colour'	Most cats show no ill effects following vaccination but some suffer a period of lethargy and poor appetite, which usually resolves within 24 hours. These reactions appear to be more common following vaccination against FeLV, but are not restricted to one vaccine type. It may be appropriate to use a different type vaccine when the next booster is due.
Mild upper respiratory signs following a modified live 'flu' vaccine	Modified live 'flu' vaccines contain viable, attenuated FCV and FHV-1 viruses, which can, in some circumstances, cause mild signs of infection. This is most likely to occur if the cat is immunosuppressed, or if the attenuated viruses enter the cat via the natural route of infection i.e. the mouth or nose. In practical terms this is most likely to occur if droplets of the vaccine are spilled onto the cat's coat at the time if injection, or if aerosol droplets of vaccine are expressed into the air when the vaccine is being prepared. In healthy cats any signs that do develop are likely to be mild and short-lived, but the attenuated viruses will be shed in saliva and may be transmitted to other cats. Killed (inactivated) vaccines may be preferred for use in large multi-cat households, and are recommended for use in pregnant queens and in immunosuppressed cats.
Shifting lameness	FCV can occasionally cause a short-lived period of pyrexia and shifting lameness, and signs may develop following vaccination although this is rare. If signs do develop they resolve within 48–96 hours.
Vaccine associated fibrosarcomas (VAFs)	It appears that, in a very small proportion of cats, administration of a vaccine may contribute to the development of a particularly aggressive form of fibrosarcoma at the site of vaccination. The problem appears to be most associated with vaccination against FeLV and rabies, and this may be due to the requirement for incorporation of an adjuvant into these killed (inactivated) vaccines. VAFs are a rare phenomenon, but when they do occur they are very aggressive and very difficult to treat.
Immune-mediated (autoimmune) diseases	Concerns have been raised that vaccinations may stimulate the development of a variety of immune-mediated diseases in humans, dogs, and potentially in other species. There is currently no strong evidence to suggest that this is the case.

Feline infectious enteritis (FIE)

FIE, also known as feline panleukopaenia or feline parvovirus, is caused by a parvovirus that is similar to the canine virus that causes severe haemorrhagic diarrhoea (see p. 72).

FIE is still a very common virus but vaccination provides good protection against this highly contagious, potentially fatal disease. It is recommended that all cats and kittens should be vaccinated against FIE.

Feline calicivirus (FCV) and feline herpesvirus (FHV-1)

These two viruses are the agents that most commonly cause the disease known as cat 'flu' (see pp. 72, 121).

Vaccination against FCV and FHV does not guarantee against infection with either of the 'cat flu' viruses but vaccination will help to reduce the risk of infection and to reduce the severity of infection if it occurs. Vaccinated cats can still become carriers and be a source of infection to other cats. For these reasons the 'cat flu' viruses remain extremely common amongst our pet cats and all cats should be regularly vaccinated against them.

Feline leukaemia virus (FeLV)

FeLV is caused by an oncornavirus, a subfamily of the retroviruses (see pp. 73, 150). An oncornavirus is a virus that is capable of causing the development of tumours.

Vaccination against FeLV is recommended for those cats at risk of being exposed to the infection, especially young cats in multi-cat households or those that are frequently involved in fights with other cats. However, vaccination offers no protection against developing the signs of disease in cats that have already picked up the virus so it may be appropriate to offer a blood test for the virus before vaccinating a cat that comes from a 'high risk' environment.

Bordetella bronchiseptica

The same bacterium that is known to cause 'kennel cough' in dogs can also infect cats, and in some cases may cause respiratory disease, most commonly sneezing and nasal discharge (see pp. 72, 122).

An intranasal vaccine is now available for use in cats and is recommended for use in multi-cat households such as breeding colonies and rescue centres that have a clinical problem with *B. bronchiseptica*.

Chlamydophila felis

This bacterial infection (previously known as *Chlamydia psittaci*) is a common cause of conjunctivitis in cats. Transmission is by direct contact between cats especially in cats and kittens in multi-cat households. It is a very fragile bacterium which does not survive in the environment (see p. 72).

Vaccination against *Chlamydophila* provides protection against severe disease but does not always prevent infection, so a mild form of the disease may still develop in cats that have been vaccinated.

Rabies

Rabies is caused by a rhabdovirus. The virus can infect many species including humans. It attacks the central nervous system and causes a range of signs including aggression, pyrexia, difficulty swallowing, facial distortion and limb paralysis. Once clinical signs develop the disease is progressive and always fatal. The virus is shed in the saliva and transmission occurs when an infected animal bites another animal. The virus does not survive well off the host, so indirect transmission does not occur.

The rabies virus has not yet been imported into the UK, but it is present in Europe, America and a number of other countries. Owners planning to take their cat abroad are advised to vaccinate their cat against rabies and, on meeting other criteria for the 'PETs Passport' scheme, may then avoid the need for quarantine on arrival back in the UK. Current regulations with regard to re-import of cats into the UK can be found at www.defra.gov.uk

Current vaccination recommendations

The Cat Group is a collection of professional organisations dedicated to feline welfare. Members include the Feline Advisory Bureau (FAB), Blue Cross, Royal Society for the Protection of Animals (RSPCA), Animal Health Trust (AHT), British Small Animal Veterinary Association (BSAVA), European Society of Feline Medicine (ESFM) and the Governing Council of the Cat Fancy (GCCF). They reviewed the subject of feline vaccination in 2003, and their findings can be accessed at www.thecatgroup.org. Their overall conclusion was to support the continued use of vaccination for pet cats, but they report that:

'...there are recent studies that have suggested that vaccine-induced immunity for some diseases may last considerably longer than 12 months . . . at present there are insufficient data available to determine optimum booster intervals in adult cats. The Cat Group encourages informed consent of owners for vaccination of their cats wherein both the risks and benefits of vaccination as well as the need for vaccination are discussed with owners and advice is provided on the basis of the best available objective data.'

The Cat Group endorses the routine vaccination of all cats to help reduce the prevalence of infectious diseases. Their recommendations are as follows:

- All cats should be routinely vaccinated for FIE, FCV and FHV-1, and these are classed as the core vaccines. They protect against viruses that are very common, that can survive in the environment and can be transferred by indirect contact.

- For the other diseases each cat should be judged on an individual basis for the need for that particular vaccine e.g. an indoor cat living in a single cat household with no access to the outside may not need to be vaccinated against FeLV as it will not come into prolonged contact with other cats.
- When vaccinations are given kittens should receive two vaccinations, 3 to 4 weeks apart, starting at 9 weeks of age. The maternal antibodies from the mother will usually last for 6 to 10 weeks in the kitten so if vaccination is carried out before 9 weeks of age there will be a poor immune response to the vaccine.
- Adult cats should have a single booster vaccination annually after the initial vaccine course.

The detailed report is available on The Cat Group's website and provides a wealth of useful information on all aspects of cat vaccinations, and will help to give an understanding of vaccination.

New developments

Vaccine manufacturers are constantly working to improve their vaccines, to develop new vaccines and to get pharmaceutical licenses for their vaccines in all countries around the world. As new vaccinations become available recommendations for their use will need to be developed. For example a vaccination against FIV is currently available in the USA, and may soon be licensed for use in some European countries, and an effective vaccination against FIP may also soon be developed. Depending on their mode of action and efficacy these vaccines may be suitable for widespread use, or they may be best reserved for cats at high risk of infection. Vaccine recommendations will need to be revised and updated as new developments are made, and as our understanding of their efficacy and duration of action improves.

2.4 MICROCHIP IDENTIFICATION

Since their introduction in the early 1990s, electronic microchips have been adopted world-wide as a form of identification, helping to reunite many lost pets with their owners as well as serving a useful function in verifying the exact identity of an animal. They provide a safe, permanent and easily traceable means to identify an animal and so have many advantages over the more traditional collar tag. Many cat owners have concerns about placing a collar on their cat for safety reasons and, as we know, free roaming cats will frequently lose their collars or ID tags. Microchips offer an easy, one off, affordable solution.

The tiny microchip is about the size of a grain of rice, and contains an identification code, similar to a supermarket bar code, which is unique to that microchip. An electronic scanner is needed to read the microchip and in the early days of the technology there were problems with incompatibility between different types of microchip and reader. However a standardised system (verified by the ISO) has now been adopted around the world and the majority of microchips can now be read with the majority of scanners. Once implanted the microchip's code number and the details of the cat and its owner are held at a central database.

The microchip is implanted using a needle (containing the microchip) fitted into either a handle ('gun') or a syringe-type implanting device (see Fig. 2.8). It should be sited under the skin between the shoulder blades (the most common site in the UK) or at the side of the neck (a commonly used site in the rest of Europe). There is a small possibility that the microchip may migrate to other places in the animal's body, e.g. the foreleg, after implantation. It is therefore important to scan the whole body when checking an animal to look for a microchip. A systematic scanning pattern should be used to cover the entire cat. Different scanners have different breadths of scanning and different sensitivities, it may take time to detect the microchip.

Microchips are the only accepted form of identification for the PETs travel scheme. They must be inserted before the rabies vaccination is administered, and must be checked at every stage of the process. The microchip should meet the ISO standard so that it is compatible with the scanners used abroad. Microchip malfunction is very rare, but it is good policy to scan an animal each time it is presented for vaccination or for examination prior to travel to ensure that the chip is still present and functioning, and to demonstrate this to the owner. Unfortunately unless the microchip can be detected and scanned at the point of departure the animal will not be allowed back into the country without undergoing quarantine.

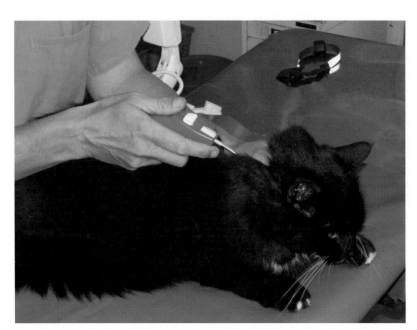

Figure 2.8 Implanting a microchip under the skin between the shoulder blades.

2.5 GERIATRIC CLINICS

Pet cats are now living healthier and longer lives than ever before due to improvements in their nutrition, their status as pets, their owners' standard of living, and the veterinary and preventative health care that is available. Care of older cats is therefore becoming increasingly important to owners and to veterinary practices, and there is increasing interest in aspects of preventive health care and early identification of disease. Geriatric clinics offer an ideal opportunity to improve the health and welfare of older cats. These clinics can be used to provide valuable advice and reassurance to owners and as a useful marketing tool for the practice.

A 'geriatric' cat can be defined as a cat that is over 11 years old, and these cats are considered to be at increased risk of developing age-related conditions and diseases. A well run geriatric clinic provides an opportunity to advise on the prevention of age-related problems and allows detection of the early stages of diseases. Owners will very often put any changes they see down to 'old age' and will not appreciate that their cat may gain substantial benefit from further investigation and appropriate management of these age-related conditions. Often owners will feel more comfortable talking to you, the nurse, about their concerns rather than 'bothering' the vet. If any abnormalities are discovered, the cat needs to be referred to a veterinary surgeon,

who will advise further investigation and treatment as appropriate. The cat will benefit from improved health care and the early detection and treatment of diseases. The practice will benefit from client loyalty and a strong bond between the client, their pet and the practice, and the nurse will benefit from a feeling of satisfaction at a responsible job well done.

Setting up the geriatric clinic

Where?
Some practices may have enough space to establish a nurses' consulting room, and this will be the ideal. Where space is tight you will have to negotiate the use of a standard consulting room. By choosing appropriate appointment times this can allow effective use of the room outside the veterinary consulting hours.

When?
Ideally at a time suitable for the client rather than a time to suit you! Ask your clients, via a questionnaire, when they would find it most convenient; then find an acceptable way to fit the clinics around the working pattern of the practice

How long?
You should allow plenty of time (minimum 20 minutes) for each consultation, to allow you to ask

questions about the cat, carry out a thorough examination and answer any questions that arise. It is better to hold fewer consultations and spend longer with the client and the cat than to miss something important because you were rushed for time. It is also important that the client feels that there is time to discuss all their concerns without feeling under any pressure.

Another advantage in allowing plenty of time is that it gives the cat time to come out of its basket, explore the room, acclimatise to the environment and relax a little before it is examined. This is always useful, and is especially important for blood pressure monitoring, the results of which can be significantly affected by stress.

Who?

A keen and enthusiastic qualified veterinary nurse with the back up of a supportive veterinary surgeon is ideal. The nurse must have good background knowledge of geriatric diseases, experience in handling and nursing cats and a willingness to recognise the limits of their knowledge.

Promoting the clinic

Once you have completed the planning stage you will need to let your clients now about this new service, what it offers, what it will cost them, and the benefits it will bring them and their cats. To avoid offending anyone, especially your older clients, try to call your clinic something other than geriatric, e.g. the 'over eleven club', the 'golden oldies' or the 'creaky club'. Once you've decided on a name spread the word as widely as you can, and try to get everyone in the practice involved.

WAYS OF PROMOTING THE GERIATRIC CLINIC
- Waiting room displays.
- Leaflets on the reception desk.
- Letters sent out with booster reminders to all cats over 11 years old.
- Word of mouth: encourage everyone in the practice to mention the clinics to clients who own cats over 11 years old: vets doing booster vaccinations; nurses running other clinics e.g. dental check ups; receptionists talking to clients on the phone.

Running the clinic

There are a lot of elements to be covered, and it is easy to forget some aspects. Establish a pattern that you will follow for every consultation, using check-lists as

necessary, to make sure that you have covered all the points, and that you have recorded all your findings. Some drug and diet manufacturers have useful support material, including prepared health check forms and questionnaires and you may like to use these, or adapt them to your own requirements.

Clinical history

It is important to start off with a detailed discussion of the cat's current health status. To use your time efficiently, and to ensure that all the necessary questions are covered it is a good idea is to ask the owner to fill in a questionnaire about their cat before attending the clinic; this gives them time to think about the answers in a relaxed manner without feeling under pressure. The questionnaire can be given to the client when they arrive in the waiting room, but remember to ask them to arrive a few minutes before their appointment time to allow them time to fill it in.

When you call the client into the consultation room you can then go through the questions and answers with the owner to gain more information. This is the ideal time to let the cat have a wander around the consulting room to acclimatise itself to the new surroundings.

Examples of questions you may like to ask include:

- How do you think your cat compares to when he/she was younger?
- Do you notice your pet sleeping more than usual?
- Does your cat have problems jumping up or going upstairs?
- Do you think your cat has gained or lost weight recently?
- Has your cat's appetite changed recently, is he/she more hungry, or less hungry?
- Does your cat have problems when eating its food?
- Has there been any change in your cat's drinking pattern?
- What diet is your cat currently being fed?
- Are there any signs of constipation, or diarrhoea?
- Is the cat on any current medication?

Don't forget to finish by asking the owner if they have any worries or concerns that have not been covered by your initial questions.

Brief physical examination

Once the cat seems calm and relaxed you can proceed to a general examination. It is always best to follow the same routine when you examine an animal, as this makes it less likely that you will miss out any important areas. It is often best to start at the head and work in a consistent pattern down the cat's body, but some cats resent having their face examined, and may be easier to handle if you start at the back end and work your way forward. Have a check list for the physical examination and record all your findings as you go along.

WEIGHT

Some cats will gain weight as they get older and less active, but many cats will tend to lose weight with age. Their bodyweight and body condition score (see pp. 68, 70) needs to be noted at each visit, and compared to the last recorded weight.

HEAD

- **Ears:** check for inflammation, smell, wax or discharge and massage the ear canals to see if the cat has ear irritation. Check if the cat is deaf by clapping your hands away from the animal to see if it responds.
- **Eyes:** check for discharge, corneal ulcers and inflammation, and look at the colour of the conjunctival membrane to check for pallor. Assess sight by dropping cotton wool in front of the cat and watching for a reaction or by getting it to walk around objects in the room.
- **Mouth:** examine the mouth for signs of dental disease (see p. 33), ulcers and tumours.

NECK

Carefully feel up and down the neck each side of the trachea to see if one or both thyroid glands are palpable; in a normal cat you should not be able to feel them.

CHEST

Watch the cat's breathing as it acclimatizes to the consulting room, looking for any evidence of an increase in respiratory effort. Run your fingers over the rib cage to feel for any 'lumps and bumps', record the site and size of any masses found. Use a stethoscope to listen to the heart and record the rate and rhythm.

Full clinical examination of the heart and lungs is a complex process and requires considerable experience. Make sure you record any abnormal findings. It is also advisable to remind the client that this is a basic physical examination and that it does not replace regular veterinary examination such as the annual health check for vaccination.

ABDOMEN

Continue to examine for further cutaneous and subcutaneous masses, including mammary tumours. These are less common in cats than in dogs, but when they do occur they are often malignant. Finish by examining the genitalia and anal area. Check if the cat has been neutered.

LIMBS

Watch the cat walking and note any stiffness or lameness. Run your hands down each leg checking for tumours and also check that the claws are not overgrown and sticking into the pads. This is a frequent problem in older cats that spend less time using scratching posts and wearing their claws down. Gently flex and extend each joint and note any joints that seem stiff, or that the cat resents having manipulated. Never over stretch any joint, and if the cat shows any sign of discomfort do not continue to examine that joint.

Further tests

URINALYSIS

Urinalysis is inexpensive and can provide valuable information, especially by showing early indications of problems such as diabetes and renal failure. The urine can be collected by the client as a free flow sample from a litter tray using non-absorbable cat litter, or a sample can be collected direct from the bladder by cystocentesis. This should be performed by a veterinary surgeon. A sample obtained by cystocentesis will be sterile with no risk of bacterial contamination.

Urinalysis should involve measurement of specific gravity, a dip-stick test and examination of the sediment (see p. 98). Bacterial culture may be appropriate depending on the initial findings, and for this a sample collected by cystocentesis will be required.

BLOOD PRESSURE

High blood pressure is a common problem of older cats and can cause significant damage to the eyes, kidneys, cardiovascular system and nervous system, but in the early stages the cat may show few signs of the problem. Geriatric clinics provide an ideal opportunity to introduce regular blood pressure screening for older cats, allowing early identification and treatment of hypertension. See page 105 for further information on measuring blood pressure in cats.

BLOOD TESTS

Providing that the cat has been fasted prior to your consultation, blood should be taken for a basic haematology and biochemistry profile. A full blood profile should be carried out on all elderly cats, but if this is not possible, perhaps for financial reasons, then the minimum requirement is to measure PCV, total protein and albumin, urea, creatinine, glucose and total T4. Other tests may also be required depending on the individual case.

Follow-up

Once you have taken a detailed history, examined the cat and performed the further tests, you will need to explain your findings to the owner. If any significant abnormalities have been identified then a vet should be called upon to arrange further examination and investigation as appropriate, but if everything appears to be normal then the next appointment should be booked for 6 months time.

2.6 ORAL HEALTH CARE

Studies have shown that 70% of cats over 3 years old have dental disease of some kind. However, it is also the case that only around 4% of the animals coming to your veterinary practice are being brought in by their owners due to oral health associated problems, e.g. difficulty in eating. These figures tell us that there are a lot of cats with dental disease that may not be receiv-

ing the treatment that they need to resolve the problem, or to prevent it from getting worse. Veterinary nurses can make a big contribution to the oral health of their clients' pets, by examining the mouth of all pets that they handle, and by discussing with their owners the condition of the teeth, the implications of the problems and the ways that they can be managed.

To help clients to manage and prevent dental disease, it is necessary to understand the problems that develop in cats' mouths, and the terms that are used to describe these problems (see Box 2.2).

Dental disease

Periodontal disease

Periodontal disease is staged according to its severity:

Stage 0: Normal healthy mouth (see Fig. 2.9).
Stage 1: Gingivitis. Gum inflammation but without loss of tooth attachment. This is due to plaque accumulation but with professional scaling and polishing it is reversible.
Stage 2: Early periodontal disease (see Fig. 2.10). Loss of up to 25% of the periodontal attachment but with minimal pocket development and bone loss.
Stage 3: Moderate periodontal disease. Loss of 25% to 50% of the periodontal attachment with

BOX 2.2   DEFINITION OF TERMS USED TO DESCRIBE DENTAL DISEASE

Plaque	An accumulation of salivary glycoproteins, polysaccharides and bacteria, which form a soft sticky paste that sticks to the tooth surface. Plaque contains a high bacterial load and if it accumulates in large amounts it pre-disposes to gingivitis and periodontal disease.
Calculus or tartar (see Fig. 2.11)	Mineralised plaque containing minerals such as calcium and phosphate from food and saliva. Calculus does not normally cause irritation but its rough surface allows plaque to form more rapidly.
Gingivitis	Inflammation of the gums (gingiva), often in response to bacteria in plaque. Gingivitis is reversible and can be treated by eliminating the plaque and bacteria.
Gingival pocket	The 'gingival sulcus' is the narrow trough between the tooth and the free gingival margin (gum edge). The normal depth in cats is 0.5 mm to 1 mm. When periodontal disease develops the gingival sulcus deepens producing a gingival pocket.
Periodontitis	If gingivitis is not treated the gums become increasingly inflamed causing gingival pockets, gingival recession and loss of gum attachment. The tooth eventually becomes mobile and will inevitably be lost. Periodontitis is usually irreversible.

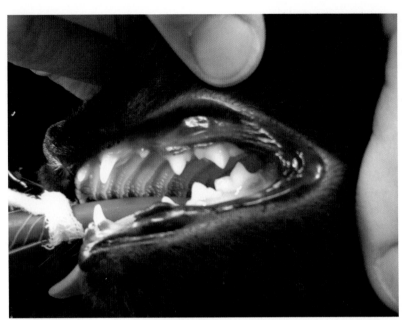

Figure 2.9 A normal healthy mouth (Stage 0).

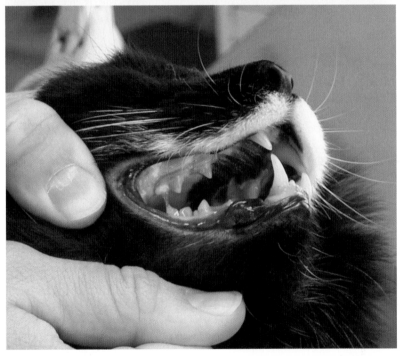

Figure 2.10 Early periodontal disease (Stage 2).

moderate to deep gingival pockets and bone loss of less than 50%. Note that gum recession can occur at the same time and therefore probing does not always reveal the deepening periodontal pockets; radiographs will help diagnosis.

Stage 4: Severe periodontal disease (see Fig. 2.11). Loss of greater than 50% of the periodontal attach-ment with severe deep pockets. Bone loss is greater than 50% and so the tooth becomes mobile and cannot be saved.

Stomatitis

This is a very uncomfortable, often painful condition of cats. Stomatitis, also known as lymphocytic-plasmacytic

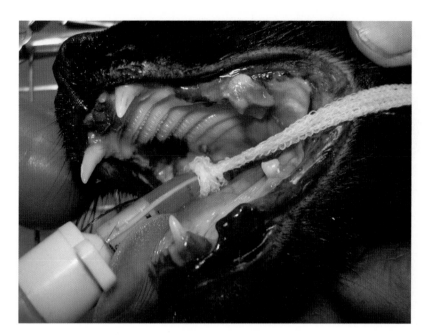

Figure 2.11 Severe periodontal disease (Stage 4) and calculus.

stomatitis, involves not only severe inflammation of the gums (gingivitis) but also of other oral mucous membranes, e.g. the buccal mucosa and glossopalatine arches (see Fig. 2.12). The tissues are often swollen, ulcerative and bleed very easily.

Stomatitis can be associated with a number of underlying diseases, and can be very difficult to treat. Cats with this problem should receive a full work-up including testing for any underlying predisposing condition, e.g. FIV, FeLV and chronic renal failure. Treatment involves professional scaling and polishing of all normal teeth, and extraction of all damaged teeth, followed by rigorous home brushing to keep the plaque under control (a major contributing factor in stomatitis). Additional antibiotic and anti-inflammatory treatment is often required.

In some severe cases and especially where homecare is not an option total extraction may be the only answer.

Feline odontoclastic resorptive lesions (FORL)

FORLs, also known as 'neck lesions', are a common dental problem in cats, currently of unknown cause. The resorptive lesion often starts at the cemento-enamel junction and often results in hyperplasia of gingival tissue covering the lesion (see Fig. 2.13). The hyperplastic gingival tissue can often be seen on visual examination of the mouth, and usually bleeds quite easily when touched. However the resorptive lesion itself may be hidden below the gum line, and dental radiography should also be performed to detect lesions in the tooth root.

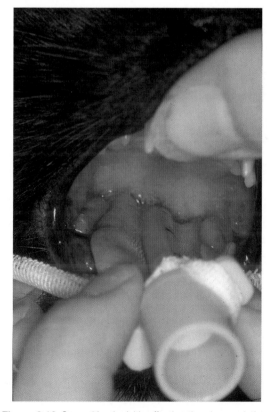

Figure 2.12 Stomatitis-gingivitis affecting the glossopalatine arches.

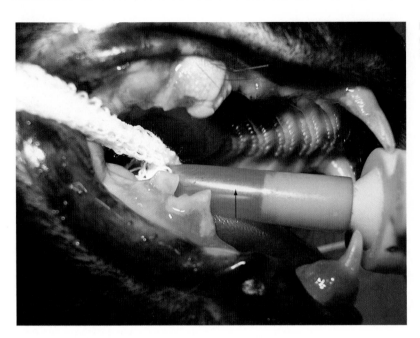

Figure 2.13 A feline odontoclastic resorptive lesion (FORL) or 'neck lesion'.

When a tooth with an odontoclastic resorptive lesion is probed under a light plane of anaesthesia the cat will often 'chatter' its jaw due to discomfort. FORLs cannot be repaired and are progressive lesions. Treatment is usually extraction of the affected tooth.

Dental care: treatment and prevention

All cats coming into the veterinary practice should have their mouths examined on a regular basis and their owners should be educated on the problems and treatment of periodontal disease. As nurses it is our job to inform and teach owners the basics of dental care, as many are still unaware that animals suffer from dental problems. It is also important to stress to owners that dental care is not just about having nice clean teeth and sweet smelling breath but also about preventative health care. Research has shown that the presence of bacteria and toxins in the mouth migrating into the blood stream can end up affecting the heart, liver and kidneys.

Dental treatment

If plaque and tartar build up are already evident then the cat should be booked in to have a general anaesthetic, oral examination (including evaluation of periodontal pocket depth), removal of plaque and tartar, polishing of the teeth surface and extractions if necessary. It is very important to explain in full to the owner what is involved in a dental scale and polish. Many owners will not realise that the cat will need a general anaesthetic and they should also be made aware of the possibility of extractions. The pricing of dentals in the clinic should also be discussed, as again owners are often unaware of the cost implications, usually comparing it to their own dentist.

When booking the cat in for a dental the owner should be informed that this is just the start of caring for their cat's teeth and that follow-up appointments and further preventative treatment will be required to prevent reoccurrence of the problem.

When performing a dental the teeth should be charted (see Fig. 2.14) and a copy given to the owner. This will show them what you have done and hopefully give them an interest in their cat's mouth and its ongoing dental care.

On discharging the cat a follow-up appointment should be made. If a large number of teeth have been extracted the mouth should be checked around 2 days later. All cats should also be scheduled for a re-visit 7–14 days after the procedure to re-examine the cat's mouth and to discuss ongoing homecare.

Dental homecare

Ongoing care of the mouth at home will make a very significant contribution to maintaining good oral health. A wide range of homecare measures may be considered, and these should be tailored to the individual client and their cat. Homecare measures must be practical for the owner to carry out and easily

Feline Dental Hygiene Record

Client identification

Name: .... Date:...

Patient File Number:..

Patient

Name:... Age: ....

Breed:................................. Sex: .... Weight:..........................

History

Main dental problem: ....

Previous treatments: ....

Current Home Care

Tooth brushing: Yes ☐ No ☐   Enzymatic Chews: Yes ☐ No ☐

Other Home-care measures:..

Oral Examination

Gingivitis:	Normal ☐	Slight ☐	Marked ☐	Severe ☐
Buccostomatitis:			Maxillary ☐	Mandibular ☐
Faucitis:			Unilateral ☐	Bilateral ☐
Bleeding Index:		1 = slight	2 = moderate	3 = severe
	Q1 ☐	Q2 ☐	Q3 ☐	Q4 ☐

Homecare: ....

....

....

Follow-up:...

....

Key to chart

LESIONS

A	abscess
C/S	calculus/slight
C/M	calculus/ moderate
C/H	calculus/heavy
ED	enamel defect
F	fistula
Fi	furcation exposure
Fx	tooth fracture
Gi	gingivitis (1-3)
NV	non vital tooth
O	missing tooth
PD	periodontitis (1-4)
PE	exposed pulp
PP	periodontal pocket
RL	resorptive lesion
W	worn tooth
X	extraction
X/S	surgical extraction

RIGHT   LEFT

103 102 101 201 202 203
104   204
106   206
107   207
108   208
109   209
409   309
408   308
407   307
404   304
403 402 401 301 302 303

Diagnosis:...

Treatment:...

Figure 2.14 A dental chart is used to record the condition of the teeth and the work that has been done. Reproduced with permission from Virbac Ltd.

tolerated by the cat otherwise they will not be maintained on a regular basis, and may not be applied at all.

TOOTH BRUSHING

This is the gold standard of tooth care and should always be recommended if practically possible. Ideally brushing of teeth is a procedure that should be introduced when the cat is a kitten as it is much more likely to be well-tolerated if started early.

There are many brushes on the market designed for cats (see Fig. 2.15), or a very soft child's brush may be used. Advise owners that the mechanical brushing action is the most important part, the dentifrice used is there really to help patient acceptance. Toothpaste should be one designed for animal use. Human toothpaste should not be used; it contains fluoride and foaming agents as well as flavourings and should not be swallowed.

Brushing must be carried out on a daily basis if it is to be effective, every other day or once to twice a week is not sufficient to keep the plaque under control.

Explain to your clients that they are not expected to go home and start brushing their cat's teeth straight away after a general anaesthetic and dental procedure.

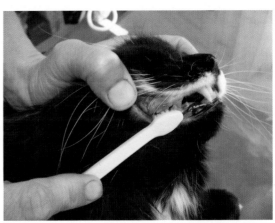

Figure 2.15 Toothbrushing is the most effective method for dental homecare.

The owner will need to build up to it slowly over a course of several weeks, starting by gently stroking the cat's mouth so that it gets used to being handled there. The next stage is to use a finger to apply the paste to the teeth (not forgetting the very back pre-molars and molars) and from here the owners could try using a facecloth, gauze swab or cotton bud as an intermediate stage before introducing the brush.

Tell owners not to worry if they notice the gums start to bleed a little, as this is a common occurrence if the gums are unhealthy and if they continue to brush the problem should resolve.

ORAL HYGIENE GELS/SPRAYS/LIQUIDS

These products are ideal for those owners who are unable to brush but are keen to provide good home-care. The products have various modes of action including prevention of accumulation of new plaque, reducing the bacterial load in the mouth, and reduction in the mineralisation of plaque into calculus by using calcium binders. Oral hygiene products containing chlorhexidine have been shown to be amongst the most effective chemical methods of plaque control available. Chlorhexidine has antibacterial activity and helps to slow down the formation of plaque; if used twice daily it can be almost as effective as brushing. The addition of zinc helps to prolong contact time in the mouth and may promote wound healing as well as having some antiplaque activity.

DIET

Certain types of diets can be used to help in controlling dental disease. They will have best effect when used in conjunction with brushing rather than as a substitute for brushing.

Standard dry diets can provide a very mild abrasive action and may encourage chewing. There are also many dry diets on the market that are formulated to promote dental care. They work in various ways from mechanical action to chemical action (reducing the mineralisation of plaque). Diets that have a mechanical action are sometimes described as 'edible tooth-brushes'. They may have a good effect on the amount of plaque and tartar accumulating above the gum line, but a significant drawback is that, due to the angle of the tooth immediately above the gum line, they cannot effectively clean within the gingival sulcus, which is a critical area for the development of periodontal disease.

CHEWS

There are now a number of commercial dental chews available for cats, many of which contain enzymes and chemicals designed to reduce plaque formation and plaque mineralisation. As with the 'dental' diets these can help to remove some plaque by a mechanical action on the crown but will not clean plaque sub-gingivally. It is thought that the chewing action may help to strengthen the periodontal ligaments over time.

Cats that will not accept commercially manufactured chews can be encouraged to chew on tough strips of cooked meat as a suitable alternative.

Follow-up

After discussion of homecare at the post-operative check, follow-up appointments should be made to continually monitor plaque accumulation and home-care. These can be made between 3 to 6 months apart, depending on the severity of the problem. When providing dental care information try to make it interesting and fun as well as informative and, as with the geriatric clinics, giving the club a groovy name may help to generate more interest from the clients.

CHAPTER 3

NUTRITION

Rebecca Giles, C&G CertSAN VN

Good nutrition is vital for health, wellbeing and longevity in the cat and feeding time is very important for cat and owner alike. It contributes to the close bond between them, and allows the owner to recognise any reduction in appetite or reluctance to eat.

Cats have very specific nutritional requirements, because they are obligate carnivores. Unlike other species such as the dog, they are not adapted to eat the wide variety of foods that are often offered to them by their human companions. Their nutritional requirements remain unchanged by evolution and are similar to those of their wild relatives.

This chapter will review the key nutritional requirements of the cat and will look at lifestage feeding, management of obesity and the principles of dietary management of medical disorders.

3.1 NUTRITIONAL NEEDS OF THE CAT

The carnivorous cat

Cats are carnivorous hunting animals and have many physical characteristics that reflect this lifestyle.

They have a short rounded skull with thick sturdy jawbones and strong masseter muscles for biting, but limited capacity for side-to-side jaw movement. These adaptations provide strength to bite and hold prey, and to tear muscle meat from bone, with limited requirement for the chewing movements that are needed to break down fibrous food. Their teeth are also developed for catching, killing and devouring prey with a large gap between the canine and carnassial teeth so the canine tooth can plunge deep into the prey. Cat's eyes are adapted for night vision, allowing effective hunting when prey animals are most active. The pupils can dilate widely and the retina has a large reflective area (the tapetum lucidum) to capture all the available light. They also have highly sensitive hearing and upright ears to pick up the high pitched sounds of their prey and have an array of very sensitive whiskers to help to locate prey and protect the face.

Their digestive tract is also adapted for a carnivorous diet, which is less varied and simpler to digest than an omnivorous or vegetarian diet:

- The feline digestive tract is shorter but the absorptive capacity is maintained because the intestinal villi are longer.
- The stomach is not used as a storage reservoir, so can be small; the capacity is around 45 ml per kg body weight, whereas the canine stomach capacity is 70 ml per kg body weight.
- The glandular portion of the stomach is also reduced because the stomach has a less significant role in the digestive process.
- The carnivorous diet is low in fibre, so the colon is shorter and the caecum is vestigial.
- The carnivorous diet is low in carbohydrate, so the cat has very limited ability to handle it (see later).

Energy requirement

Energy is provided by the intake of protein, fat and carbohydrate. Protein and fat are essential but carbohydrate is not essential for cats and in fact they have quite a low tolerance for carbohydrate in the diet.

A cat's daily energy requirement is based on its resting energy requirement plus any extra energy required to account for its activity level, its life-stage or physiological state and any requirement for weight loss or weight gain. Calculating the amount of energy that is needed is an approximation, because all cats are different, but the following principles and calculations are applicable:

1. Resting energy requirement (RER) is the amount of energy used by an inactive animal, in a thermoneutral environment, 12 hours after eating. It is very similar to the 'basal energy requirement' (BER), but is easier to measure. RER can be calculated using the formula:

$$RER \text{ (kcal)} = 70 \times (\text{body weight}^{0.75})$$

2. If the cat weighs more than 2 kg, this equation can be simplified, and a reasonably accurate estimate of RER can be found using the calculation:

$$RER \text{ (kcal)} = (30 \times \text{body weight}) + 70$$

Table 3.1 shows worked examples of how these calculations are used to estimate a cat's resting energy requirement.

3. Maintenance energy requirement (MER) is the amount of energy required by an animal to maintain its current daily activity level without gaining or losing body condition. It does not include the energy that is needed for growth, healing, pregnancy or lactation.

4. For cats with an 'average' activity level MER can be calculated using the formula:

$$MER \text{ (kcal)} = RER \times 1.4$$

5. Daily energy requirement (DER) is the actual energy needed per day, taking into account life stage, physiological state, and activity level. For example a growing kitten has a higher DER than an adult cat; a pregnant cat has a higher DER than a neutered cat; and an inactive indoor cat has a lower DER than an active cat with a large territory.

Table 3.2 indicates the approximate DER for cats in various life stages and physiological states. It must be remembered that all animals are individual and that their energy requirements will vary.

Table 3.1 Calculating a cat's resting energy requirement (RER)

For cats over 2 kg in body weight:

RER (kcal) = (30 × body weight [kg]) + 70

e.g. For a 3.5 kg cat: RER = (30 × 3.5) + 70
                                   = 175 kcal

For cats under 2 kg:

RER = 70 × (body weight$^{0.75}$)

e.g. For a 1.5 kg cat: RER = 70 × (1.5$^{0.75}$)
                                   = 94.9 kcal

NB: If you are using a standard calculator, you will need to know that 1.5$^{0.75}$ can be calculated by taking the square root of 1.5 twice then cubing the result:

$\sqrt{1.5}$ = 1.2247
$\sqrt{1.2247}$ = 1.1067
1.1067 × 1.1067 × 1.1067 = 1.3555
70 × 1.3555 = 94.9

Table 3.2 Approximate daily energy requirements in different physiological states

Physiological state	Approx DER
<3 months old (growth)	2.5–3 × RER
3–6 months old (growth)	3–2.5 × RER
6–12 months old	2.5–2 × RER
Inactive neutered adult	1.2–1.4 × RER
Obese adult	0.8–0.9 × RER
Pregnancy[a]	1.6–2.0 × RER
Peak lactation[b]	3.0–5.0 × RER
(3–6 weeks post partum)	

DER, daily energy requirement; RER, resting energy requirement.
[a] For more information on nutritional requirements during pregnancy see p. 45.
[b] For more information on nutritional requirements during lactation see p. 45.
Adapted from Hand, Thatcher, Remillard and Roudebush (2000). Small Animal Clinical Nutrition, 4th edn. Mark Morris Institute, Topeka.

Energy content of food

INTERPRETATION OF PET FOOD LABELS

The ingredients listed on a pet food label are expressed as a percentage of the total product. You will notice that the carbohydrate level is not indicated – this can be calculated by adding up the amounts of the other ingredients (including water) and subtracting the total from 100.

Example: Calculating the carbohydrate content of a wet food:

1. Information provided on the packaging of the food

   Protein, 8.0%
   Oil, 4.5%
   Ash, 2.5%
   Fibre, 0.3%
   Moisture, 82%

2. Sub-total of all the listed ingredients = 8 + 4.5 + 2.5 + 0.3 + 82 = 97.3%

3. Carbohydrate content = 100 − 97.3 = 2.7%

Alternatively, or if the label does not provide sufficient information, the pet food manufacturer can be contacted for more information.

CALCULATING THE AMOUNT OF FOOD REQUIRED

It is now possible to calculate the metabolisable energy value (ME) of this food. The ME value is the most accurate expression of how many calories the cat will be able to absorb (remember all foods have a calorie content, but how useful it is depends upon how digestible it is). It is important to use this value when calculating the volume of food to give the cat over 24 hours. All pet food manufacturers can supply the ME value of their products, usually a quick phone call to the company is all that is needed to get this information. However, it is quite a simple calculation and it is worth knowing how to do it.

The calculation involves adding up the useable energy (in kcal/g) provided by each energy giving component in the food i.e. protein, fat and carbohydrate. Table 3.3 indicates the ME value of the different nutrients. These values, combined with the information regarding the nutrient content, can be used to calculate the ME of any pet food.

Each nutrient contributes a proportion of the overall ME, equivalent to its ME value multiplied by the amount of that nutrient present in the food.

Example: Calculating the metabolisable energy of a wet food.

1. Protein: ME of protein = 3.5 kcal/g

   Protein content of the food = 8.0%
   ME contributed by protein = 3.5 × 8.0 = 28 kcal per 100 g wet food

2. Fat (oil): ME of fat = 8.7 kcal/g

   Fat content of the food = 4.5%
   ME contributed by fat = 8.7 × 4.5 = 39.15 kcal per 100 g wet food

3. Carbohydrate: ME of carbohydrate = 3.5 kcal/g

   Carbohydrate content of the food = 2.7%
   ME contributed by carbohydrate = 3.5 × 2.7 = 9.45 kcal per 100 g wet food

4. Total ME: Add all the individual contributions together:

   Total ME = 28 + 39.15 + 9.45 = 76.6 kcal per 100 g wet food

Table 3.3 Metabolisable energy values for different nutrients	
Nutrient	ME content of nutrients
Protein	3.5 kcal/g
Fat	8.7 kcal/g
Carbohydrate	3.5 kcal/g

Once the DER of the cat and the ME value of the food are known then the amount of that food that is required to be fed each day can be calculated.

Example: Calculating the food requirement of a 5 kg, normal weight cat.

1. Daily energy requirement = 1.4 × RER

   RER = (30 × body weight) + 70 = (30 × 5) + 70 = 220 kcal/day
   DER = 1.4 × 220 = 308 kcal/day

2. The ME value of the food is 76.6 kcal per 100g
   ME per gram of food = 76.6 ÷ 100 = 0.766 kcal/g

   To meet the DER of 308 kcal/day the cat must eat 308 ÷ 0.766 = 402.09 g/day.
   If the food comes in 100 g sachets, four sachets of the food should be fed daily.

COMPARISON OF FOODS

When comparing nutrient levels of pet foods it is very important to allow for the differences in water content between different types of food. By using 'dry matter' values, rather than 'as fed' values an accurate comparison between different food types can be made.

If dry matter values are not given on the label, they can be calculated from the other information that is supplied.

Example: Calculating the protein content of a wet food, on a dry matter basis.

1. Information provided on the packaging of the food

   Protein, 8.0%
   Moisture, 82%

2. Total dry matter = 100 − Moisture content = 100 − 82 = 18%

3. Protein content as fed = 8%

   Dry matter protein content = protein content as fed ÷ total dry matter × 100
   = 8 ÷ 18 × 100
   = 44.4% protein on a dry matter basis

To compare this wet food with a dry food, the dry matter protein content of the dry food must also be calculated:

1. Information provided on the packaging of the food
   Protein, 23%
   Moisture, 10%
2. Total dry matter = 100 − moisture content = 100 − 10 = 90%

3. Protein content as fed = 23%

Dry matter protein content = protein content as fed ÷ total dry matter × 100
= 23 ÷ 90 × 100
= 26% protein on a dry matter basis

As you can see it is essential to use the dry matter comparisons: using only the 'as fed' values the dry food would appear to contain more protein than the wet food, but in fact the reverse is true.

Nutrients

Feeding a balanced diet is essential for good health. Table 3.4 summarises some of the key nutritional requirements of adult cats.

Water

Water is an essential requirement for life. About 70–80% of lean body mass is water, with older or fatter animals having proportionately less than younger animals. It is essential for all body functions, including:

- Carriage of nutrients, enzymes, hormones, blood cells etc to their destinations within the body.
- Heat regulation.
- Maintenance of cell integrity.

Water is obtained from food and from drinking of water, but is also created by the breakdown of fat, protein and carbohydrate during digestion – this is known as metabolic water. Metabolic water contributes about 5 to 10% of the daily water requirement.

Daily water requirements depend on the amount of water lost by urination, defecation, perspiration and evaporation. Other factors that affect water requirements include lactation, illness, type of food fed e.g. wet or dry, and body surface area.

In general water requirement is estimated at 50 ml/kg body weight per day.

The type of food fed to the cat greatly influences the amount of water drunk. Cat owners who feed a wet food may rarely see their cat drink, while those who feed a dry diet may see their cat drink more regularly. Despite this, most cats that are fed a dry diet do not increase their water intake sufficiently to compensate for the absence of water in the food and in some cases this can encourage the formation of urinary crystals or bladder stones.

It is vitally important that clean, fresh water is available to cats at all times, although some cat owners have noticed that their cats prefer to drink water from less conventional sources such as watering cans or even the toilet! Filtering water may improve its palatability by removing some of the chemicals used in the processing of water, or collecting rainwater may be a practical alternative. Cats can also be encouraged to drink more by the addition of small amounts of a palatable flavour to water such as 'catmilk' or water from canned fish. Some cats prefer to drink from a source of running water, so another way of encouraging the cat to drink is to provide a water fountain, which constantly re-circulates the water.

Protein

Proteins are organic compounds made from one or more polypeptide chains of amino acids linked together with peptide bonds. There are 23 naturally occurring amino acids and, as they may be joined together in any combination, there is a huge variety of proteins possible.

Protein is needed for:

- Tissue growth and repair.
- Healthy tissue and immune function.
- Transport and storage of oxygen and other nutrients.
- Enzyme production.
- Hormone production.
- An energy source.

Protein deficiency can lead to:

- Poor growth.
- Weight loss.

Table 3.4 Key nutritional factors for adult cats at maintenance	
	Amount required[a]
Energy density (kcal ME/g)	4.0–5.0
Protein (%)	30–45
Fat (%)	10–30
Crude fibre (%)	<5
Calcium (%)	0.5–1.0
Phosphorus (%)	0.5–0.8
Ca/P ratio	0.9:1–1.5:1
Sodium (%)	0.2–0.6
Potassium (%)	0.6–1.0
Magnesium (%)	0.04–0.1
Chloride (%)	>0.3

[a] Dry matter basis.
Adapted from Hand, Thatcher, Remillard and Roudebush, (2000). Small Animal Clinical Nutrition, 4th edn. Mark Morris Institute, Topeka.

- Impaired immunity.
- Delayed wound healing.
- Poor coat condition.

Table 3.5 Essential amino acids for the cat	
Phenylalanine	Histidine
Valine	Arginine
Tryptophan	Leucine
Threonine	Lysine
Isoleucine	Taurine
Methionine	

Dietary protein can be of animal or vegetable origin, but cats have a high requirement for protein of animal origin. The term 'biological value' is used to describe how useful a protein is with regard to its suitability and the amount of amino acids it contains. For example, egg has a high biological value of 100% whereas leather is also a protein but is inedible and has a biological value of 0. Biologically useful proteins are metabolised into their component parts: amino acids (see later), carbon skeletons and nitrogen. The carbon skeletons are used as an energy source and the nitrogen may be synthesised into non-essential amino acids or other nitrogenous compounds.

Cats have an unusually high requirement for protein because they use it as an important source of energy, whereas (non-carnivorous) humans use carbohydrate as their main energy source. Cats need to derive at least 10% of their energy from protein in order to stay in a positive nitrogen balance, i.e. to prevent the use of the body's own tissues for energy production. They are unable to adapt their metabolism to use alternative energy sources if protein is lacking in their diet. This absolute requirement to use protein as an energy source means that cats have a constant need for protein in the diet.

Amino acids can be divided into two groups: essential and non-essential.

Essential amino acids cannot be manufactured within the body, so they must be present in the diet. Non-essential amino acids are needed for growth and metabolism, but they can be manufactured in the body by metabolism of other amino acids if they are lacking in the diet.

The essential amino acids for cats are shown in Table 3.5; this list is the same as the list for the dog, with the important addition of taurine. Taurine is found only in animal derived protein and without sufficient quantities of dietary taurine cats may suffer from blindness due to central retinal degeneration, heart failure due to dilated cardiomyopathy, and reproductive failure.

Arginine is also an essential amino acid that has particular importance in the cat. It has a very important role in the urea cycle, which is central to the metabolism, re-use and detoxification of proteins. Arginine is therefore a particularly important amino acid for a species that relies so heavily on protein metabolism and catabolism. A deficiency of arginine rapidly results in a build up of toxic ammonium in the blood, which can cause severe neurological signs. Fortunately arginine is present in almost all protein sources, so it is very difficult to induce arginine deficiency in cats fed normal diets, however, cats fed unusual diets, e.g. baby foods or protein deficient vegetarian diets can develop encephalopathy within hours. Arginine has also been shown to have beneficial effects in times of illness, stress and trauma by supporting the immune system.

Carbohydrate

Carbohydrates provide the body with energy and may also be converted into body fat. All animals have a metabolic requirement for glucose, which can be supplied either by synthesis within the body or from dietary sources. Carbohydrates are of little value to the cat: they derive all the glucose they need from protein metabolism, and lack significant levels of the enzymes required for carbohydrate digestion and absorption. Feeding a diet that is too high in carbohydrate can cause diarrhoea as the sugars are not digested and therefore pass through the body.

Amylase, the enzyme that initiates starch digestion, is not present in feline saliva (unlike dog and human saliva). Cats also have limited ability to manufacture pancreatic amylase and are unable to increase its production in response to a high carbohydrate meal.

Other enzymes that are responsible for the absorption of glucose into the bloodstream are present in much lower levels than in the dog.

Glucokinase is an enzyme produced in the liver that converts glucose into a form that can be stored for future use by the tissues and cells. Dogs and humans respond to a high carbohydrate meal by increasing their production of glucokinase to allow removal of the carbohydrate from the blood stream and storage in the liver. Cats are unable to manufacture glucokinase and so cannot handle high carbohydrate meals well.

Lactase is the enzyme required for digestion of the milk sugar lactose. Cats have difficulty digesting milk because, after weaning, their ability to produce lactase falls to a very low level.

While we can see that carbohydrates are of less value to the cat than the dog, they still have some importance to the species. Carbohydrates may be of value as an energy source during lactation when energy requirements are particularly high, or if dietary protein is in short supply.

No preparatory cat food will be free of carbohydrate (although it is not a requirement to list the carbohydrate content on the packaging). Some diets will have higher levels than others – and in general dry foods will have a higher carbohydrate content than tinned foods, for processing reasons. Reputable pet food companies are aware of the nutritional needs and limitations of the cat and allow for this when manufacturing their cat foods.

Fat

Fat is a valuable energy source for cats. It delivers twice as many calories as an equivalent weight of protein or carbohydrate and it is also a vital source of essential fatty acids (EFAs) and a carrier of fat-soluble vitamins. Fat also enhances palatability.

Dietary fats consist mainly of triglycerides, made up of one molecule of glycerol and three molecules of fatty acids. Triglycerides can be synthesised from non-fat sources such as carbohydrate or protein during times of positive energy balance. However, some biologically active lipids cannot be synthesised and a dietary source of these is required. These are known as essential fatty acids and a dietary deficiency can produce signs of disease.

Fatty acids are important for:

- Muscle contraction.
- Regulation of blood pressure, body temperature and blood clotting mechanisms.
- Control of inflammation.

There are three essential fatty acids:

- Linoleic acid.
- Arachidonic acid.
- Linolenic acid.

Arachidonic acid is synthesised from linoleic acid in dogs but not in cats and so must be present in the diet of the cat. Arachidonic acid is only found in fats of animal origin – more evidence that the cat is an obligate carnivore. Essential fatty acid deficiency may result in impaired wound healing, impaired reproductive performance, a dry coat and scaly skin.

Fat in food can become rancid (oxidised) if stored incorrectly, especially in warm or humid conditions. Oxidised fatty acids lose their nutritional value and produce harmful free radicals. This process can be prevented by the inclusion of anti-oxidants such as vitamin E. It also helps to store dry food in a cool, dark place; to use smaller bags to ensure freshness and to seal them between use.

Vitamins

Cats are unable to convert beta-carotene to vitamin A (unlike dogs and humans) and therefore require a supply of pre-formed vitamin A in their diet. Pre formed vitamin A is only found in animal tissues. Cats can only convert a limited amount of vitamin D from sunlight so they need a dietary source, which is only found in animal fats.

Feline food preferences

Cats are thought to be fussy eaters compared with dogs. To some extent this is true – cats instinctively test out food before eating. In the wild they will catch prey and consume it immediately, so they have a preference for food which is at body temperature. Cats are reliant on many senses in order to assess food that is offered to them. Firstly they will sniff the food; they react more favourably to food with strong aromas. Texture is also very important – cats prefer a texture similar to that of flesh, they are not attracted to food with powdery, sticky or very greasy textures. Cats that are accustomed to a specific texture, e.g. moist or dry may refuse foods with a different texture and it can be helpful to offer a variety of food types from an early age to avoid this.

Introducing dietary changes

If a cat's food is being changed this must be done gradually as cats are less tolerant of dietary changes than dogs. Ideally any changes should be made over 7 days. During this time the cat should be observed very closely in case the food is rejected, as a major reduction in calorie intake or a period of starvation could lead to hepatic lipidosis. The new food should be introduced gradually by mixing in small amounts with the previous food and increasing the amount of the new food daily or at each meal time until the new food is the only food given. Alternatively, some of the new food could be offered in a bowl next to the old food so that palatability can be assessed. If acceptability is a problem then the food could be warmed to

Table 3.6 Some common feeding mistakes and the problems they cause

Mistake	Problem	Action
Diet too high in fresh meat such as chicken or beef muscle meat.	Muscle meat is too high in phosphorus and too low in calcium. Causes nutritional secondary hyperparathyroidism, resulting in low bone density, bone pain and pathological fractures.	Young, growing cats are especially at risk. Ensure weaning kittens are introduced to a well-balanced kitten diet at an early stage. Only feed fresh meat as a complementary food, not as the main constituent of the diet.
Predominantly raw fish diet.	Raw fish contains an enzyme called thiaminase, which breaks down thiamine, a B vitamin important for neuromuscular function. Initial signs are anorexia, weight loss and depression progressing to neurological signs of ataxia, paresis and eventually seizures.	Treatment involves changing the diet to a well-balanced commercial pet food. Additional thiamine supplementation is required until the neurological signs disappear.
Too much liver.	Liver is very palatable to cats and is very high in vitamin A. Excessive amounts cause 'Hypervitaminosis A', resulting in liver damage and painful bone disease. The effects of vitamin A on bone growth and remodelling result in the development of bony outgrowths, especially of the cervical vertebrae and the long bones of the forelimb causing pain and reduced mobility. Hypervitaminosis takes years to develop, but once the bone changes have occurred the damage is permanent.	Only feed liver as an occasional treat.
Feeding baby-food or powdered soups to anorexic cats.	These foods contain onions and onion powder which contain chemicals that damage cats' red blood cells and can cause severe anaemia.	Cats should never be fed any foods that may contain onions or onion powder, even if just as a treat.
Vegetarian diets.	As we have seen it is practically impossible to formulate a vegetarian diet that will meet the nutritional needs of a cat.	Feed cats a balanced, carnivorous diet.

body temperature (if wet) or dry food could be soaked in boiled water and then mashed up and offered while still warm, though not too hot.

In summary the temperature, texture and aroma of food is very important to cats. Many cats prefer to eat on a little and often basis, this may be because in the wild they will consume between 10 and 20 small meals a day.

Feeding problems

When choosing a cat food it is important to consider the cat's age, the completeness of the diet, its palatability and also its cost. Cat owners love to please their cats and as such sometimes make mistakes that can lead to serious problems in the long term.

The first opportunity to make a mistake is when weaning kittens as it is at this time kittens can get focused on one type of food and it can be difficult to get them to eat other more suitable foods. Kittens and growing cats are particularly vulnerable to dietary problems, but adult cats can also suffer the consequences of being fed an inappropriate diet (see Table 3.6).

BOX 3.1   KEY POINTS

- Cats are obligate carnivores.
- Cats have a higher requirement for protein than dogs.
- Cats are less able to tolerate carbohydrates in their diet.
- Cats need a dietary source of:

    Taurine: an essential amino acid in the cat – only found in animal tissue.

    Arachidonic acid: an essential fatty acid in the cat – only found in animal fats.

    Pre-formed vitamin A – only found in animal tissues.

    Vitamin D – only found in animal fats.

3.2   FEEDING THE PREGNANT AND LACTATING QUEEN

A pregnant queen has an increased caloric requirement from the time of conception. She uses the additional calories to build energy stores that will allow her to cope with lactation, as well as to support the growing foetuses. The pregnant queen actually gains weight herself, as well as carrying the additional weight of the pregnant uterus, so once the kittens are born only 40% of the weight gain during pregnancy will be lost leaving 60% as energy stores for the queen to use during lactation. This is not the case in pregnant bitches; they only gain small amounts of weight in the first two-thirds of pregnancy and then go back to their previous weight immediately after parturition.

Before breeding the queen should be on a good quality energy dense food, in preparation for the forthcoming pregnancy. Queens that are obese or undernourished should not be used for breeding.

Pregnancy

Dietary changes during pregnancy should be avoided as they may cause diarrhoea which reduces the availability of nutrients for the queen and the developing foetuses.

Feeding a diet with a metabolisable energy of 4.0–5.0 kcal per gram of dry matter will provide adequate energy throughout the pregnancy. In late pregnancy the queen will have less room in her abdomen so feeding an energy dense diet will be beneficial here too. Ad-lib feeding is appropriate for most breeding queens as long as they are observed for any signs of obesity (however this may be difficult to do in a pregnant cat). Feeding between 1.6 and 2 times RER should ensure that energy and nutritional needs are met during pregnancy.

Nutritional requirements remain very much the same as for non-breeding cats but provision of a balanced diet becomes even more important. Nutritional imbalances may manifest as suboptimal breeding efficiency, or may cause deformities and still births, for example taurine deficiency may cause foetal death and deformities, and delayed growth and development. However, as long as a good quality cat food is being fed there is no need to give extra supplements, and they should be avoided as over-supply of some nutrients may cause unwanted complications.

Eclampsia (pregnancy hypocalcaemia) is a potentially fatal condition that can arise if an inappropriate diet is fed during pregnancy. It is rare in cats but if it does occur it is likely to happen in the last three weeks of pregnancy, whereas in bitches it more commonly develops during lactation.

Lactation

Lactation is highly energy demanding and nutritional needs are higher during lactation than during pregnancy, reaching a peak requirement at 3–4 weeks post-parturition. The queen should continue to be fed a high quality energy dense diet throughout her lactation and ad lib feeding is essential; feeding kitten food is ideal as the kittens can be weaned on to this too.

There is also an increased fluid requirement to meet the needs of milk production so plenty of fresh water must always be available.

Carbohydrate is a non-essential nutrient for cats, but it is does provide some real benefits during lactation when energy needs are very high. By using carbohydrate as an energy source the queen can divert more of her protein intake to the kittens and to her own essential requirements (a 'protein sparing' effect). Carbohydrate can also be used to produce the milk sugar lactose.

Table 3.7 shows the nutritional requirements of the queen during pregnancy and lactation.

Table 3.7 Nutritional requirements of the queen during pregnancy and lactation	
Nutrient	Required amount[a]
Protein	At least 35% DM
Fat	At least 18% DM
Calcium	1.0–1.6% DM
Calcium:phosphorus ratio	1:1 to 1.5:1
Carbohydrate (for lactation)	At least 10% DM

DM, Daily energy requirement; [a] Dry matter basis.
Adapted from Hand, Thatcher, Remillard and Roudebush (2000). Small Animal Clinical Nutrition, 4th edn. Mark Morris Institute, Topeka

3.3 FEEDING KITTENS

Kittens should weigh between 90–100 grams at birth and gain 50–100 grams per week over the first 5–6 months.

During the first 24–72 hours the queen will produce colostrum (first milk) and it is very important that the kittens receive this within the first 12 to 16 hours of life. Colostrum contains all the nutrients that the kittens will need as well as maternal antibodies (immunoglobulins), growth factors and digestive enzymes. During the first 12 to 16 hours of life the kittens are able to absorb maternal antibodies through their small intestines, but after that time an 'intestinal barrier' develops to prevent absorption of harmful substances and this also prevents absorption

of maternal antibodies. After the first 12 to 16 hours the queen's milk will continue to provide immunoglobulins that will have a local effect on the intestinal tract but absorption of intact antibodies cannot occur.

The queen's milk will continue to change in its composition throughout lactation to meet the changing needs of the growing kittens. A good indicator that the queen is coping and providing enough milk for her kittens is that the kittens should be contentedly sleeping and warm rather than noisy, distressed and cold. Kittens will feed from their mother for the first three to four weeks and then the mother will start the weaning process at about this stage. Soft, palatable food should be made available to the kittens so that they can learn to feed gradually, and a good quality kitten food is the ideal choice. It is important to keep the feeding area clean and not to allow the food to go stale. The kittens will walk through the food but the mother will usually clean them up. Weaning will be completed by about 6–8 weeks, and at this time the mother will start to reject the kittens when she feels they are being too demanding. It is helpful for the kittens to spend some time away from their mother every day during the weaning process to give her a break and to ensure that she eats and drinks enough herself. Eventually the mother's milk will cease and weaning will be complete.

At this stage the kittens should be consuming a good quality proprietary kitten food. This may either be wet food, or dry food which has been soaked to soften it; at this age the kittens' teeth will be too fragile to deal with dry food. They should be given between 4 and 6 meals a day and fresh water should be available to them at all times. The kittens' lactase activity will now be decreasing so giving milk will not be helpful and will be unnecessary if a good quality kitten food is fed.

Hand rearing newly born kittens

In some circumstances hand rearing of kittens is necessary because of loss of the mother, rejection of the kittens or lack of milk production from the mother. Hand rearing of kittens is very difficult and problematic but can be rewarding when successful.

Kittens need warmth, fluid, food and stimulation. A boxed in area with clean, dry bedding should be provided – at this stage the bedding should be smooth (e.g. cotton sheet) as their tiny claws can easily become tangled in fleece type bedding.

It is very important to keep the environmental temperature fairly constant because kittens are unable to regulate their own body temperature until they are about two weeks old. Normal body temperature at this stage is 35–35.5°C (95–96°F). Care must be taken when providing warmth; the neonatal kittens cannot move out of range if they get too hot, so they can rapidly become over-heated if they are placed too close to a direct heat source such as a heat lamp. A thermostatically controlled heat pad would be the ideal, using a thermometer safely secured to the wall of the kittens' area to monitor the environmental temperature, which should be 30–34°C (86–93°F) for kittens of this age.

The kittens should be bottle-fed using a preparatory feline milk replacer. Table 3.8 shows the nutritional requirements of newborn kittens. Suitable milk replacers are available from veterinary practices and some pet shops. They come as powder for reconstitution, and it is important that the instructions supplied with the powder are followed carefully.

Hand-reared kittens are particularly prone to infections so it is very important that all feeding equipment is sterilised and then rinsed and dried thoroughly after use. Bacteria thrive in a warm, damp environment and any food residues will provide an ideal growth medium for bacteria. Basic rules about safe food handling and storage must be applied. If the total daily food requirement is made up in the morning it should be kept refrigerated until required and gently warmed before being given to the kitten.

Care should be taken to ensure the food is neither too hot nor too cold when hand feeding. Feeding with a dropper bottle rather than a syringe is preferable as it encourages the kittens to suck (see Fig. 3.1). Syringe plungers can be unpredictable and can deliver the milk too quickly which will increase the risk of aspiration pneumonia. Newly born kittens will probably need feeding hourly and they will not sur-

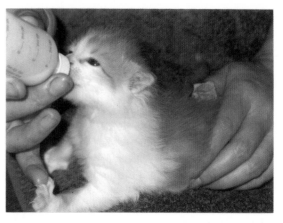

Figure 3.1 Bottle feeding a kitten. Reproduced with permission from Annette Miller.

vive for long if their intake of fluid/food is inadequate. A kitten that is cold, hungry or too hot will cry; weight gain and contented sleep are good signs that the kitten is getting everything it needs. After feeding, newly born kittens will need help with passing urine and faeces; usually the queen does this by washing the kittens rear ends, but this action can be mimicked using a dampened cotton bud or cotton wool ball. Again, great care should be taken to prevent infection of the urogenital area.

Kittens over the age of two weeks are more active and are increasingly able to control their own body temperature. They will start to show interest in solid food at 3–4 weeks of age (see p. 47) and the frequency of bottle feeds can be reduced in line with the increased intake of solid food by the kittens.

Supplemental feeding

Occasionally older, semi-weaned kittens will need some supplemental feeding if the queen's milk supply is reduced e.g. due to sickness, accident or the development of mastitis. In this instance proprietory milk replacers can be used as previously described. All the usual rules regarding good hygiene should be followed. Supplemental feeding may need to be continued until weaning is complete.

3.4 OBESITY

Obesity is becoming a common problem amongst pet cats, and veterinary practices are seeing increasing numbers of overweight cats with obesity related

Table 3.8 Key nutritional requirements of new-born kittens	
Nutrient	Requirement
ME density	>4.5 kcal/g
Protein	>35%[a]
Fat	>21%[a]

[a] Dry matter basis.

conditions. Cats are termed as obese when they are 15% or more above their ideal weight, or have a body score of 5 out of 5 (see p. 68).

Obesity occurs if caloric intake exceeds usage. Obesity can be caused by feeding the cat too many calories. This is more of a problem when feeding dry food and when using ad libitum feeding. On the other hand, cats may not use as many calories as they are given because of inactivity and because neutering reduces caloric needs.

Achieving successful weight reduction in cats can be more of a challenge than in dogs because of the differences in lifestyle between dogs and cats. Prevention is better than cure, so a chat with the nurse at a critical stage in the cat's development, e.g. at neutering time, may educate the owners into the prevention of obesity.

Recognising obesity

Assessing the development of fat deposits in the cat is more difficult than in the dog because fat accumulates intra-abdominally first and then builds up peripherally e.g. over the ribs. Using body condition score systems is helpful (see pp. 68 and 70), and if the cat is body condition scored and weighed at every visit to the practice this can help keep track of any changes and hopefully identify any problems early on, before other clinical signs develop.

Health risks associated with obesity in cats

Many owners perceive that 'a fat cat is a happy cat'; however obesity is associated with a number of significant health problems, and will have a major negative impact on the cat's quality of life.

Diabetes mellitus

Obesity is a risk factor for diabetes mellitus in many species, not just cats, but insulin resistance due to obesity is an especially common cause of diabetes in cats. Weight reduction may greatly increase insulin sensitivity and therefore reduce the dose of exogenous insulin required. Occasionally, the need to give insulin may cease after successful weight reduction.

Feline lower urinary tract disease (FLUTD)

Obese cats are known to be at increased risk of developing FLUTD, and there may be a number of expla-

nations for this. Firstly, the consumption of a high proportion of dry food is a recognised risk factor for both conditions. It may be that increased consumption of minerals is a factor, added to the fact that many cats don't increase their water intake enough to compensate for the lack of water in dry food, which in turn can lead to the production of too highly concentrated urine. In addition obese cats tend to be less active, they may visit the litter tray less often and so retain urine for longer allowing crystal formation and aggregation.

Osteoarthritis

Excess body weight puts increased strain on the joints. The increased wear and tear contributes to the development of arthritis in older age.

Hepatic lipidosis

Hepatic lipidosis is a serious condition, which is characterised by accumulation of triglycerides in the liver. An imbalance between uptake and removal of triglycerides by the liver leads to reduced hepatocyte function and eventual liver failure. Affected cats develop severe anorexia, depression and jaundice and the condition is often fatal. The risk of hepatic lipidosis is greatly increased in obese cats that suffer a period of anorexia. Illness, stress or a change of diet can trigger the anorexia, but hepatic lipidosis can also be triggered by aggressive attempts to get the cat to lose weight. This is why care must be exercised when creating a weight reduction programme for cats. Hepatic lipidosis is treated by assisted feeding (naso-oesophageal or preferably gastrostomy tube feeding) and supplementation of arginine, taurine, vitamin E and L-carnitine. The assisted feeding must meet the cat's energy requirements and will need to be continued until the cat voluntarily eats adequate calories, which may take several weeks. With early intervention and good nutritional support, cats can recover from hepatic lipidosis.

Other adverse effects of obesity
- Anaesthetic complications and poor wound healing.
- Decreased heat tolerance and stamina.
- Respiratory difficulties.
- Dystocia.
- Poor skin and coat quality.
- Decreased immune function.
- Reduction in the pet's quality of life.

Weight reduction plans

The best way to treat obesity is to reduce the caloric intake and to increase exercise. Restricting food intake alone will often not be very effective, as the body will reduce its metabolic rate to compensate for the reduced food intake so weight loss may not occur. Care must also be exercised when reducing a cat's caloric intake because of the risk of inducing hepatic lipidosis. It is also very important to rule out other reasons for weight gain, such as the presence of tumours or ascites, before embarking upon a weight reduction plan. Care should be taken when trying to reduce weight in growing animals, pregnant or lactating queens or cats with a history of hepatic lipidosis, and veterinary advice must be followed closely in these cases.

Setting the target weight

Calorie restriction should be initiated with care and the target weight should not be less than 85% of the present weight. Setting the first target for weight loss at 15% (even if the cat is much more obese) gives the owner an achievable target over a reasonable time scale, and should avoid the temptation to reduce calorie intake further to speed up the process. Once the first target weight is reached, a new target weight can be set if necessary and the energy requirement recalculated.

What to feed

The cat's food should be changed to a proprietary weight reduction food which is formulated to be low in energy but will have increased nutrients to avoid any deficiencies occurring. Manufacturers can supply veterinary practices with comprehensive feeding guides for ease of use.

L-carnitine is a co-factor in fatty acid metabolism and supplementation may be beneficial in obese cats and those that are on a weight reduction plan. It may lead to slightly faster weight reduction and help prevent hepatic lipidosis. A suggested dose rate is 250 mg per cat per day; some preparatory weight reduction diets are supplemented with L-carnitine.

Recent work suggests that feeding a low carbohydrate (<10%), high protein (45%) diet to obese cats will help preserve lean body mass. Lean body mass is important as it is involved in the basal metabolic rate (BMR). A reduction in lean body mass lowers the BMR and therefore may lead to weight gain once more.

Any change to the cat's diet should occur over a transitional period of about 7 days, since cats are less able to tolerate dietary changes than dogs. If the cat refuses to eat any of the appropriate weight reduction diets, then significant calorie restriction may not be possible without risking hepatic lipidosis. For these cats the owner may need to rely on cutting out all 'extras', making a small reduction in the amount of the current food being fed, and on increasing activity levels. This will probably achieve some weight reduction but it is likely to be a much slower process.

How much to feed

It is usual to restrict calories to no less than 60% of the maintenance energy requirement at target weight, and a restriction to 70% of MER may be preferable in the first instance.

Example: Calculating target weight and daily food intake (see pp. 39–40 for definitions of terms).

1. Present weight: 6.5 kg

   First target: 15% weight loss
   $= 6.5 - (15\% \times 6.5) = 5.53$ kg

2. MER at target weight $= 1.4 \times$ RER at target weight

   RER $= (30 \times 5.53) + 70 = 235.9$ kcal/day
   MER $= 1.4 \times 235.9 = 330.3$ kcal/day

3. For controlled weight loss, daily energy requirement $= 70\%$ MER

   DER $= 330.26 \times 70\% = 231$ kcal/day

4. The dry food to be fed has a metabolisable energy value of 283 kcal per 100 g as fed
   ME per gram of food $= 283 \div 100 = 2.83$ kcal/g

   To meet the DER of 231 kcal/day the cat must eat $231 \div 2.83 = 81.69$ g/day. Therefore the amount of food needed daily can be rounded down to 80 grams per day.

Increasing exercise

Many cat owners are surprised to be asked to increase their cat's activity. It is commonly believed that cats, especially adult cats, are more self-sufficient than dogs and do not need encouragement to exercise. However, as in all species, inactivity can lead to obesity and an increase in activity will increase the metabolic rate and therefore help with weight reduction. The general rule with cats is 'the cheaper the toy the more fun it is'! Paper bags, boxes and newspaper are well received, and some cats really enjoy playing with fishing rod toys. Providing other forms of environmental enrichment, such as giving additional food and water bowls and litter trays, plus grooming the cat may also be of benefit. Dividing the daily food ration, using a feeding ball, and 'hiding' the food around the house will encourage cats to move around during the day.

Monitoring progress

It is important to monitor the patient closely during the weight reduction programme. An early check is required to ensure the cat is eating the diet and that the amount given is suitable for the cat. The owner should be instructed to revert back to the previous diet if the cat refuses to eat the new diet within a reasonable time (2 days), hopefully the transition period will be smooth and the cat will accept the new diet. Thereafter fortnightly visits will allow for a chat with the owner, and a check for the cat to ensure all is running smoothly. Aiming for 1–2% weight loss every fortnight is realistic. Once the owner and cat are happy with the new regime and diet, the number of visits to the practice may be reduced to once a month to avoid stress to the cat through travelling. As the weight reduction plan develops it is important to give owners encouragement and support. 'Rewards' help to keep the client motivated:

- Take before and after photographs.
- Make a weight chart to record progress.
- Arrange for the clients to come in to the clinic at the same time as other owners with overweight pets so that they can compare notes.
- Give gifts to successful dieters.
- Publicise the 'dieter of the month' on a waiting room notice-board.

What problems could occur?

WEIGHT LOSS TOO RAPID

- Check your calculation and the amount of food given.
- Body score the patient as the difference in weight may also be due to an empty bladder and empty colon.
- Has the cat's activity level increased greatly?
- Is the cat actually eating the prescribed food (very important in cats)?

TOO LITTLE WEIGHT LOST

- Re-check your weight reduction calculations.
- Body score the patient as the difference in weight may be due to a full bladder or colon.

- Make sure the owner is weighing the food correctly.
- Find out if there has been interference with the diet, e.g. children feeding table scraps, treats.
- Is the cat getting too little exercise?
- Is there any underlying medical cause?

If all the above points have been considered and addressed, but the cat is still not losing weight, then it is likely that cat has a particularly slow metabolism, and so needs fewer calories than would be assumed from the standard calculations based on the requirements of an 'average' cat. Further reduction in calories may be needed but with great care because of the risk of hepatic lipidosis; start with a further reduction of 5–10% and closely monitor the cat's progress.

Obesity clinics are very rewarding for veterinary nurses and for owners. Achieving the target weight will maximise quality of life for the pet and will lead to positive health benefits.

BOX 3.2 KEY POINTS

- Owners must be informed of the importance in dieting obese cats.
- They must be made aware of feline hepatic lipidosis.
- The cat should be given a proprietary food designed for weight reduction. Weight reduction plans should not be carried out using the existing food.
- Fresh water should always be available (not milk – calories!).
- Owners should ensure that their cats receive more exercise (as long as this is not contraindicated).
- Owners and cats need support throughout the weight reduction plan and beyond.

3.5 NUTRITIONAL REQUIREMENTS IN DISEASE

Nutrition can play an important part in the treatment and recovery from disease and trauma. Altering the levels of different nutrients in the food can have a beneficial effect leading to faster recoveries and improvement in quality of life. For example, the reduction in phosphorus levels in diets for cats affected by renal disease is known to delay progression of the disease and prolong survival. Today there are many diets that are produced to assist in the treatment of disease and the pet food companies also produce literature to help in the correct use of these diets. When using special diets it is important to have an understanding of the reasoning behind it, the requirements of the patient and any situations in which the specialised diet would be inappropriate. The effectiveness of any diet will be limited by the cat's acceptance of the new diet and/or its ability to digest and absorb the diet.

Caloric requirements may be substantially altered in sick cats compared to healthy cats. There is usually an increase in energy requirement due to the disease process and the need for tissue repair and this must be taken into account when assessing their nutritional requirements. However, care must be taken when applying generalised rules, and it is particularly important to closely monitor the individual cat; sick cats are often less active and may even be restricted to a cage for the duration of their illness which will reduce their energy requirement. They may also have problems dealing with any nutrients that are given in excess of their needs. The calculated energy requirement must be used only as a starting point, and it is important to monitor the bodyweight daily using accurate scales. Adjustments can then be made to the caloric intake if an undesirable trend in the weight of the patient is noted.

Hospitalised and sick cats are likely to be anorexic due to pain, stress, nausea, dehydration etc., and many will need encouragement to eat (see Fig. 3.2 and Box 3.3). At this time it is easy to induce food aversions because the cat may associate certain foods with the discomfort that it is feeling. It is important to alleviate pain, dehydration and stress in the hospitalised cat so that it is more likely to eat and therefore not deteriorate. Once the negative symptoms of illness and hospitalisation have been minimised it is time to encourage the patient to eat.

The type of food offered will depend on the cat's ability to digest and absorb nutrients and the suitability of the food for the condition that is being treated. However, it is worth remembering that in most cases getting the cat to eat something is much better than leaving it to refuse to eat a diet that is deemed more 'suitable'. Remember how we ourselves feel when we are ill but need to eat despite feeling under the

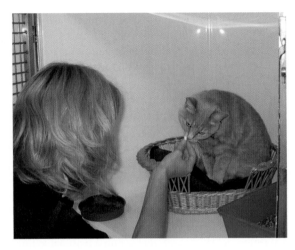

Figure 3.2 Encouraging a hospitalised cat to eat.

weather, and use similar approaches to feeding hospitalised cats.

Find out what the cat prefers to eat at home, including the type of food (dry versus wet), and feed this type to the cat. Always offer small amounts, as it is easy to get overfaced by large amounts of food, and more can always be offered if all is eaten.

Giving a choice of food is a good idea but restrict the choice to two foods as being surrounded by many food bowls will overwhelm the cat and may delay progress.

BOX 3.3   HINTS ON TEMPTING APPETITE

- Use small amounts of food initially.
- Warm food to body temperature – cats eat freshly killed prey so this is their preferred food temperature.
- Foods with strong odours, e.g. sardines may help get the cat eating again.
- Offer only two types of food at any one time.
- Remove uneaten food after 1 hour.
- Give the cat a 'rest' from food in the cage especially if it is nauseous.
- Mash up food.
- Tempt to eat by hand feeding – many cats respond well to this.
- Remember to offer some dry food too as some cats have a preference for this type.

Foods with strong odours will help tempt cats especially if they have problems with their sense of smell (e.g. due to upper respiratory disease). Cats rely heavily on their sense of smell in order to eat, and are much more selective about food types than dogs.

The type of food bowl used will also have some influence on food acceptance, using shallow bowls is preferable to ones with steep sides which can mean that the whiskers are affected, leading to possible discomfort. Ceramic or plastic bowls may be preferred to metal bowls.

Once a food preference has been established this should be continued, although some cats may require variety in order to keep interested in eating. If a 'prescription' type diet is required then this can be very gradually phased in as previously described (p. 44).

For cats with low food intake the veterinary surgeon managing the case may choose to use appetite stimulants. These drugs may be very useful but it is worth remembering that using appetite stimulants will be unlikely to make the cat consume its daily RER and that they are for short-term use only.

Commonly used appetite stimulants include:

- Cyproheptadine (Periactin; Merck, Sharp and Dohme): an antihistamine. Dose 2 mg per cat, per os once or twice daily. It may take up to 24 hours to take effect. Use for approximately one week and then taper the dose.

- Diazepam: given intravenously this can have a dramatic effect that is very short-lived (just a few minutes) so it is very important to have the food ready before the drug is given! This can be useful when assessing ability to eat, jaw movement etc in cases with a history of dysphagia. When given by mouth diazepam has little, or no, appetite stimulant effect.

Finally, if the cat has not eaten, or has been consuming less than its resting energy requirement, for three days then it is important to intervene with assisted feeding techniques (see p. 111). The method of assisted feeding will depend upon the cat's condition and anticipated length of illness/anorexia. The least invasive method is via a naso-oesophageal tube. This is easily placed without sedation or general anaesthesia and, once secured, may be kept in place for up to seven days. Other feeding tubes such as oesophagostomy, gastrostomy and jejunostomy tubes require a general anaesthetic and endoscopic or surgical placement.

Further reading

Agar S 1993 The Waltham book of companion animal nutrition. Pergamon, Oxford.

Agar S 2001 Small animal nutrition, Butterworth Heinemann, Oxford.

Hand MS, Thatcher CD, Remillard RL and Roudebush P (eds) 2000 Small animal clinical nutrition, 4th edn. Mark Morris Institute, Topeka.

THE HOSPITALISED CAT

CHAPTER 4

Valerie Pollard, DipAVN(Surgical) VN
Susan Howarth, DipAVN(Surgical) DipAVN(Medical) VN

4.1 HOSPITAL ENVIRONMENT

A cat ward should be self-contained and not included in the same area as the dog ward, as the requirements of cats and dogs are very different. The cat generally appreciates a quiet and subdued environment. The cat ward should be designed in a way that allows the feline patient to be observed unobtrusively and quietly. If space does not allow for a separate ward, an area at one end of the dog ward should be kept for cats only, keeping them as far away as possible from noisy boisterous dogs. Low-level back ground music in the ward often helps the cats relax.

Many feline patients do respond well to human interaction. Taking time to play, stroke and groom the cat will reduce the patient's stress levels and may even improve its general demeanour. However, if a particular patient is feral or unused to human contact then any kind of interaction may well be extremely stressful.

Design of the cat ward

When designing and building a cat ward you need to think about the requirements of the feline patient as well as the requirements of the veterinary team.

Cats do not appreciate being placed in close proximity to other unknown cats. Some cats will show physical aggression toward other patients if they can see them, the more nervous cat may attempt to hide but will be unable to escape from the aggressor, increasing stress levels. To reduce the stress visual contact between patients needs to be prevented. This can be achieved by placing the cages, with solid sides, adjacent to each other and having them in one bank only. The addition of a pheromone plug-in diffuser (Feliway™) will also help to minimise stress.

Having the cages in one bank will also minimise the risk of spread of respiratory infections, although patients suspected or diagnosed with an infectious disease should be placed in an isolation ward. The sneezing distance of a feline is about 60 cm, so if your ward has cages facing each other, there needs to be at the very minimum 60 cm distance between them; 1 m would be much more suitable.

The cage level should be at a safe height for personnel. The ideal base level for a cage is waist high. The cat is fully visible and can be retrieved easily without needing to use steps and without placing your head into the cage. However due to the general lack of space in most practices, cages are often banked up, with up to three stories of cages and with the base of the top cage at most nurses' head and shoulder height. This not only prevents good observation and creates difficulties in cleaning, but also poses a serious health and safety issue to personnel. To try and retrieve a cat from one of these cages without any kind of step, which in itself is a health and safety issue, would be dangerous. You can't get hold of the cat correctly, which undoubtedly will cause it to struggle. The lowest level cages placed several inches off the ground are not much better. You can observe the patients well, but you have to bend down to remove the cat, placing your face in the danger zone. Cats also feel more secure at higher levels. The lower cages should be raised off the ground by at least 30 cm. The empty space above and below the cages can be used for storage.

The cattery area needs to have central heating to provide an ambient temperature of around 18–23°C. Some manufacturers of cages are able to supply under-cage heating.

Adequate ventilation is also important. Windows are good for providing natural light, but if they are going to be used for ventilation, bars should be placed in front to prevent patients escaping. A system of ducting or extractor fans should be in place to provide a minimum of 10 changes of air per hour.

The materials that the ward is constructed from need to be hard wearing, non-porous and cost-effective. Most cattery cages will be seated on a plinth and this tends to be made of concrete or wood. Wood is extremely porous and may rot if not properly treated, but is relatively cheap and easy to work with.

Concrete can also be porous, though not to the same degree as wood, and requires coating. Once coated it is a good permanent structure with no risk of harbouring bacteria.

The floor also needs to be considered carefully. Older style hospitals may have sealed concrete or tiled floors with a central drain to allow for any waste to drain away. This is of more use in a kennel environment where dogs may eliminate in their kennels and everything can be washed away easily. The floor should be easy to clean, non-absorbent, slip-proof and sealed at the edges, running up the wall for at least 10 cm. This prevents dirt and bacteria getting trapped in the corners and skirtings.

Electric sockets for heat blankets, drip pumps, clippers etc, should be placed at convenient points around the ward. The provision of a workstation area with examination table, sink unit and storage, will minimise the need for carrying the feline patient around the hospital. All of the above should be replicated on a smaller scale for an isolation unit.

Design of the cat cage

Most cages are constructed of either stainless steel or fibreglass. Stainless steel kennels can stain with some disinfectants, feel quite cold to the touch and may even conduct heat away from the cat; they are also quite dark and noisy. White fibreglass cages give greater visibility, those with a glossy finish reflect light and are easier to clean.

The front of a hospital cage must also be easy to clean, allow good observation and prevent any kind of escape. Generally two types are used in practice: the stainless steel mesh gate, and the toughened glass door. A glass door (see Fig. 4.1) allows very good visibility of the patient, without any bars obscuring the view, reduces the risk of airborne spread by sneezing, and reduces the chance of the patient putting paws through bars and opening the door or causing injury to themselves.

There are no legal restrictions on the size of a hospital cat cage because usually the patient's stay in hospital is short-term, often just a day. This does not mean that they should be squeezed into the smallest available space! At the very least the cat should have adequate space for a litter tray, bedding and food/water bowls. These bowls should be placed as far from the litter tray as possible (see Fig. 4.2). Placing the litter tray in one corner and the food/water in the diagonal corner, allows for the greatest distance between them. Most cats will not want to eat if the bowl is in close proximity to

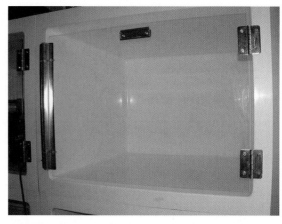

Figure 4.1 Laminated cat cage with toughened glass door.

their toilet. The ward should contain a mix of cage sizes for the long and short-stay patient. The cat that requires hospitalisation for longer than 24 hours should have a larger space allowing some degree of free movement.

Most cats like to have the opportunity to hide, so the provision of some kind of den will help to reduce stress. An 'Igloo' type bed can be used, but these are easily soiled and may get misplaced after washing. An old cardboard box is a cheap and easy option. Placing the box on its side with the open end either to the side or back of the cage, will allow the patient some degree of privacy. The cat can be observed without disturbance by making slits in the side of the box.

Cats also enjoy being in a high position as it makes them feel safe and out of harm's way. Ideally a shelf is available, providing this is not contraindicated, for instance if the animal has a fracture. Bedding can be placed on the shelf, but an alternative should be offered on the lower level as well.

It is best to provide the cat with the same litter it uses at home. Examples of litters available are clay-based ones, recycled newspaper or wood pellets. Wood-based litters are pellets that fluff up when used and release a pine smell, which some cats do not like. Natural peat-based litter and sand are very soft for the cat to stand

BOX 4.1   IDEAL REQUIREMENTS FOR A FELINE WARD CAGE

- Temperature controlled.
- Hygienic: non-staining, easy to clean, without sharp corners or joints (retain dirt and bacteria).
- Moulded.
- Minimal vibration, drumming etc.
- Escape proof.

BOX 4.2   SUGGESTED CAGE SIZES

	Height	Width	Depth
Day patient/ overnight	610 mm	610 mm	762 mm
Long stay	700 mm	1000 mm	1000 mm

on. Kittens may try to eat some litters, so bulking litters should be avoided, to prevent intestinal problems.

The choice of cat litter will also depend on the reason for hospitalisation. For instance if you require a urine sample you may need to use non-absorbent litter. Non-absorbent litter comes in two varieties: the re-usable gravel type, or disposable beads. The latter is easier to use and does not give false urine test results due to contaminants from previous patients or detergents from cleaning. Cats with open wounds or draining catheters should not have litter that is dusty or composed of small granules that may attach to the wound. It

may even be preferable in these cases not to use litter at all and shredded paper may be a better alternative.

A cat that refuses to use the litter tray will be uncomfortable and this can increase its amount of pain and discomfort. So the choice of litter is important not just for practical reasons but also for the patient's comfort. It is important to clean the litter tray soon after it has been used and at least twice daily.

If a sterile urine sample is required (cystocentesis) the litter tray needs to be removed to avoid the cat emptying its bladder.

Cleaning and disinfecting

It is important always to practise good hygiene, as this will prevent both nosocomial (hospital acquired) and zoonotic (from animal to human) infections. The cat ward needs to be cleaned on a daily basis. Thorough cleaning with non-abrasive materials needs to be done first, followed by the use of disinfectant. No disinfectant

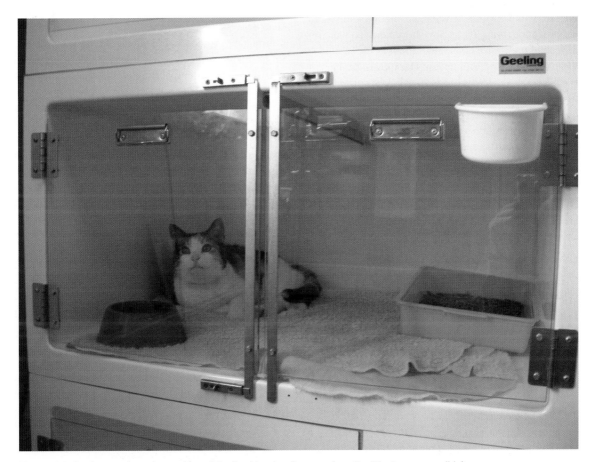

Figure 4.2 Cat in cage (note the position of the food bowl as far away from the litter tray as possible).

will be able to reach microorganisms that are hidden in dirt.

If stainless steel food and water bowls are used they can be sterilised between each patient to prevent cross contamination, which is very useful in the isolation unit. Your choice of bedding material can also be a factor in cross-contamination/infestation. Towels and blankets have the potential to harbour parasites but acrylic will not.

All equipment and tabletops need to be cleaned and disinfected between patients. Cats cannot metabolise phenols, so any disinfectant containing these (for instance Jeyes Fluid, Izal, Stericol, Clearsol, Dettol and Ibcol) should not be used anywhere near a cat ward, as even the fumes can be toxic to them.

Disinfectants are designed for use on either the environment or the skin, and occasionally both. It is important to be aware of the properties of the different types, and not to misuse any disinfectants. All pre-diluted solutions must be clearly labelled. Inappropriate use of disinfectants could result at best in an inadequately disinfected tabletop and at worst in chemical burns to either you or your patient. You should ensure that you have read the instructions fully, as well as the manufacturer's Control of Substances Hazardous to Health (COSHH) sheet. All disinfectants will have correct dilution rates, active temperature, contact time requirements and time taken to deteriorate. More does not necessarily mean better; the mixing of detergents and disinfectants can reduce the effectiveness of one or both of them.

There are many disinfectants on the market, divided into a number of categories. Table 4.1 shows the disinfectant categories and their properties, followed by a list of more commonly used trade names and their specific properties.

When deciding on the protocol for the practice several questions need to be answered:

- What area is the product to be used in?
- How much 'traffic' is there in this area?
- Is this a high-risk area (isolation, theatre etc)?
- Is it likely to be heavily soiled?
- Does this area accommodate patients, if so what species?
- How often will it need cleaning?
- What material is the surface/equipment etc made of? (Some materials may be damaged by the cleaning solution.)

These questions emphasise that each area will have specific needs and that different agents will be needed in different areas, rather than using a 'general purpose cleaner' throughout the practice. A cleaning/disinfecting protocol can be drawn up for the practice, which includes the type of detergent/disinfectant to use, dilution rate, temperature of use, contact time and frequency of cleaning for each area of the practice.

When cleaning cages and surfaces with a spray it is best to use single-use disposable paper towels. Cloths such as 'J-cloths' will harbour bacteria even if regularly changed and can transfer bacteria from one cage to another.

The detergent used to clean hands in between patients also needs to be considered carefully. The necessary contact time and action on bacteria, fungi and viruses does vary.

BOX 4.3   DEFINITIONS OF TERMS USED IN CLEANING MATERIALS/DISINFECTANTS

- **Asepsis:** State of being free from pathogenic organisms.
- **Antiseptic:** Chemical compound that has the power to kill microorganisms on living tissue, but not effective against bacterial spores.
- **Disinfectant:** Chemical compound used to remove or destroy pathogenic microorganisms but not necessarily bacterial spores on non-organic material.
- **Bactericidal:** Chemical compound that kills bacteria.
- **Bacteriostatic:** Chemical compound preventing bacteria multiplying.
- **Sterilisation:** Removal or destruction of all living microorganisms.
- **Detergent:** Facilitates removal of dirt.

BOX 4.4   THE IDEAL DISINFECTANT

- Highly effective against a wide range of microorganisms.
- Effective in low concentration.
- Safe.
- Non-staining.
- Biodegradable.
- Not inactivated by organic material.
- Good wetting and penetrating powers.
- Stable in storage.
- Readily available.
- Relatively inexpensive.
- Easy to apply.

Table 4.1 Disinfectant groups

Disinfectant	Brand names	Use	Dilution strength	Active against	Effectiveness	Inactivated by	Notes
Alcohols	Ethanol, surgical spirit	Trolley tops, thermometers and skin	No more than 70% proof, can be mixed with chlorhexidine or iodine	B & F	Good B & F No activity against spores Variable against viruses	Poor penetration of organic material	Expensive, and highly flammable
Aldehydes: Formaldehyde Gluteraldehyde	Parvocide Gigasept, Formula H	Cattery cages and non-autoclavable equipment e.g. endoscopes	Follow manufacturer's instructions (depends on microorganisms present)	B, F & V	Excellent for B, V and F but slow to work		Expensive. Irritant and toxic properties extremely hazardous
Ampholytic Surfactants	Virkon	Cattery cages, floors, bowls etc	Made up from powder to a 1% solution, also a detergent	B, F & V	Excellent for B, V and F Odourless and non-toxic	Large amounts of organic material	Built in colour indicator. Stains steel and rusts brass (contact 48 hrs)
Chlorhexidine	Hibitane, Hibiscrub	Skin	Use neat or diluted 10% sol. May have detergent added	B & F	Average B and Good F		Expensive
Halogens Hypochlorites	Domestos, Bleach	Environment	12–24 ml in 1 litre water	B, F & V	Excellent	Organic material	Alkaline, corrosive. Chlorine gas
Iodine Iodophors	Pevidine	Skin	Use neat or diluted 1:20 for mucous membranes 1:50 for eyes	B & F	Excellent Can be used with alcohol		May be irritant to skin and may stain.

B, bacteria; F, fungi; V, viruses.

(Continued)

Table 4.1 Disinfectant groups—cont'd

Disinfectant	Brand names	Use	Dilution strength	Active against	Effectiveness	Inactivated by	Notes
Phenol compounds Black, white, clear and chlorinated phenol Chloroxylenol	Jeyes fluid, Izal, Stericol and Clearsol. Dettol	Floors Undiluted for sinks and drains	10–20 ml in 1 litre water	B & F	Very good	Rubber and plastic, detergents and organic material	Cheap, odorous, irritant. TOXIC TO CATS
Quaternary ammonium compounds	Cetavlon	Surfaces and skin	As disinfectant 10 ml in 100 ml water (1–2 ml in 100 ml for skin)	B	Good if solution fresh	Soap	No fungal action
Quaternary ammonium compounds plus detergent	Savlon, Trigene, Sanivet	Skin	As disinfectant 10 ml in 100 ml water (1–2 ml in 100 ml for skin)	B	Good if solution fresh	Soap	No fungal action

B, bacteria; F, fungi; V, viruses.

Allergic reactions to skin scrubs can occur and you may need to have a choice of agents available within the practice.

The drying of hands is also very important to prevent cross-infection and the use of disposable paper hand towels is again recommended. There are now several alcohol-based wipes and foams available for hand-washing, which have been used in the human field. These can speed up the process and will also be quick drying. They also have the advantage of not requiring water, so can be used anywhere.

BOX 4.5   SUMMARY: DISINFECTION

- Assess each area's disinfection requirements; not all areas will have the same requirements.
- The importance of cleaning cannot be over emphasised, as the presence of organic material will inactivate most disinfectants.
- Standardise the disinfectant protocol and make sure it is available to all personnel.
- Make sure disinfectant is easily accessible; if people have to go looking for it, it will not get used!

4.2   CAT HANDLING AND RESTRAINT

As stated before, good hygiene should always be followed in the hospital but especially when dealing with the patients, as the stressed/ill patient is more susceptible to a nosocomial (hospital-acquired) infection. Always wash your hands before handling a cat and try to treat non-infectious patients before infectious patients, thus reducing the risk of transmission.

Transferring cats

When admitting cats to the hospital they should be transferred from the owner's carrier into a practice basket. This ensures the cat is in an escape-proof basket, ideally a top loader for easy access. This basket should also provide adequate space and visibility.

The carriage of cats around the hospital should always be done in an escape-proof basket as described above.

Transfer from basket to cage (see Fig. 4.3)
1. Check all doors/windows are closed.
2. Cattery kennel open and prepared with bed, litter tray, water bowl etc.
3. Gently open the basket with one hand and place your hand in and toward the cat, thus preventing the cat from jumping out, calming the cat with your voice all the while.
4. With the lid fully open, place one hand on the back of the cat's neck firmly but reassuringly, while sliding the other hand under the cat's abdomen and thorax.
5. Gently hold the scruff with one hand and lift the cat out with the other hand. The scruff can then be firmly grasped if the cat starts to panic or become aggressive.
6. Immediately bring the cat close into your body holding the hindquarters into your body with your elbow and extending your arm under the abdomen, resting the thorax on your palm. For added security you can also grasp the forelegs between your fingers.
7. Now place the cat gently into the cattery kennel, allowing the cat to find its feet and gently release your hold.

Cats on drips can have the line run out of the top of the basket without occlusion. Cats wearing Elizabethan collars fit comfortably into most baskets. Even cats with external fixators or Robert Jones dressings can be placed in baskets without causing any discomfort.

Restraining cats

Restraint for physical examination
Minimal restraint is generally required for the physical examination; lots of fussing and talking helps to calm the cat. The general aim is just to prevent the cat moving around too much on the examination table. This is achieved by holding the cat into your body or gently around the shoulders and neck (see Fig. 4.4).

Restraint for procedures
The restraint of cats for procedures should again initially start out with the minimal hands-on approach. Most cats prefer not to be pinned down or handled roughly, especially if they are in any kind of respiratory difficulties. A calm and peaceful patient can turn quite uncooperative if an overly firm approach is made initially.

If you do find that a cat is getting stressed, it is worth trying to loosen your hold first rather than the natural response of tightening your grip. If the cat does turn fractious or aggressive, it is important to stop handling and approaching the cat for a few minutes. This is the time the cat needs to settle down again. Another attempt can be made and either body wrapping the cat in a towel or using a cat muzzle will allow handling of most cats (see Figs 4.5, 4.6).

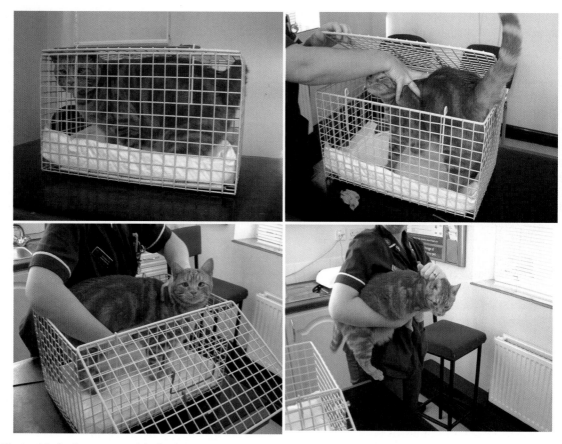

Figure 4.3 Getting a cat out of the basket.

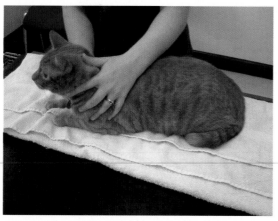

Figure 4.4 Gentle restraint for physical examination.

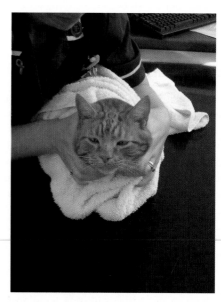

Figure 4.5 Cat wrapped in towel.

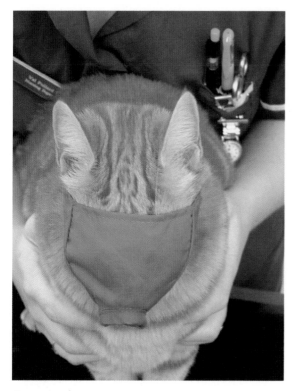

Figure 4.6 Cat wearing cat muzzle.

A common need for restraint is for venous access. Whether it is for blood samples or catheter placement, the position of restraint depends on the preference of the veterinary surgeon or nurse taking the sample. (The methods described here are for right handed persons. If a person is left handed, left needs to be replaced by right and vice versa.)

Restraint for jugular vein access (sternal recumbency) (see Fig. 4.7)
1. The patient is placed onto a non-slip table surface with the handler standing to the patient's left.
2. Place your right arm around the cat's body holding him/her into your side with slight pressure from arm and elbow, and grasp both front legs in the right hand.
3. With your left hand the patient's head is held up and the angle of the head is adjusted to help visualise the vein.

Some veterinary surgeons/nurses may request that the cat be bought to the very end of the examination table and the forelegs be drawn down and over the end.

Restraint for jugular vein access (dorsal recumbency) (see Fig. 4.8)
1. The handler sits down and the cat is placed into the handler's lap.
2. The handler grasps all four legs in one hand.
3. The handler extends the cat's neck with the free hand and restrains the head with the same hand.

In the method described above the person taking the sample raises the vein and takes the sample. Another way of restraining the cat is for the nurse to hold the legs and raise the jugular vein and for the

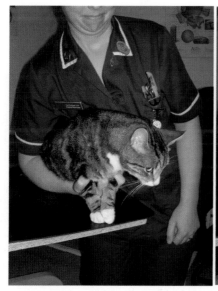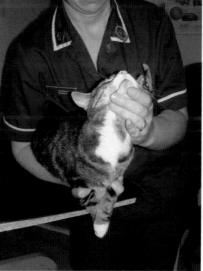

Figure 4.7 Restraint for jugular vein access (sternal recumbency).

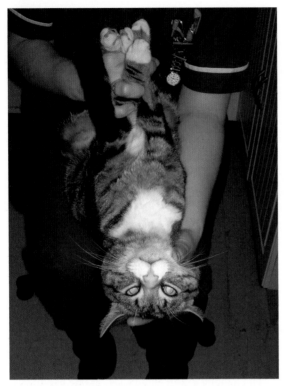

Figure 4.8 Restraint for jugular vein access (dorsal recumbency).

person taking the sample to hold the head and take the sample.

Restraint for cephalic vein access (see Fig. 4.9)
1. The patient is placed onto a non-slip table surface with the handler standing to the patient's left.
2. The handler's right arm is placed around the patient's body and grasps the right leg in the right hand and extends it forwards.

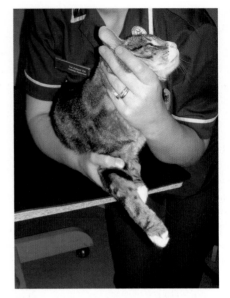

Figure 4.9 Restraint for cephalic vein access.

3. With your left hand, gently hold the head of the cat into your body and away from the sample taker. If the cat fidgets or becomes fractious, then change the head hold to a firm grasp of the scruff.
4. If the cat continues to fidget a second pair of hands can be used to gently hold and put pressure on the hindquarters, this will give added security.

Restraint for lateral recumbency (see Fig. 4.10)
Some procedures, such as ECGs, ultrasound examinations, placement of jugular and femoral vein catheters etc, require the cat to be held in lateral recumbency. On the whole most cats tolerate this surprisingly well, if handled gently and given a lot of verbal reassurance. It is always useful to have a second pair of hands available to stroke the head and offer more reassurance.

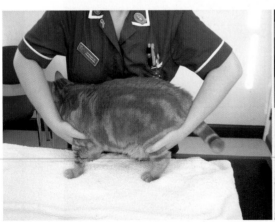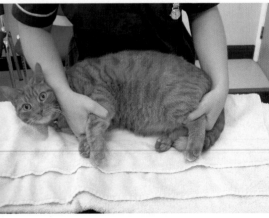

Figure 4.10 Restraint in lateral recumbency.

To place the cat in right lateral recumbency (see Fig. 4.10):

1. Stand the cat on a table, the right hand side of the cat's body flat against your body. If not interfering with the procedure, it is good practice to place a soft cover on the table.
2. Place your arms over the cats back and hold the forelegs in your right hand and back legs in your left hand.
3. Gently lift, and slide the back of the cat down your body and lie the cat down.
4. Place a little pressure with your right arm across the cat's neck to prevent too much movement.
5. If further support is required, quickly release the fore legs and grasp the scruff firmly. For most cats this is enough to subdue them.
6. If the cat is not immobilised enough for the procedure, one person will need to hold the frontlegs and head/neck and another person will need to hold the back legs.

If the cat is particularly restless and only the abdomen needs to be in lateral recumbency (for instance for an abdominal ultrasound) the following technique can be used. Grip the cat by the scruff of the neck, offer its fore-paws to the edge of the table and then draw the cat away from the edge – most cats will 'latch on' to the table, thus securing their fore-paws, and leaving your other hand free to grasp both hind-limbs at the level of the hocks. Gently stretch the cat out and rotate the abdomen in lateral recumbency.

Handling aggressive cats

Aggressive cats can be more complex to deal with than the aggressive dog; they may give very little warning that they are about to explode! The experienced nurse should be able to spot this and take evasive action. Ears will become flattened and the cat will become increasingly vocal: from hissing and spitting to a low throaty growl that increases in intensity and volume. An aggressive cat will feel like a pent-up bundle of energy in your hands becoming tense and literally ready to explode.

If you have any suspicion that the cat you are handling is in any way fractious, having a towel on standby and wrapping them prior to restraint can be enough to subdue them. Proprietary cat bags are sold for use instead of a towel, and a limb or head can be extended through pre-made holes. However, there is space in the bag for the cat to move around, despite the best attempts at restraint. The unzipping of the specified hole and fishing round for the limb can be almost farcical! For this reason the use of a large thick towel is recommended (Fig. 4.11).

Especially when a procedure may be uncomfortable, having another person around to try and distract the cat by talking or rubbing or tapping the head with an implement like a pen (to reduce the risk of injury to fingers) can be enough to allow an injection or examination to take place. Cat muzzles (preferably muzzles with Velcro fastening) are useful in that the cat is unable to see and it will not be able to bite

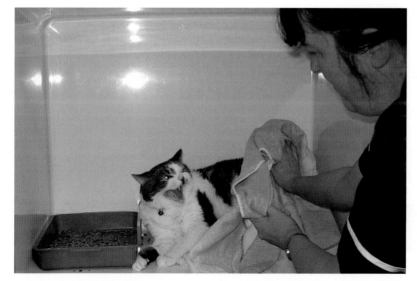

Figure 4.11 Cat showing marked aggression.

(see Fig. 4.6). Elizabethan collars can also be used to prevent the handler getting bitten, while still allowing the face to be observed.

In the case of feral or extremely nervous cats, a decision to handle them as little as possible should be taken. This avoids causing them greater stress and reduces the risk of injury to both nurse and patient. The basic equipment for handling these is again a towel to throw over the cat so they cannot see where you are. A pair of good leather or suede gauntlets should be worn when grasping the cat from the basket or cage, to prevent injury from biting or scratching. Place the cat directly into a crush basket to allow safe administration of sedatives prior to further examination (Fig. 4.12). The cat should be left in the basket while sedation takes effect. This should be covered and placed somewhere quiet, but you should continue monitoring in case of adverse reactions to the sedative.

4.3   ASSESSING THE FELINE PATIENT

Any patient in hospital should be assessed by a nurse at least twice daily and by a veterinary surgeon at least once daily. It is important to perform each assessment in a systematic fashion. This prevents subtle changes being missed.

Experience is important in assessing the cat and by doing this frequently and systematically, experience

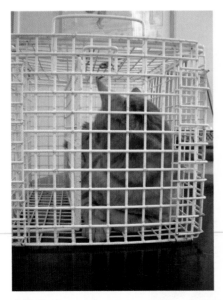

Figure 4.12 Cat in a crush cage.

will be gained and will it be possible to differentiate normal variations from abnormal.

It is important to note if the cat has been eating or drinking and if it has urinated and defaecated. This should be noted on the kennel chart, commenting on normal or abnormal appearance (Fig. 4.13).

General demeanour

Observe the cat first, while it is in the cage or basket. When observing the cat an assessment can be made whether it is bright, alert and responsive. Any change in consciousness should be noted as this is a sign that needs prompt investigation as to the underlying cause. Any abnormal behaviour, sounds and body posture should be noted. There may be obvious signs of stress or aggression at this point, which should be noted as this may change how you approach the cat. Typical signs of stress are hiding, hissing, or sitting in the litter tray. Ideally the cat should be coming forward for attention and be alert, following the activity in the cat ward.

Respiratory system

The respiratory rate and pattern is best assessed before the cat is handled. The normal respiratory rate in the cat is 20–40 breaths/minute with a regular rhythm and breathing should be without any visible effort. It is important to realise that as soon as there is any visible increase in respiratory effort, a veterinary surgeon needs to be consulted immediately as this could be a potential life-threatening situation.

You should then 'introduce yourself' to the cat, verbally reassuring and stroking to relax it. Cats generally respond much better if time is taken to do this.

The basic examination should be performed in a quiet and calm environment to reduce stress-induced abnormalities.

Pulse

Pulse quality is formed by a combination of the strength of the contractility of the heart, the volume of blood ejected with each heartbeat and also the compliance of the peripheral artery. The normal pulse is easily palpable in the cat.

The pulse is best assessed using the femoral artery. Experience is essential to get familiar with a 'normal' pulse and to be confident about reporting changes in pulse quality, pulse rate, rhythm and pulse deficits.

THE FELINE HOSPITAL
HOSPITAL RECORD

DATE:	CONTACT NUMBER:	
Owner Name	Clinical Summary	Special considerations
Species	Breed	Colour		
Sex	Age	Weight	Clinician	

Nutritional requirements

AM		PM	
Temp		Temp	
Pulse		Pulse	
Resp		Resp	
Ate		Ate	
Drank		Drank	
Take out		Take out	
Urine		Urine	
Faeces		Faeces	

Fluid requirements & Meds

Procedures

Comments / Client communication

Figure 4.13 Hospital record sheet.

The pulse rate in the cat is normally between 120–180/minute and should be regular without pulse deficits. Any irregularity or either slow heart rates (bradycardia) or fast heart rates (tachycardia) should be reported to the veterinary surgeon immediately.

Mucous membranes

The oral mucous membranes are assessed for colour and moistness. The normal mucous membrane colour is light pink (Fig. 4.14). Abnormalities found include pale (Fig. 4.15), cyanotic (blue-grey) and jaundiced (yellow) mucous membranes (Fig. 4.16). There also may be signs of increased bleeding tendencies, such as echymoses or petechial haemorrhages.

Temperature

Body temperature is commonly taken with a rectal ther-mometer. Infra-red ear thermometers and thermo microchips are now available. These make the process less stressful for all concerned. The ear thermometers are not always reliable. Whichever method you choose you must continue to use the same method throughout the patient's stay in the hospital, to give consistent results.

Weight and body score

Cats will sit happily in the perfectly sized baby weigh-ing scales, which are much more sensitive for the smaller patient. The patient can also be weighed in a basket on the standard large practice scales, and the weight of the basket subtracted. Either way the patient should always be weighed on the same weighing scales to accurately assess weight gain or loss.

The basic principle of body-scoring is to assess the patient's body condition by site and manipulation. Ideal is just being able to feel the spinal processes and the ribs with minimal amount of pressure over the coat, having a 'waist' when viewed from above, and tucking up of the abdomen towards the hind limbs when viewed from the side (see Fig. 4.17).

There are several methods for body-scoring patients. Either a scale of 1–5 is used, with 3 being an ideal body score or a scale of 1–10 is used with 5 being the ideal body score. Whichever body score is used, it should be standard within the practice.

To arrive at a figure you must use both your eyes and hands to physically assess the patient. For instance if using the system in Figure 4.17, a 5 would be a very obese cat. Start by viewing the cat standing from the side; this cat would have a very saggy abdomen and from above no 'waist', possibly even a barrel type fig-ure. When the cat is palpated the ribs and spinous processes are not palpable without a degree of pres-sure. A very thin/emaciated/cachectic cat gets a score of 1. All bony prominences are easily palpable with an extremely tucked-in waist as viewed from the side and above.

Urinating and defaecating

If the animal has not urinated, the bladder can be checked by palpation. The bladder is located in the caudal abdomen and normally feels like a round, smooth ball, not more than the size of an orange. Care should be taken not to use too much pressure when palpating the bladder (Fig. 4.18).

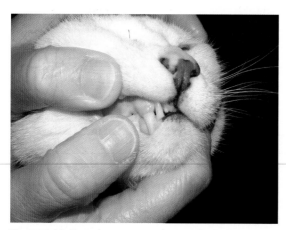

Figure 4.14 Normal mucous membrane colour.

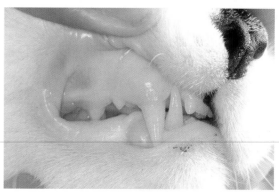

Figure 4.15 Pale (oral) mucous membranes. Reproduced with permission from Sarah M. A. Caney.

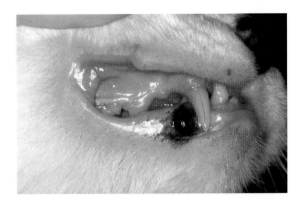

Figure 4.16 Jaundiced oral mucous membranes.

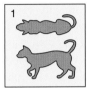
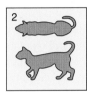
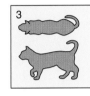
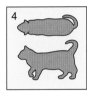
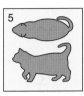

Figure 4.17 Body scoring system: 1 = emaciated; 2 = underweight; 3 = normal, 4 = overweight, 5 = obese. Reproduced with permission from Hill's Pet Nutrition.

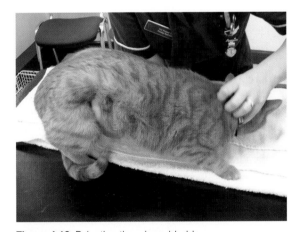

Figure 4.18 Palpating the urinary bladder.

If the animal has not defaecated it is worth palpating the abdomen to check for faeces in the colon. Normal faeces in the colon are easily compressible.

Pain assessment

Recognising signs of pain in the feline patient is a little more difficult than in the canine patient. Cats are generally more private creatures and will quite often retreat to the back of the kennel or attempt to hide as a normal behaviour, but it could be stress related.

This is why it is important to understand from the history and owners what is normal behaviour for the individual patient. By knowing this you will pick up subtle changes in behaviour, which could denote pain. There are also different types of pain with different intensities.

The treatment of pain with adequate analgesia can often be overlooked or underestimated in the whole treatment plan. The type and amount of analgesia should be constantly re-assessed to ensure adequate pain relief is being supplied. Analgesia can be provided in many different ways, not just pharmacologically. The importance of good nursing cannot be over-emphasised.

The provision of a low-edged litter tray for cats with limb or pelvic pain can help them to use the tray. Cats with fractures should be provided with adequate immobilisation by correctly applied dressings. A badly applied dressing at best can increase pain and at worst can result in the loss of a limb. These patients should have adequately padded bedding; with the use of incontinence sheets or bedding that draws urine away from the patient (Vetbed) if he/she is unable to use a tray.

Cats will require less medical pain relief if they are provided with a stress-free environment. Measures that can be taken in the cat ward have been discussed

BOX 4.6 KEY POINTS: PHYSICAL EXAMINATION

- Work methodically.
- Take time to reassure the cat.
- Perform all examinations that can be influenced by stress first.
- Make a record of all findings, normal as well as abnormal.

BOX 4.7 SIGNS OF PAIN

Physical	Behavioural
Inflammation	Inappetence
Tachycardia	Depression
Rapid pulse, not weak	Aggression
Tachypnoea	Vocalisation on
Pyrexia	movement
	Self-mutilation

BOX 4.8 KEY POINTS: ANALGESIA

- If it would hurt you, then it will hurt the cat!
- Multimodal approach, NSAIDs/opiates/local anaesthetic/nursing care.
- Monitor frequently.
- Know your patient's normal behaviour and note changes from that.

earlier and it may also help to provide some home comforts and if possible allow owners time to visit and groom the cat.

Make sure the bladder is emptied regularly. A full bladder is uncomfortable in itsewlf; combined with other pain it can increase analgesia requirements.

4.4 NURSING THE INFECTIOUS CAT

As a veterinary nurse, it is important that you gain a clear understanding of the most common infectious and contagious diseases in the cat and how these are transmitted. Only then are you able to nurse these patients effectively without risk of transmission of infection to other patients in the surgery. It is also important to know about any zoonotic potential of the infectious organisms.

Isolation area

This facility is vital in the management of infectious diseases. The area should be designed to incorporate the following features:

- A self-contained room, preferably with a separate entrance. A foot-bath containing suitable disinfectant should be placed outside (see Section 4.1 for suitable disinfectants).
- Appropriate protective clothing should be available such as, aprons/disposable suits, gloves, face-masks and shoe covers.
- Everything needed for inpatient care: food, bowls, litter, litter trays, grooming equipment, waste disposal facilities. Also a range of commonly used medications and equipment, e.g. needles, syringes, catheters, drips etc, will prevent unnecessary crossing over to the rest of the hospital.
- Own water supply for washing and disinfection. The cleaning utensils should be clearly marked 'for isolation only'.
- The cages should be arranged in such a way that they will reduce the risk of transmission by aerosol spread (see Section 4.1).
- The ventilation system should be of an appropriate design. Ideally an 'active' ventilation system should be used, which draws air out of the isolation ward to replace it with clean air. This method of ventilation is often incorporated into an air-conditioning unit and can be temperature controlled. Active ventilation can greatly reduce the number of airborne pathogens in the environment. If air conditioning is used the filters should be cleaned and disinfected on a regular basis, according to the manufacturer's instructions, as dirty filters can be a potential source of environmental contamination.

Strict cleaning and hygiene protocols should be put in place and adhered to by everyone. This is the main way to reduce the numbers of infectious agents present in an isolation facility. The number of staff entering the isolation area should be strictly limited to persons designated for care of isolation patients only.

Barrier nursing

This is the method of nursing that should be used when nursing a patient with an infectious disease.

- There should be one/two nurses designated to the care of the patient to prevent cross contamination.

- Protective clothing should be worn, and discarded immediately after use.
- Personal hygiene must be strictly adhered to, this prevents cross contamination and infection with zoonotic agents.

This technique can still be used in the absence of isolation facilities. One area or corner of the practice, away from the thoroughfare of other people and patients can be dedicated to a patient with a possible infectious disease when necessary. Small portable cages can be used and are easily disinfected and stored when not in use. Food bowls, litter trays, blankets and bedding should be kept separate and labelled. It is often a good idea to colour code the equipment that is for isolation use only.

Common feline infectious diseases

There are a number of infectious agents to which feline patients are susceptible. The diseases are dis-

drugs) are more likely to develop clinical signs after exposure to the dermatophyte.

'Cat flu' (feline upper respiratory tract disease)

These terms describe infection with either one or both of the upper respiratory viruses: feline calicivirus (FCV) and feline herpes virus (FHV).

Clinical signs are mainly restricted to the upper respiratory tract and include sneezing, nasal discharge and in the more severe cases anorexia and pyrexia (for more details see Chapter 6). Calicivirus may also be associated with chronic gingivitis.

Both viruses are highly contagious and are spread by aerosol transmission, and by direct and indirect contact.

Cats recently infected with FCV become convalescent carriers and shed the virus while recovering from infection; this period of viral shedding can persist for months, and in some cases years.

Cats recovered from a FHV infection become life-long carriers that *appear* to be free from infection, until times of stress, such as a period of illness or hospitalisation. The stress may induce the return of clinical signs and shedding of the virus. This should be considered when nursing a 'stressed' feline patient in any part of the hospital, as these cats could potentially become sources of infection.

Any virucidal disinfectant (see Section 4.1) can be used to disinfect contaminated areas.

Bordetella

Bordetella bronchiseptica is a Gram-negative bacterium. It can act as a primary pathogen in cats, but more commonly its involvement in upper respiratory tract disease is as a secondary infection in association with the respiratory viruses. Many cats carry the agent without developing any signs of disease, but these cats may be a potential source of infection to other 'in contact' cats.

Clinical signs, when they occur, typically include fever, sneezing, nasal discharge, submandibular lymphadenopathy, and occasionally rales on auscultation of the chest. Disease is usually mild and self-limiting, unless there is concurrent infection with other agents.

Transmission is via intimate contact or by droplet infection. *Bordetella* does not survive for long periods outside the host and is readily killed by many common disinfectants. In a heavily contaminated environment it may survive long enough for indirect transmission to occur, especially if the bacteria are contained in infected mucus.

The disinfectant of choice is a reliable bactericidal agent such as Virkon.

Chlamydial conjunctivitis

The causal agent is *Chlamydophilla felis*, previously known as *Chlamydia psittaci*. Clinical signs include persistent conjunctivitis, mild nasal discharge, sneezing and coughing.

Transmission is by direct contact and the agent is mainly shed into the ocular discharges. The disinfectant of choice is Virkon.

Feline infectious enteritis (FIE)

The causal agent is a feline parvovirus, also known as feline panleucopenia virus, due its ability to cause severe depletion of the white blood cells. Clinical signs include pyrexia, lethargy, vomiting, watery diarrhoea and dehydration.

The virus is shed into the saliva, vomit, faeces and urine. It will spread by direct or indirect contact and can survive in the environment and on fomites for up to a year. Vertical transmission, via the placenta or milk, can also occur. Any virucidal disinfectant can be used to disinfect contaminated areas.

Salmonella

This is a potentially zoonotic infection caused by the bacterium *Salmonella typhimurium*. Cats are generally quite resistant to this infection, but debilitated or immunosuppressed animals may become infected and develop clinical signs. The most common source of infection is infected meat, which is eaten by the cat. The bacterium may then establish a gastrointestinal infection and can be shed in the faeces.

When clinical signs do occur they are usually restricted to the gastrointestinal tract and include acute or chronic diarrhoea, weight loss, lethargy and pyrexia. The disinfectant of choice is Virkon.

Toxoplasma

The causal agent is a protozoan *Toxoplasma gondii*. Most infected cats show no signs of disease. If clinical signs do occur they may be relatively non-specific, such as lethargy, vomiting and anorexia, or may be related to the specific organs which are infected.

T. gondii has a complex life-cycle involving several host species. Cats have a central role in the spread of infection as they are the only 'definitive' host species, i.e. the only host which supports completion of the life-cycle. Ingesting intermediate hosts such as mice and wild birds, or through being fed uncooked infected meat, infects the cat. Once the infection is established the cat will shed oocysts in its faeces for a short period of time. A further 1 to 5 days later the oocysts will sporulate and become a potential source of infection to new hosts. Sporulated oocysts can remain viable in the environment for many months.

Toxoplasma is a potentially zoonotic disease and human infection with *T. gondii* is common. Humans can become infected via ingestion of sporulated oocysts in contaminated soil (gardening) or water, or by eating undercooked meat that has come from an infected animal. Direct contact with an infected cat is not thought to be a significant source of infection due to the delay between passage of oocysts and sporulation to the infectious stage. Daily cleaning of litter trays will also prevent contact with sporulated oocysts. In most cases infection is subclinical or causes mild, self-limiting signs of fever and malaise; however severe disease can occur in immunosuppressed individuals. If a pregnant woman is infected for the first time during her pregnancy the infection can cause abortion, or serious damage to the unborn foetus.

This organism is generally not susceptible to disinfectants, so good hygiene routines are essential to limit the spread of oocysts.

Feline infectious anaemia (FIA)

The causal agent is a *Mycoplasma*. There are at least two distinct genotypes *Candidatus mycoplasma haemofelis* (large form) and *Candidatus mycoplasma haemominutum* (small form). *M. haemofelis* is more pathogenic, but not very prevalent in the UK. Clinical signs include acute haemolytic anaemia, pyrexia, weakness and collapse.

Mycoplasmas are unlikely to exist outside a carrier animal and are thought to be spread by insect vectors such as fleas. It is therefore important that all hospitalisation wards, including isolation facilities, are routinely treated with an insecticide preparation.

Feline leukaemia virus (FeLV)

The causal agent is a retrovirus. Clinical signs are varied, and are associated with diseases of the haematopoietic system, infiltration of the different organs with neoplastic lymphocytes or a gradual depletion of the immune system making the cat more prone to secondary infections.

The virus is shed mainly in the saliva, but also in urine and faeces. It can only be transmitted by direct contact between cats and prolonged contact with the infectious agent is required, for instance through mutual grooming, sharing of litter trays or food bowls, and occasionally through bite wounds. Vertical transmission between a queen and her young can also occur, via the placenta or in the milk.

The virus is very fragile and has very limited ability to survive outside the host. It is easily killed by a virucidal disinfectant such as Virkon. As long as there is no direct contact between hospitalised cats there is little risk of this virus being transmitted in the hospital environment.

Feline immunodeficiency virus (FIV)

The causal agent is a retrovirus. The disease causes immunosuppression and increased vulnerability to secondary infections with other organisms. It also causes a predisposition to certain neoplastic diseases.

The virus is shed in the saliva and transmission is by direct contact such as via biting, and possibly through prolonged social contact and sharing of food bowls in multi-cat households. The virus is easily destroyed in the environment and by virucidal disinfectants such as Virkon. As with FeLV, good hygiene and lack of direct contact between hospitalised cats will prevent transmission within the veterinary practice.

Feline infectious peritonitis (FIP)

The causal agent is a feline coronavirus (FCoV), but most cats infected with FCoV will not go on to develop FIP.

The virus can cause various clinical signs depending on the immune response of the cat. Signs can range from mild diarrhoea in cats with strong immunity, or 'dry' FIP (affecting the central nervous system, eye, abdomen, liver, kidneys) in cats with less of an immune response. In cats with an inadequate/nonprotective weak immune response 'wet' FIP (ascites, pleural effusion, pericardial effusion) can develop.

FCoV is very contagious and is mainly shed in the faeces, but is also present in saliva for a short period early in the course of infection. Transmission to other cats occurs through close contact with infected cats, and by indirect contact, mainly through shared litter trays.

Prevention of transmission of FCoV in the hospital environment is achieved by good hygiene practice especially in relation to litter trays. The virus is readily killed by virucidal disinfectants such as Virkon.

4.5 NUTRITIONAL SUPPORT

This aspect of patient care is often overlooked and it often falls to the veterinary nurse to take the lead in the nutritional management of hospitalised patients.

It is vital that the correct nutrition is maintained during a cat's stay in hospital to improve the general health of the cat, aid recovery and to reduce the time spent in hospital.

Making sure a cat eats can prove a challenge even when the patient is a 'well' cat, as cats can be very capricious in their eating habits. It is important to realise that the hospitalised 'well' cat can be overlooked and that the stress of the hospital environment may increase their energy requirement. This factor coupled with the fact they are not eating as much or as often as they do at home can lead to the patient becoming undernourished during its stay in hospital.

Encouraging the 'well' cat to eat

- It is important that information regarding the cat's normal diet is obtained from the owner as soon as the patient comes into the hospital. Ideally the cat should be fed the same variety and texture of food.
- It is advisable to remove the cat's litter tray at feeding time as cats are generally quite fastidious creature and prefer not to eat when a litter tray is about.
- Cats generally prefer fresh food to stale food, so if the food is not eaten within 20–30 minutes, remove the food and try again a short time later with some fresh food.
- Cats find food that has been warmed to body temperature more appealing than food straight from the fridge.
- Cats prefer to feed from a shallow bowl or saucer, rather than a large, deep-sided bowl, especially when in unfamiliar surroundings.

If all the above fails to encourage the cat to eat, the cat's favourite treats, or freshly cooked chicken or fish can often help to 'kick-start' the patient's appetite, but it must be remembered that these alone do not constitute a balanced diet.

Monitoring

The veterinary nurse plays a vital part in updating the patient's hospitalisation records and the nutritional state of the patient is no exception. Daily checks including measuring body weight are essential.

Care should be taken to accurately measure how much food is eaten by the patient rather than relying on estimates, as one person's spoonful can be very different to another. Careful record keeping allows the cat's nutrition intake to be accurately calculated, rather than simply recording whether it is eating or not. Observations of how the cat eats its food are also important to record, as this can give a good indication on the patient's general state of health.

By maintaining accurate hospitalisation records any deterioration in the patient's condition can soon be noted and steps to rectify this can be initiated. For further details on nutrition see Chapter 3.

4.6   DRUG ADMINISTRATION

When administering drugs to the feline patient it is important to use the appropriate restraint (see Section 4.2). Depending on the patient you may not require assistance, but on the whole it is easier and less stressful if an assistant is used.

It is important to have all you require to hand to minimise the time needed to restrain the patient, which may include:

- The correct medication, with dose rate already calculated and prepared.
- All aids available: damp cotton wool, surgical spirit, scrub, paper towel, cotton towel for restraint if required, pill popper, gloves, apron, goggles, mask etc.
- Hospital record sheet and pen.
- Drip stand.
- Watch/clock.

Medication and drugs can be administered by a number of routes: orally, optically, aurally, subcutaneously (s.c.), intramuscularly (i.m.), intravenously (i.v.) or via inhalation and it is important to use the appropriate route of administration for the drug used.

Oral medication

Oral medications will be prepared in tablet, powder, capsule, liquid or paste form. All have slightly different techniques required for administration.

Giving the hospitalised cat tablets or capsules in food is not to be advised. More often than not the medication has an unpleasant odour and is detected by the patient, so is not eaten. This may even put it off from eating further meals. If you do not actually see the cat eat the medication you cannot be completely

sure that it has. Also if the cat does not eat its food immediately the dosing interval will be affected. The easiest option if the cat has a good appetite is to place the tablet in a treat type pocket and feed it as a treat, although this is only useful in a minority of cats.

In most cases cats need to be restrained when giving oral medication. Start off with the assistant restraining the patient as described in Section 4.2 for examination, ensuring that the forelimbs are adequately under control. If the cat is in any way wriggly or lively, it is often best to go straight for the towel restraint technique. This is preferable as the medication is often administered first time without the need for repeat attempts. It is much less stressful than using inadequate restraint and multiple attempts at administering the medication.

TABLETS AND CAPSULES (see Fig. 4.19)
1. With the cat adequately restrained stand with the cat on the examination table to your less dominant side.
2. With your less dominant hand grasp the cat's head gently but firmly, with your thumb and second finger on either side of the jaws, at the temporo-mandibular junction; your third and ring finger either side of the base of the ear and your little finger tucked back supporting the base of the skull.
3. Gently lift the cat's head upwards until it is looking at the ceiling and the neck is straight.
4. At this point the lower jaw should gently drop open about 5 mm.
5. Grasp the medication in your dominant hand between thumb and second finger. Gently prize open the cat's mouth with your middle finger.
6. Once the cat's mouth is open reasonably wide, pop the tablet quickly to the back of the mouth beyond the base of the tongue. Do not release the tablet/capsule until you have it at that point.
7. Quickly remove dominant hand from the cat's mouth but still holding the head with your other hand until you are sure the medication has been swallowed. Some people advocate rubbing the throat to encourage swallowing, but if you have placed the tablet in the right place it should automatically be swallowed. Cats usually start licking their lips once they have swallowed the medication. The tablets/capsules should be given with some liquid or butter to help passage through the oesophagus and prevent oesophagitis.

If you are unable to get the medication into the cat's mouth due to inability to open the mouth wide enough,

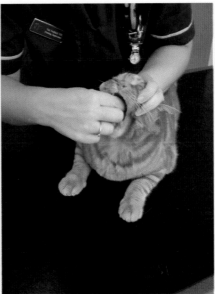

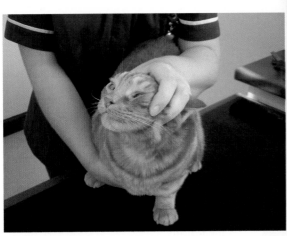

Figure 4.19 Giving tablets or capsules.

or risk of being bitten, then 'pill poppers' are very useful. The technique is the same but instead of using your hands to place the tablet, the 'pill popper' is placed at the back of the throat and the plunger depressed to release the medication. There is no need to open the mouth further than it already opens when the cat is looking upwards.

LIQUID MEDICATION (see Fig. 4.20)
1. Restrain the cat and hold the head as for administration of tablet/capsules.
2. Tilt the head so the side nearest you is slightly elevated. Move your thumb rostrally and gently raise the upper lip.
3. Hold the syringe or pipette in your dominant hand and place the nozzle into the side of the mouth, between canine and premolar teeth.
4. Gently dribble the medication into the mouth little by little, allowing time for the cat to swallow.
5. If the cat gets distressed or is dribbling the medication, stop restraining the head, wipe away any excess and allow the cat to calm down.
6. Repeat as above holding the head in a more upright position to encourage swallowing, until the whole dose has been administered.

POWDER/GRANULES
These can be quite difficult to administer to cats. Placing the medication in the fridge before administering can reduce the odour of a lot of powders or

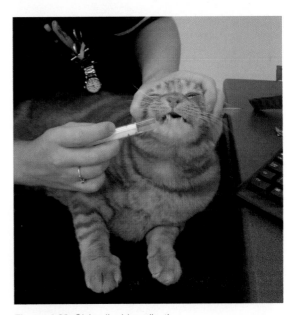

Figure 4.20 Giving liquid medication.

granules. The best option may be to dissolve the medication in a small amount of water and syringe the solution into the cat's mouth. It is also possible to purchase empty gelatine capsules into which powders or granules can be placed.

Eye medication (see Fig. 4.21)
Ocular medications are normally presented as drops or ointment and therefore require slightly different tech-

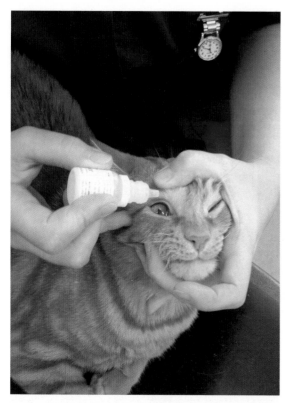

Figure 4.21 Administering eye drops.

niques for administration. With both types of preparation the nurse will probably be able to administer them without assistance in most cases. Some patients will resent the application, as the eye being treated may be painful due to bruising or inflammation, and some medications can cause discomfort on application. Before administering any treatment, the eye should be cleaned gently to remove any discharge or dried-on residue from previous treatments.

1. It is usually easiest to have the cat out of the cage and backing into the person administering the medication.
2. With your hand on the cat's head gently raise the upper eyelid of the affected eye.
3. Gently squeeze a drop from the bottle, holding it 1–2 cm from the orbit.
4. If an ointment, gently squeeze the tube dispensing from medial to lateral canthus.
5. After either type of application, rub the upper eyelid over the orbit to help disperse the medication.
6. Be aware that some medications can cause salivation as the medication drains into the oral cavity via the tear ducts.

Ear medication (see Fig. 4.22)

Ear medication usually comes in liquid form. Most cats will allow this type of treatment without restraint, although it can be useful to have an extra pair of hands to prevent the cat from head shaking and covering everything and everyone with a mixture of ear drops and ear discharge!

1. With the cat restrained on the examination table, take firm hold of the affected pinna and gently elevate away from the skull. This straightens out the ear

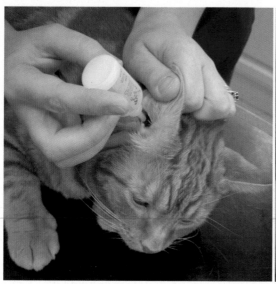
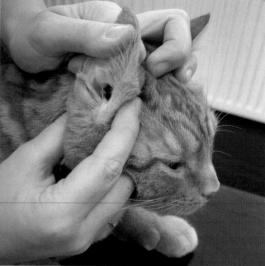

Figure 4.22 Administering ear drops and rubbing the base of the ear afterwards.

canal allowing medication to drain down to the horizontal canal and not just sit in the vertical canal.

2. Place the nozzle into the entrance of the ear canal, but do not force it. Ensure that the drops will penetrate into the ear canal and not just sit in the folds at the base of the ear.
3. Squeeze the bottle dispensing the required number of drops into the ear.
4. Still holding the pinna with one hand, massage the base of the ear with the other. This ensures all surfaces within the ear are coated with the medication.
5. Cats will invariably shake their heads after the medication has been given.

Inhalation therapy (see Fig. 4.23)

Inhalation therapy is useful for cats with certain respiratory diseases. It allows the cat to be medicated with anti-inflammatories and bronchodilators without systemic absorption and subsequent side effects. Most cats tolerate inhalation therapy very well and it is often easier than giving cats tablets or liquid medication.

The cat is placed on your lap with its back towards you. The metered dose inhaler (MDI) is placed on the inhalation chamber (Aerokat™), which is connected to a clear facemask. The appropriate number of puffs from the MDI are given into the inhalation chamber and the mask is placed over the cat's mouth. The cat is allowed to take 7–10 breaths with the facemask in place and that will be sufficient to inhale all the medication in the chamber.

Subcutaneous injections (see Fig. 4.24)

The administering of medications by injection requires some training. Owners can be given lessons

Figure 4.23 Inhalation therapy. Photograph courtesy of Annette Litster.

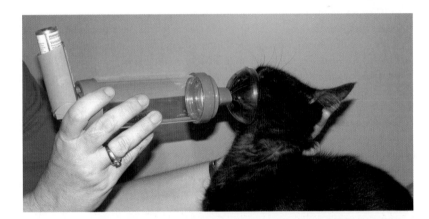

Figure 4.24 Subcutaneous injection.

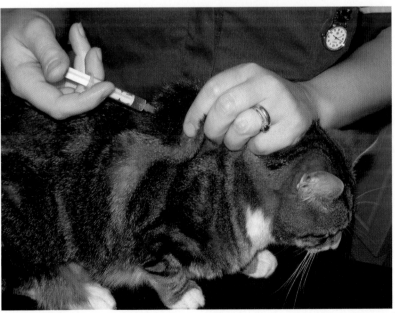

on injections by the subcutaneous route, which is essential if they have to treat their diabetic cat with insulin. For the comfort of the patient use the smallest gauge needle possible, but not so small that it is difficult to expel the medication from the syringe.

Subcutaneous (s.c.) injections are generally administered in the scruff of the neck, as the skin is fairly loose with minimal nerves present. Unless the cat is aggressive there should be no need for a second pair of hands for restraint.

1. With the cat sitting in a basket, cage or on the examination table, facing away from you, grasp the scruff with your less dominant hand.
2. Gently lift the skin up and away from the body wall and form a triangle of skin at the caudal edge of the scruff.
3. Find the centre of this triangle with a finger from your other hand locating the point at which the needle will enter.
4. With your dominant hand place the needle gently but firmly into triangle. You should feel a little resistance as the needle passes through the dermis into the subcutis.
5. Once in the correct position you can release the scruff a little and draw back on the syringe to confirm your position.
6. If your syringe fills with air you probably have gone all the way through the skin fold and out the other side. Withdraw the needle a little and draw back again. If you still get air then come out completely and start again.
7. If you get blood back, you may have caught a small skin vessel, withdraw and start again.
8. Once sure of your position depress the plunger of the syringe administering the medication, withdraw the needle quickly and cap your needle.

Intramuscular injections (see Fig. 4.25)

Only fully trained staff should use the intramuscular and intravenous routes. Under the Veterinary Surgeons Act 1966, alongside veterinary surgeons, listed qualified veterinary nurses and student veterinary nurses under direct supervision are permitted to administer medical treatment via these routes.

Intramuscular (i.m.) injections will more often than not require a second pair of hands to restrain the cat. This route is uncomfortable and depending on the amount and type of drug may be painful. To help reduce the discomfort it is important to ensure your

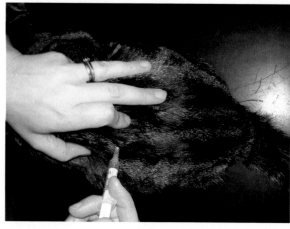

Figure 4.25 Intramuscular injection (lumbar muscles).

needle is sharp and as small a gauge as possible. The main sites used are the lumbar muscles and the muscles of the quadriceps group. It is easiest to use the lumbar muscles and uptake of medication is reliable and quick.

1. With your patient suitably restrained locate the lumbar spine by palpation.
2. Then grasp the lateral edge of the lumbar muscle so it is held between your thumb and the spine.
3. Place the needle firmly into the centre of the muscle belly at right angles to the skin. Draw back as described for the subcutaneous route; if you get blood then withdraw and replace.
4. Depress the plunger of the syringe administering the medication.

Intravenous injections

Intravenous (i.v.) injections are useful when large volumes of a drug are required or the speed of effect needs to be rapid. The average time for intravenous drugs to be distributed is 1–2 minutes compared with 20–30 minutes for intramuscular and 30–45 minutes for the subcutaneous route An intravenous bolus should be administered slowly as emesis may be induced, even anti-emetic drugs given too rapidly via the intravenous route will cause emesis.

The cephalic, saphenous and jugular veins can be used for intravenous injections. The sublingual vein can also be used but only in the anaesthetised or comatose patient. If the cat needs repeated intravenous injections, or if the drug causes side effects if given perivenously, an intravenous catheter must be placed. The main site for use is the cephalic vein; this should be clipped and cleaned for both injection and catheter placement. The cat should be restrained as described previously. The skin should be prepared and the vein raised as described in Chapter 5. The hypodermic needle should be of a small gauge and also sharp, so if it has passed through a rubber stopper two times it should be replaced with a new needle. To check if the needle is in the vein, the plunger should be withdrawn slightly to create negative pressure, so a little blood will enter the syringe. This will confirm position of the needle in the vein. The drug can then be given. After this the needle should be withdrawn and pressure should be applied to avoid haematomas.

The main problems encountered with the intravenous injection are the misplacement of the needle or the needle moving out of the vein once placed (see Box 4.9). Administration should be stopped immediately and you should inform the veterinary surgeon as soon as possible of the type and amount of drug that was administered. Depending on this, first aid measures may need to be taken. In cases of non-irritant substances it may be sufficient to gently massage the leg to disperse the drug into the rest of the tissues. In the case of a tissue-toxic drug, a diluent may need to be injected into the periphery, or cold compresses applied to prevent further distribution of the drug via the peripheral vascular system.

Chemotherapeutic agents

Chemotherapeutic agents are any drugs used in the treatment of cancer and are known as cytotoxic, as they inhibit cell growth or destroy cells. Several routes may be used for administration and it is extremely important that you know which route is used for which drug. If the wrong route is used the patient may develop severe side effects, even death. It is very important that all these drugs are administered with great care to both patient and staff. All personnel handling cytotoxic drugs should wear protective clothing to prevent absorption of the drug through skin or mucous membranes. Any practice using chemotherapy should have 'Local Rules' for the handling and use of cytotoxic drugs, under the COSHH regulations.

Protective clothing used should include goggles, mask, hat, double gloves and a gown.

Most protocols will include an agent that has to be administered via the intravenous route. As most of these drugs should be calculated on body surface area an accurate and up-to-date body weight is required. Standard tables are then available to allow conversion from body weight to surface area.

Some drugs come in a powder form and require reconstituting with water for injection. This should be done in a fume cupboard. Maintaining equal pressure inside and outside the vial will minimise the risk of aerosolisation. This is done by injecting small amounts of air to replace the fluid that is removed from the vial. The veterinary nurse can practise this with other noncytotoxic drugs, such as antibiotics. All drugs should be prepared, labelled and put on absorbent paper.

Intravenous cytotoxic drugs should not be administered without the use of an intravenous catheter. If the vein is punctured and the catheter not placed correctly that vein should be left and another site used. To continue to use the same site after repeat punctures could result in the drug 'leaking' around the vein. With most chemotherapy drugs this can cause damage to the peripheral tissues, creating necrosis and sloughing with the very real risk of limb loss.

The choice of room or area to start chemotherapy administration is important to ensure first time placement of the catheter. It should be quiet, free from other animals and the doors locked if possible to prevent anyone disturbing at the most vital moment.

Dispose of all sharps immediately; do not re-cap needles to prevent needle stick injury. All waste should be labelled as cytotoxic and clinical waste should be double bagged.

Once the agent has been administered or is being administered, the patient should be monitored closely for signs of immediate side effects or reaction. Allergic reactions have been reported and monitoring temperature, pulse and respiration is advisable. The nurse needs to continue wearing protective clothing to prevent any contact with the cytotoxic drug. The development and monitoring of side effects is ongoing. The owners need to be aware of this and look for signs. The drug may affect other rapidly growing cells,

BOX 4.9 SIGNS OF PERIVASCULAR INJECTION

- Resistance when injecting the drug into the vein.
- Swelling immediately around the vein at the site of the needle.
- Swelling above the site of the needle.
- Patient showing signs of resentment or pain.

e.g. the gastrointestinal tract. Signs of vomiting, diarrhoea, cystitis etc should be reported straight away. The veterinary surgeon will want to monitor the patient's red and white cells regularly (before each treatment), in order to look for signs of infection or a depleted cell count. Some agents such as doxorubicin will continue to be excreted by the patient for at least 24 hours, so protective clothing should continue to be worn when handling the patient's bedding etc. If the patient is returned home at this time, the owners will need to be informed and educated on how to handle their pet.

4.7 FLUID THERAPY

Fluid therapy is an extremely important part of veterinary medicine. It is vital that a veterinary nurse is able to recognise when a patient requires fluid therapy and how to correctly calculate, administer and monitor a patient during its treatment. It is also important that a veterinary nurse is familiar with the various types of fluids that are available in practice and the most effective route by which they should be administered.

Recognising dehydration

Many methods can be used for assessing or estimating the level of dehydration in a patient, but none of these methods are 100% accurate when it comes to estimating existing deficits and ongoing losses. Therefore constant monitoring of a patient that is receiving fluid therapy, or that may need fluid therapy, is vital. Fluid overload or electrolyte imbalances are common problems in cats that are being treated with intravenous fluids.

Clinical history
The clinical history may give a clue as to whether it is likely that a patient is dehydrated. For instance a cat that has been anorexic and has been vomiting is likely to have a fluid deficit. The amount of fluid the patient is believed to have lost should be taken into account when calculating the replacement volume (see later).

Clinical examination
This can also provide information about the patient's hydration status (see Table 4.3). Clinical signs such as loss of skin elasticity or 'skin tenting', peripheral pulse weakness, prolonged capillary refill time, dry mucous membranes, sunken eyes, lethargy and weakness can all indicate various degrees of dehydration. In older cats 'skin tenting' is not very reliable as the skin elasticity reduces with age.

Monitoring changes in body weight can also be useful in calculating the amount of fluid a patient has lost, providing that an accurate body weight has been recorded recently. For instance an acute loss of 100 g of body weight can be equated to a loss of 100 ml of body fluid.

Laboratory analysis
There are a number of laboratory tests that can be carried out 'in house' to help to determine the level of patient dehydration.

- Urine specific gravity – will generally increase with dehydration; provided that renal function is normal and there are no other pre-existing conditions that can affect urinary concentration, such as diabetes mellitus or hyperthyroidism.
- Packed cell volume – will generally increase with all types of fluid loss, with the exception of acute haemorrhage. Every 1% rise in PCV is equivalent to a loss of 10 ml of fluid per kilogram of body weight.
- Total plasma protein – will generally increase with dehydration, unless the patient has a pre-existing low plasma protein level.

Laboratory results should be used alongside clinical history and clinical examination to achieve an overall assessment of the patient.

Routes of fluid administration

Fluid therapy may be administered by the following routes:

The alimentary route
The alimentary route has many advantages. The fluids need not be sterile and fluid composition is not as critical, as selective absorption will occur in the intestines. Large volumes can be administered, especially if a feeding tube is used.

For this route to be effective however, the alimentary tract must remain capable of absorption. Therefore this is not the route of choice for cases with vomiting or diarrhoea or patients with circulatory shock.

The subcutaneous route (see Fig. 4.26)
Relatively large volumes of fluid can be administered subcutaneously, using a standard giving set and

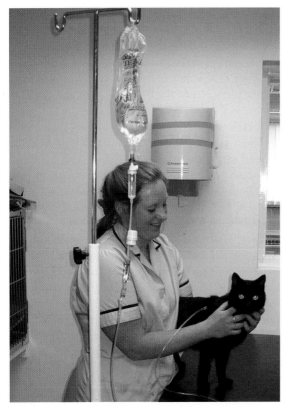

Figure 4.26 Administration of s.c. fluids using needle, standard giving set and fluids.

hypodermic needle. This should be done aseptically using sterile isotonic fluid. Only crystalloid fluids can be administered via this route.

Absorption depends entirely on adequate circulation and perfusion to the subcutaneous layers, so this route is not appropriate for use in cats with circulatory collapse or vasoconstriction of the subcutaneous vessels e.g. in hypothermia. It is also unsuitable for correction and replacement of large fluid volumes or for acute losses, as it takes more than 45 minutes for the fluid to be absorbed.

Advantages of this route are that a limited amount of equipment is required for administration, which make this route relatively inexpensive in comparison to other routes. Volume overload is unlikely due to the slow rates of absorption into the circulation.

This route is really only practical for short-term administration of crystalloids to patients that are reasonably well hydrated. Repeated administration can be painful, and may lead to local infection and in severe cases skin sloughing.

The intravenous route

This is the route of choice when rapid rehydration is required, e.g. in cases of circulatory shock. It is the only route suitable for administration of colloids, plasma, whole blood and parenteral nutrition. Fluid can be placed directly into the circulatory system, which often gives a rapid improvement in a patient's condition. This is also the route of choice when long-term fluid therapy is required.

It is important to maintain strict asepsis when placing the intravenous catheter in order to prevent complications (see Chapter 5). It is often possible to place an intravenous catheter even in the smallest kitten, although it may be necessary to use the jugular vein. The use of local anaesthetic skin creams can help.

A sterile isotonic solution is used, and should be warmed to body temperature before infusion into the patient. This is especially important in smaller patients receiving relatively large volumes as the rapid administration can contribute to hypothermia.

Intravenous fluid therapy requires specialised, sterile equipment and constant monitoring of the patient. The immediate entry to the circulatory system can lead to circulatory overload if the fluid that is administered is not effectively redistributed or excreted. Care should be taken with cats that are suffering from cardiac disease or anuric renal disease, as these cats are at high risk of developing circulatory overload and pulmonary oedema.

The intraperitoneal route

The peritoneum has a high capacity for absorbing fluids and vessel constriction to this area occurs relatively late in the course of circulatory collapse. This route can be used in small kittens where venous access is difficult.

The solution that is administered should be, sterile, isotonic and close to body temperature to promote maximum absorption and comfort. Aseptic technique is essential to prevent peritonitis.

The intraosseous route

This route can be utilised in small kittens or cats that are presented in a state of collapse, where venous access cannot be achieved. The placement of the intraosseous needle is painful and local anaesthesia will be required, but the ongoing administration of fluid is generally well-tolerated. This technique requires specialised sterile equipment and strict asepsis should be adhered to during placement and maintenance to avoid local infection and osteomyelitis. This technique is often only utilised in the short term, until venous access can be gained.

Fluid types (Table 4.2)

The veterinary surgeon will base the choice of fluids on the patient's condition. The veterinary nurse's role is to monitor the patient's condition for signs of progress or deterioration and to keep accurate hospital records as this can give valuable information as to if and when the fluid type needs to be changed.

Most fluids used will be isotonic fluids with the same osmotic pressure as plasma. Hypotonic (lower osmotic pressure) and hypertonic (high osmotic pressure) fluids are only used in specific circumstances. It is important to realise that most fluids are low in potassium and that inappetent cats on fluid therapy will become potassium depleted quite rapidly. To prevent this from happening it is often necessary to add potassium chloride to the fluids.

Crystalloids

Crystalloids pass readily through the cell membrane and are rapidly distributed throughout the entire body.

In general around one-third of the fluid supplied will remain in the circulatory system, and around two thirds will diffuse into the cells and interstitial spaces. The movement of the crystalloids into the interstitium and body cells is influenced by hydrostatic pressure, oncotic pressure and the lymphatic system.

Colloids

Colloids contain large molecules that remain trapped within the circulatory system. This increases the plasma's osmotic pressure, which helps to prevent fluid from diffusing out of the circulation, so these fluids are referred to as plasma volume expanders.

These fluids can be used to cause rapid volume expansion in cases where there has been severe haemorrhage, but they will not replace any blood components such as blood cells and clotting factors. Colloids can also be used to replace the circulating volume if there is severe dehydration, but they must be used with care to prevent volume overload.

Whole blood

Whole blood is indicated in cases of anaemia, severe blood loss, or less frequently for patients with clotting

Table 4.2 Fluids for intravenous use			
Solution	Type	Use	Examples of indications
Hartmann's (Ringer's lactate)	Isotonic	Replacement of water and electrolyte losses	Acidosis, vomiting, diarrhoea
Ringer's	Isotonic	Replacement of water and electrolyte losses	Vomiting
0.9% NaCl	Isotonic	Replacement of water and electrolyte losses	Vomiting, urinary obstruction
5% Dextrose	Isotonic	Replacement of water	Primary water deficits
0.18% NaCl + 4% dextrose	Isotonic	Replacement and maintenance	Primary water loss and ongoing losses
Haemaccel/Gelofusin	Isotonic	Restoration of circulating volume	Haemorrhage, severe dehydration
Dextrans	Hypertonic	Restoration of circulating volume	Haemorrhage, severe dehydration
Hypertonic saline	Hypertonic	Restoration of circulating volume	Severe haemorrhage, hypovolaemic shock
Plasma	Isotonic	Restoration of circulating volume, proteins and clotting factors	Hypoproteinaemia, burns, Warfarin poisoning
Whole blood	Isotonic	Replacement of RBCs, platelets, clotting factors restoring circulating volume	Haemorrhage, anaemia, platelet and clotting factor deficiencies

or platelet deficiencies. Whole blood can be separated to provide blood fractions, such as packed red blood cells or plasma, which may be indicated in some cases. Cross matching of the donor and recipient is essential prior to transfusion (see later).

Calculating fluid volume

The amount of fluid that is supplied to the cat must compensate for the amount of fluid that has already been lost (fluid deficit), the additional fluid that will be lost (ongoing losses), and the ongoing day to day needs of the cat while it is being treated (maintenance fluid).

Fluid deficit

First the amount of fluid deficit needs to be calculated. This can be done on the basis of acute weight loss (providing the original weight was known), but is more usually calculated by assessing the percentage dehydration (Table 4.3). The fluid deficit, measured in millilitres, can then be calculated from the formula:

$$\text{Deficit (ml)} = \text{body weight (kg)} \times \text{percentage dehydration} \times 10$$

For instance if a 1 kg kitten is 10% dehydrated, the fluid deficit is approximately 100 ml.

Table 4.3 Estimating dehydration from clinical signs

Dehydration (%)	Clinical signs
Less than 5	None detectable
5–6	Subtle loss of skin elasticity
6–8	Dry mucous membranes
	Slightly prolonged capillary refill time
	Slightly sunken eyes
	Marked loss of skin elasticity
10–12	Dry mucous membranes
	Capillary refill time >2 seconds
	Sunken eyes
	Tented skin stands in place
12–15	Shock
	Collapse
	Death imminent

Fluid maintenance

On top of the fluid deficit the cat will require maintenance fluids, if it is not maintaining its own requirements by eating and drinking. The maintenance requirement in the cat is between 40–60 ml/kg/24 hours.

Ongoing fluid losses

Finally, the patient's ongoing losses should be taken into account. A cat with renal failure or diabetes will be producing more urine than normal, and extra fluid must be supplied to compensate for the polyuria. Similarly a cat suffering from diarrhoea will be losing additional fluid each time it defaecates, and this must be replaced.

The amount of additional fluid lost can be estimated by measuring the volume of urine passed, or by weighing soiled litter and bedding to give an estimate of the weight of urine, faeces and vomit that has been lost. Alternatively an estimate can be made by assuming that each episode of vomit of diarrhoea amounts to around 4 ml/kg body weight, e.g. a 1 kg kitten that has vomited twice would require a further 8 ml of fluid to be administered.

Fluid rate

Once the total amount of fluid that is required has been calculated, the rate at which it is to be supplied must be established. This is a task for a veterinary surgeon.

There is no set rule as to how quickly or slowly fluid should be administered. If the fluids are administered too slowly there is a danger of hypovolaemic shock but if the fluids are administered too fast there is the possibility of fluid overload, especially if the kidneys or heart are not functioning properly. As a general rule the rate of replacement should mirror the rate at which the fluid was lost.

Acute fluid replacement

A cat that experiences an acute loss of blood from its circulatory system would require rapid replacement of a suitable fluid in order to correct its hypovolaemia and hypoperfusion. In this instance fluid can be replaced relatively rapidly.

As a guide:
- Mild hypoperfusion 10–20 ml/kg in the first hour.
- Severe hypoperfusion 30–40 ml/kg in the first hour.

Response to this fluid should be assessed after the first hour. It is worth keeping in mind that only 5% of body weight equates to circulating volume or plasma water, so in a 1 kg kitten this will only be approx 50 ml of fluid. Failure to respond to fluid therapy could be due to ongoing haemorrhage. If this is uncontrolled internal haemorrhage care should be taken with these aggressive rates of fluid replacement, as increasing the blood pressure can result in further bleeding. Rapid fluid replacement requires extreme care in patients with respiratory, cardiac and renal problems.

Chronic fluid replacement

A cat that has been inappetent for a number of days will be experiencing a chronic loss of fluid, due to lack of fluid intake and continued normal losses. This chronic fluid loss can be replaced more gradually. The fluid will then be able to move from the vascular space, which is usually adequately maintained by the body's mechanisms for dealing with dehydration, into the cellular spaces, which will have given up fluid to maintain the circulating volume and blood pressure. It is usually appropriate to aim to replace half of the deficit in the first 6–8 hours of fluid therapy and the rest over the remaining 24 hours.

Replacing like for like will help ensure that fluid overload is avoided. This is especially important when dealing with cats, because of their small size. At this point it is important to remember that every patient is an individual and even when great care is taken to calculate estimated fluid volumes and rates of administration, complications can occur. It is therefore important to monitor the patient's vital signs and general demeanour during treatment. Any changes should be noted and reported to the veterinary surgeon and the fluid therapy adjusted accordingly.

From the calculation in Box 4.10, it can be seen that small volumes and slow drip rates are required for smaller feline patients. This can be difficult to achieve using normal giving sets that deliver 20 drops per ml, so the use of a *paediatric* giving set, which delivers 60 drops per ml is recommended in all cases. Alternatively a paediatric burette can be used; these can be fitted on to a normal fluid bag to provide a limited volume of fluid through a giving set that delivers 60 drops per ml (Fig. 4.27).

In small patients, or when accurate supply of fluid is required, an infusion pump provides the ideal, and safest solution to the problem (Fig. 4.28). These automated pumps can be programmed to deliver a set amount of fluid over a given time. They are normally fitted with an alarm to alert personnel to any obstruction to flow or to indicate when the bag of fluid is empty or when the required volume has been supplied. Use of an infusion pump ensures that only the desired volume of fluid is delivered, at a constant and pre-determined rate that is not affected by the position of the cat's limb,

BOX 4.10 EXAMPLE OF FLUID REPLACEMENT REQUIREMENT

1 kg kitten; 10% dehydrated, off food and vomiting approximately twice daily
Deficit = body weight (kg) × % deficit × 10 = 100 ml
Maintenance = 50 ml/kg/day = 50 ml
Additional losses = approx 8 ml/day
Total volume to replace = 158 ml

First 6 hours
Half of the deficit = 79 ml
79 ml ÷ 6 hours = 13.2 ml/hour
13.2 ml ÷ 60 minutes = 0.22 ml/minute
0.22 ml × 20 drops = 4.4 drops/minute for 6 hours
(For standard giving sets 20 drops = 1 ml, paediatric giving sets provide 60 drops/ml)

Next 18 hours
Remaining half of deficit = 79 ml
79 ÷ 18 hours = 4.4 ml/hour
4.4 ml ÷ 60 minutes = 0.07 ml/minute
0.07 ml × 20 drops = 1.5 drops/minute for next 18 hours

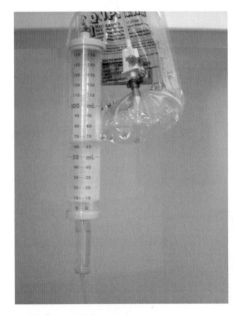

Figure 4.27 Paediatric burette.

or by flexion of the elbow, a common cause of obstruction to flow when using a standard giving set.

Syringe drivers and spring-loaded syringes are also designed to administer a pre-determined amount of

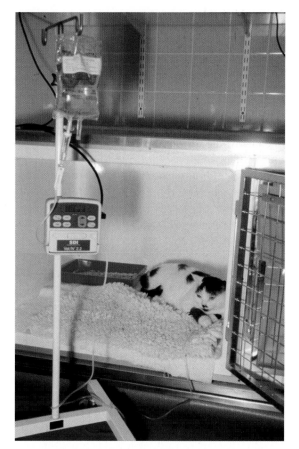

Figure 4.28 Fluid pump.

fluid over a given period (Fig. 4.29). The total volume is limited by the capacity of the syringe, which usually varies between 20 and 120 ml. These devices are particularly useful when dealing with tiny kittens as only small volumes of fluid are needed.

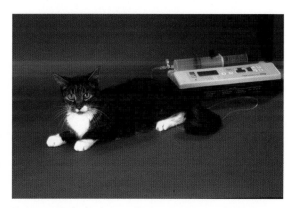

Figure 4.29 Syringe driver. Reproduced with permission from Sarah M.A. Caney.

Monitoring fluid therapy

Any patient receiving fluid therapy should be closely monitored for signs of over-infusion and to assess if the fluid therapy is having the desired effect.

Signs of over-infusion

Over-infusion of any patient is life threatening, and can happen very quickly in smaller feline patients.

It is important that a veterinary nurse becomes proficient at recognising any signs of over-infusion and reports them to the veterinary surgeon immediately.

BOX 4.11   SIGNS OF OVER-INFUSION

- Depression.
- Tachypnoea.
- Dyspnoea.
- Pulmonary oedema.
- Rasping/crackly chest noise/serous nasal discharge.
- Congestive heart failure.

Blood transfusion

A blood transfusion may be indicated if a patient's PCV has fallen to below 20% in a short space of time, or in cases of major haemorrhage. The volume transfused can be calculated using the patient and donor's PCV and is usually around 10–20 ml/kg.

To avoid serious, potentially fatal, transfusion reactions both donor and recipient cats must be blood typed or cross-matched, to make sure they are compatible before the transfusion is started. It is also important to screen the donor cat for infectious diseases such as FeLV, FIV and *Mycoplasma haemominutum*.

Inherited antigens present on the red blood cells' surface membrane determine blood types. An A-B system is used in cats; there are three basic types, A, B and AB. Commercial test kits can be used in-house to determine the blood type. Certain blood types are more common in certain breeds (Table 4.4).

A serious, usually fatal blood transfusion reaction will occur following transfusion of Type B cats with Type A blood. If a Type A cat receives Type B blood the transfusion reaction will be milder and less acute, but the transfused blood will not last longer than a few days. Type AB cats are rarely encountered; they should receive blood from a Type A donor.

The initial signs of a major transfusion reaction may include urticaria, erythema or pruritus, vomiting,

Table 4.4 Blood types		
Blood type	Cat breed	Prevalence in population
A	Domestic short hair, Domestic long hair	Majority of population
	Siamese, Burmese, Tonkinese, Oriental short hairs, Maine Coon, Manx	>90% of population
B	Abyssinian, Persian, Exotic, Himalayan, Somali, Burmese, Scottish Fold, Sphynx	10–25% of population
	British short hair, Ragdoll, Rex and Birman	>25 % of population
AB	No specific breed association, but more common in breeds with higher proportions of type B cats	Uncommon

vocalisation, pyrexia, depression, dyspnoea, tachypnoea or coughing. Signs progress to include tachycardia or bradycardia, tremors or convulsions, shock and cardiopulmonary arrest. Jaundice will also develop if the cat survives the initial crisis.

Even when the cats have been typed, minor incompatibilities could still be present and the cats may show some of the above signs to a lesser extent. It is therefore important to monitor the cat during transfusion.

The ideal donor cat should be a large (>5 kg) young to middle-aged cat that is FIV, FeLV and *Mycoplasma haemofelis* negative. Between 10 and 20% of the total blood volume can be collected (50–66 ml for a 5 kg cat) but if more than 10% of the donor cat's circulating volume is collected intravenous fluids should be supplied to prevent hypovolaemia. Blood is collected from the jugular vein into a suitably sized syringe pre-loaded with a citrated anticoagulant (1.3 ml anticoagulant for every 10 ml of blood to be collected). It is preferable that the donor cat is not sedated unless absolutely necessary.

According to RCVS guidelines, blood should only be taken from a donor for a specific patient rather than to be stored and used on any patient in the future. However, if the correct ratio of a citrated anticoagulant has been used, any surplus blood can be stored in a refrigerator for up to 30 days. Stored blood must be well-mixed, and gradually warmed to body temperature before transfusion.

When supplying blood to a patient it is essential that the correct administration set be used. Blood transfusion sets must be fitted with filters, which filter any clots. They also have wider tubing to allow the blood to flow more easily as it is much more viscous than any other fluid types.

CHAPTER 5

TECHNIQUES

Perdi Welsh, BSc(Hons) DipAVN(Surgical) CertED VN

5.1 BLOOD SAMPLING

Introduction

Blood samples may be obtained from a feline patient to diagnose various diseases and monitor a patient's response to treatment. The veterinary nurse's (VN's) responsibilities can include:

- Restraining the patient to facilitate collection of the sample.
- Obtaining the blood sample from the patient (qualified, listed VN).
- Handling the sample (using correct blood tubes, separating blood etc).
- Performing basic in-house blood tests.
- Storing and/or sending the sample to an external laboratory.

Each practice will need to weigh up the advantages and disadvantages of in-house testing based on a number of factors (see Table 5.1).

Various components of blood can be examined in-house by means of relatively basic and inexpensive equipment (Table 5.2). It is vital that good sample handling, correct sample storage and regular quality control checks are carried out to ensure reliability of results.

Table 5.1 Advantages and disadvantages of commercial versus in-house laboratories		
Commercial laboratory	**Advantages**	Specially trained staff and better equipment, therefore more likely to achieve accurate results. Convenience – someone else does all the work. Many laboratories provide a high level of diagnostic interpretation with the results.
	Disadvantages	Results are not immediate, may take 2–3 days for the results. May be more expensive to the client.
In-house laboratory	**Advantages**	Increased availability of testing equipment making it easier and more affordable for practices to run many in-house tests. Meets with increased client expectations. Faster results especially important for treating critically ill patients. May be more cost-effective – particularly if only one test is required.
	Disadvantages	Technical staff require training and need a sufficient throughput of cases to remain competent and confident at performing tests to ensure accurate results. Some tests are too expensive or too specialised to perform e.g. histopathology. May be expensive to run – equipment initially expensive to purchase and requires regular maintenance. Stringent health and safety regulation requirements.

Table 5.2 Examples of some commonly performed in-house blood tests

Haematology
- Measurement of packed cell volume (PCV).
- Examination of blood smears (differential white blood cell count, blood parasites, reticulocyte count).
- Total white cell counts.
- Total blood cell counts.

Biochemistry
- Many practices now have 'dry' chemistry systems whereby a range of biochemical tests can be performed relatively easily and inexpensively. The sample is added to pre-calibrated reagent slides and results are rapid. Equipment costs are relatively low, but reagent slides are relatively expensive, and results may not be accurate in all cases.
- 'Wet' chemistry systems are also becoming available for in-house use; the equipment is more expensive to buy, but reagent costs are much lower. Test results are very reliable if the machine is properly maintained and used.
- Total protein may be measured if a refractometer is available and hand-held glucose meters are available for measurement of blood glucose (note however, that most of these instruments are for human use and so care should be taken with interpretation of results). Blood dipsticks are available to measure blood urea nitrogen (BUN).

Virology
- Commercially available ELISA (enzyme-linked immunosorbent assay) test kits are available for various infectious agents e.g. FeLV, FIV. ELISA kits detect either antigen or antibodies in serum samples.

Obtaining samples

For most tests, the patient should be starved for 12 hours before sampling to reduce the risk of a lipaemic sample and aberrant results. It is especially important not to stress the feline patient during collection of the sample as test results, especially glucose and PCV, may be affected by stress. It is also important to avoid creating too much negative pressure within the syringe when collecting blood as this will cause haemolysis, which will affect the test results.

Sampling sites

For most cases the sample is best obtained from the jugular vein, although personal preference and familiarity with technique play a part in the selection of the sample site. The main advantage of jugular samples is that larger volumes of blood can be obtained more rapidly resulting in better quality samples, which are less likely to clot. Some cats that resent restraint for jugular puncture will be much more tolerant of sampling from the cephalic vein. If only a single drop of blood is required, e.g. for use in a glucometer, a sample can be obtained from the peripheral ear vein, or from the capillaries of the ear (see p. 90). This technique is well tolerated and only requires a single person to collect the sample. Table 5.3 reviews some of the advantages and disadvantages of each site.

Collection technique

To minimise stress to the patient, restraint should be firm but gentle. Many cats appear to tolerate the restraint methods for jugular samples better than for cephalic sampling, especially when they are placed in dorsal recumbency on the handler's lap (see Chapter 4, p. 63).

The site of venipuncture needs to be clipped. Scissors can be used but care has to be taken not to damage the skin. Ideally electrical clippers are used, although the noise of the clippers can be a stress factor. To reduce stress the clippers should be turned on at a distance from the cat to get it used to the noise, and talking to the cat will help to muffle the sound. The best option is to invest in clippers that produce the minimum of noise.

The skin then has to be prepared aseptically using cotton wool and a skin disinfectant followed by surgical spirit.

Table 5.3 Advantages and disadvantages of different sampling sites

	Advantages	Disadvantages
Jugular	• Large quantities obtained. • Rapid collection – less time restraining patient and less risk of sample clotting. • Larger needle used – less risk of haemolysis. • Cephalic vein left undisturbed if catheterisation required. • Many cats tolerate restraint for jugular sampling better than for cephalic sampling methods. • Easier to obtain sample in very small cats or patients with circulatory collapse.	• Requires practice – both in obtaining the sample and in restraining the patient. • Not well-tolerated by some cats with muscle or neck pain, or with oral pain.
Cephalic	• A familiar technique therefore handlers and operators are often more comfortable taking samples this way. • The vein may be more easily seen. • Some fractious cats are more easily restrained this way and can be wrapped in a towel for better restraint.	• Smaller quantities obtained. • Longer collection time – increased risk of clotting. • Smaller needle used – increased risk of haemolysis. • May affect the vein for subsequent catheterisation.
Ear	• Allows sample to be collected by one person. • Quick to perform. • Well-tolerated.	• Only produces a single drop of blood. • Requires practice.

JUGULAR SAMPLES (see Fig. 5.1)

The patient can be restrained either in an upright 'sitting' position or in dorsal recumbency, as described in Chapter 4, p. 63.

1. The collector raises the vein with the thumb of the left hand placed over the thoracic inlet. The skin around the site can be stretched slightly with the fingers of the left hand to help visualise the vein. The collector may raise and release the vein to aid visualisation of its position (if it cannot be seen, it is often palpable).

2. The collector inserts the needle into the vein, taking care not to advance the tip of the needle through the vein and out the other side (see Fig. 5.1).

3. Gentle negative pressure is applied by withdrawing the syringe plunger a small distance. As blood flows into the syringe the negative pressure is maintained by continuing to withdraw the syringe plunger at the same rate as the blood is flowing into the syringe. Take care not to withdraw the needle as you pull back on the plunger.

4. Once an adequate volume of blood has been collected the thumb raising the vein is released and the needle removed.

5. The handler places immediate gentle pressure over the needle insertion site to prevent further leakage of blood from the vein. Note that some people find bending the needle slightly (using the needle cover) helps to ensure the needle enters the vein at the correct angle.

CEPHALIC SAMPLES (see Fig. 5.2)

The cat is restrained as described in Chapter 4.

1. The handler raises the vein, by wrapping their thumb around the humerus, just above the elbow and twisting the skin slightly laterally (see Fig. 5.2). The rest of the hand is behind the elbow to avoid the cat retracting the leg. Alternatively a tourniquet

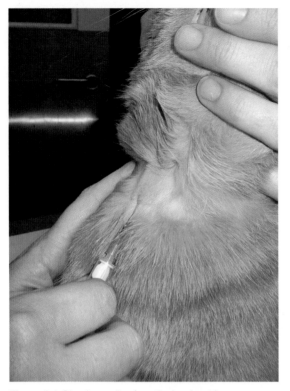

Figure 5.1 Blood sampling from the jugular vein.

can be placed in that area to raise the vein allowing the handler to concentrate on restraining the cat.

2. The collector stabilises the vein with the left thumb placed alongside the vein.
3. The needle is inserted through the skin and into the vein and the sample is obtained.
4. The handler releases the vein and the needle is removed.
5. The handler places immediate pressure over the vein.

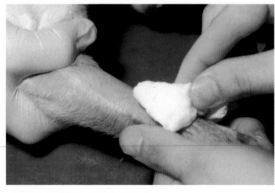

Figure 5.2 Preparing site of the cephalic vein for blood sampling or placement of an intravenous catheter.

EAR SAMPLES

1. Gently apply a warm pad to dilate the blood vessels in the ear.
2. Place the cotton wool on the inside of the pinna and prick the outside ear margin when using a needle or automatic lancing device. When using a lancing device that creates a vacuum, place the lancing device on the inside of the pinna, lance and then keep the device in place sufficiently long to allow the vacuum to form.
3. Allow a drop of blood to form on the ear.
4. Touch the sample strip to the drop of blood. The blood will be drawn up by capillary action. Ensure that the sample strip contains a sufficient amount of blood.
5. Move the cotton wool over the ear-prick and apply gentle pressure for a few seconds to stop further bleeding. Ear vein samples are most often used for glucometer readings.

The technique for collection of the sample is as follows:

1. A glucometer that accepts strips filled by capillary action, and that is unaffected by the angle at which it is held.
2. Warm heat pad, e.g. gel-pad or warm, wet wash-flannel in a plastic pack.
3. Cotton wool ball – provides protection to the fingers while pricking the ear and acts as a pressure bandage after pricking the ear.
4. Automatic lancing device, ideally one that creates a vacuum, or a 25 G needle.

Sample handling

It is important to know which tests the veterinary surgeon wants to run before the sample is taken as the handling of the sample is critical in obtaining accurate results. For instance samples for haematology must be placed in an appropriate anti-coagulant immediately, while other assays, e.g. parathyroid hormone measurement, require immediate centrifugation and freezing of the sample. The sample should be clearly labelled with the time, date and patient's details.

Some sample tubes contain an anticoagulant. The choice of anticoagulant will depend on the test being performed. It is important to use the correct anticoagulant as an incorrect choice may invalidate the results. When blood is stored in a tube containing anticoagulant it is important that the sample and anticoagulant are

Table 5.4 Sample tubes and anticoagulants for blood testing

Sample tube	Standard tube colour	Blood test
Ethylene-diamine-tetra-acetic acid (EDTA)	Pink	Anticoagulant of choice for haematology profiles. Appropriate choice for some virus tests.
Heparin	Orange	Anticoagulant of choice when plasma is required. Suitable for general biochemistry.
Plain tube	No colour, red (brown = gel)	Required when serum is required e.g. hormonal assays and some antibody assays (viral or bacterial). ELISA testing.
Fluoride oxalate	Yellow	Glucose.
Citrate	Purple	Coagulation screen.

gently mixed together as soon as the sample is placed into the tube, otherwise small clots will form, which will invalidate many test results. As soon as the tube has been sealed, roll it between your fingers, or gently invert it several times to ensure good mixing. Never shake the tube as this can damage the red blood cells causing haemolysis. Watch the sample for a few seconds to ensure that no visible clots form. Table 5.4 shows which storage method is preferred for commonly performed tests.

For most routine tests (if the test is not to be performed within two hours of collection) the sample may be refrigerated for up to 48 hours. Before any tests are performed, the sample should be returned to room temperature and for whole blood samples mixed thoroughly by inverting the tube several times or rolling it gently between your hands.

Plasma and serum are obtained by centrifuging the sample (see Boxes 5.1 & 5.2).

Before using the sample to run any tests it is important to check that it is an appropriate sample, has been stored correctly and that there is no evidence of a

BOX 5.1   PLASMA SEPARATION

1. Collect the whole blood sample into a heparin sample tube.
2. Centrifuge at 2000–3000 rpm for 10 minutes, or according to the instructions supplied with the centrifuge.
3. Remove the separated plasma by pipette and transfer to a plain tube.

BOX 5.2   SERUM SEPARATION

1. Collect the whole blood sample into a plain sample tube.
2. Leave sample to clot at room temperature (approximately 30 minutes).
3. When the clot has retracted, run a small stick (e.g. capillary tube) around the wall of the container to loosen the clot.
4. Replace the lid of the sample container and centrifuge at 2000–3000 rpm for 10 minutes, or according to the instructions supplied with the centrifuge.
5. Using a pipette suck up the serum taking care not to draw up any of the clot.
6. Transfer the serum into a plain, labelled container.
7. The sample may be refrigerated or frozen until required.

Table 5.5 Common sample problems

Problem	Appearance	Source	Cause
Haemolysis	Plasma/serum appears red.	Breakdown of red cells within the sample.	Sample collected through too small a needle. Too much negative pressure applied at time of sample collection. Rough handling of sample after collection. Prolonged storage of the sample.
Lipaemia	Plasma/serum appears white.	Excess fat in the plasma.	Recent meal. Some endocrine disorders, e.g. diabetes mellitus.
Blood clot in anticoagulated sample	Dark red gelatinous mass within the liquid blood.	Insufficient contact with anticoagulant.	Delay between collecting blood and placing into storage tube. Inadequate mixing of blood and anticoagulant.
Icterus/jaundice/ hyperbilirubinaemia	Plasma/serum appears yellow.	Excess bilirubin in the sample.	Haemolytic anaemia, liver disease or obstruction of the bile duct.

problem with the sample that would invalidate the results of the test you are about to run (see Table 5.5). If the serum appears abnormal check with a veterinary surgeon that it is still acceptable to use the sample for the tests that are planned.

Fresh smears for haematology (see Box 5.3)
Blood smears can be stained with various agents to allow the red and white cells to be examined under a microscope. The morphology (structure) of the cells (see Fig. 5.5) can be evaluated, differential

BOX 5.3 TECHNIQUE FOR MAKING A SMEAR

1. Prepare equipment – microscope slides, 'spreader' slide, blood sample (in EDTA), alcohol, capillary tubes, disposable gloves.
2. Wear gloves.
3. Clean the slide with alcohol to degrease it and ensure it is dry.
4. Place the slide on a pale background (bench paper or tissue).
5. Gently mix the blood sample.
6. Using a capillary tube, draw up a small amount of blood from the sample tube.
7. Place a small drop of blood at one end of the slide.
8. Hold the slide steady with one hand and with the other, hold the spreader slide firmly on the slide just in front of the drop of blood at a 45° angle.
9. Draw the spreader slide back to the drop of blood and allow the blood to spread out along the edge of the spreader slide (Fig. 5.3).
10. Move the spreader slide forward in a single, smooth fairly rapid motion.
11. Air-dry the smear by waving the slide quickly through the air.
12. Check the quality of the smear. The resulting smear should be pale in colour, with an even distribution of blood, diminishing as it advances across the slide. If it is good, label the slide and stain immediately, if in house staining is requested.

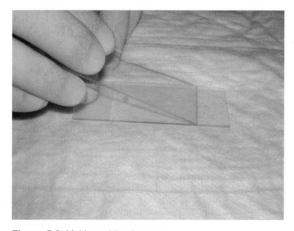

Figure 5.3 Making a blood smear.

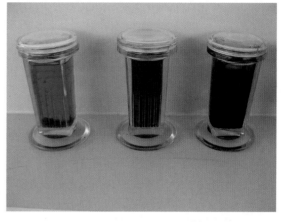

Figure 5.4 Coplin jars filled with Diff-Quik™ solutions.

white cell counts and platelet counts performed and blood parasites can be detected. PCR tests are now available for more accurate diagnosis of *Mycoplasma* infections.

The aim is to spread a drop of blood evenly across the slide so that the cells form a 'monolayer' i.e. the blood film is only one cell thick so the cells do not lie on top of each other. Blood films should be prepared immediately, allowed to dry naturally, and kept at room temperature.

Staining is useful to show up the cell morphology. The Diff-Quik™ staining system, which is commonly used in veterinary practice, provides quick and acceptable results (see Figs 5.4, 5.5 and Box 5.4).

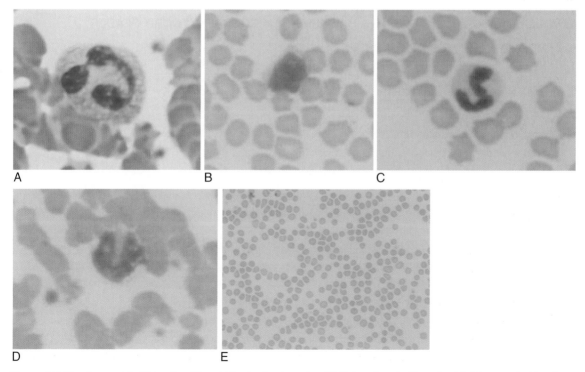

Figure 5.5 Blood smear identifying the different blood cells: A, eosinophil; B, lymphocyte; C, neutrophil; D, monocyte; E, red blood cell (courtesy of IDEXX Laboratories).

BOX 5.4 DIFF-QUIK™ TECHNIQUE

1. Wear gloves.
2. Prepare the staining solutions by dispensing into Coplin jars or similar (see Fig 5.4).
3. Dip the prepared, dried smear into the fixative (solution A, light blue methanol) five times for one second each time.
4. Remove and allow excess fluid to drip back into the jar.
5. Dip the slide into the first red stain (eosin) as before.
6. Dip the slide into the second purple (thiazine) stain seven times (which helps to stain the platelets).
7. Rinse the slide with buffered distilled water and leave upright to air dry.

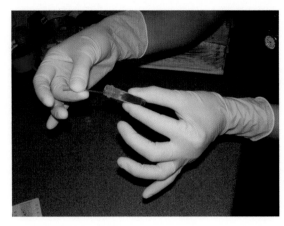

Figure 5.6 Filling microhaematocrit tube.

It is important that the stain bottles that are used for blood smears are not used for staining any other samples that would contaminate the stain, e.g. skin scrapings, ear wax smears and faecal smears.

Packed cell volume (PCV) (see Box 5.5 & Figs 5.6–5.8)

Measurement of PCV assesses the percentage of the blood that is occupied by red blood cells. It is useful for assessment of anaemia or dehydration. The normal PCV for the cat is 0.26–0.45 l/l.

BOX 5.5 MEASURING PCV USING A HAWKSLEY™ MICROHAEMATOCRIT READER

1. Prepare equipment (blood sample in EDTA tube, microhaematocrit (capillary) tubes, centrifuge, Cristaseal™ or similar, Hawksley™ microhaematocrit reader or similar, tissues and disposable gloves).
2. Wear gloves.
3. Gently mix the blood sample by inverting the tube several times.
4. Hold the sample tube at the 45°angle.
5. Fill one capillary tube three-quarters full with blood (Fig. 5.6).
6. Place a finger over the top of the tube to prevent the tube emptying.
7. Wipe the outside of the tube with tissue.
8. Seal the end of the tube with Cristaseal™ (Fig. 5.7).
9. Repeat the procedure to fill the second tube.
10. Place the two tubes into the centrifuge opposite each other with the sealed ends facing outwards.
11. Secure the safety plate if present.
12. Centrifuge for five minutes at 10 000 rpm, or according to the instructions supplied with the centrifuge.
13. Place one tube into the groove on the Hawksley™ microhaematocrit reader.
14. Place the bottom of the RBC column (top of the Cristaseal'™ plug) on the baseline of the scale.
15. Move the sample along the scale until the top of the plasma is level with the upper sloping line.
16. Adjust the movable line so that it is at the top of the RBC column (Fig. 5.8).
17. Read and record the percentage value on the scale.

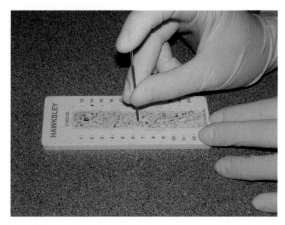

Figure 5.7 Sealing microhaematocrit tube.

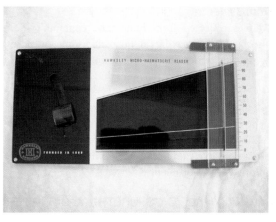

Figure 5.8 Measuring PCV, using a Hawksley™ microhaematocrit reader (in this case the PCV is 26%).

5.2   URINE SAMPLING

Introduction

Relatively simple in-house testing of urine can provide information regarding the urinary tract and other systemic diseases. The VN needs to be aware of the methods available for collecting urine, how to handle and store urine samples and how to perform standard in-house tests, for example, measurement of urine specific gravity, urine biochemistry using dip-sticks, and microscopic examination of urine.

Collection techniques

The method of collecting a urine sample will depend on the patient and the reason for testing the urine. Urine may be collected from a free flow sample, from a litter tray, or by catheterisation or cystocentesis.

Free flow

Free flow samples are obtained either as the patient urinates or by manual compression of the bladder. It is almost impossible to catch a sample while the feline patient is urinating, so free flow urine samples are more commonly obtained by manual expression of the bladder (see Box 5.6). The bladder needs to contain at least 10–15 ml of urine for this to be possible. Gentle constant pressure is applied to the bladder to encourage the patient to urinate. Urine must never be collected by this method if urethral obstruction is suspected, and extreme care must be taken if the bladder has been subjected to trauma or neoplasia is suspected, which may result in the bladder or urethra rupturing.

An important consideration of free flowing sample collection is that the sample contains the first flow of urine, which may be contaminated with cells and bacteria from the distal genital tract and vaginal or prostatic fluids. This makes these samples unsuitable for bacteriology and quantitative protein analysis.

BOX 5.6   TECHNIQUE FOR MANUAL COMPRESSION OF THE BLADDER

1. Collect all equipment – disposable gloves, sterile universal container, clean, dry kidney dish.

2. Assistant restrains the patient in standing position on the table.

3. Clean external genitalia to decrease contamination of the sample.

4. Locate the bladder by palpation of the caudal abdomen (see Chapter 4, p. 69).

5. Exert gentle constant pressure on the bladder (note: it may take a few minutes for the bladder sphincter to relax and enable the patient to urinate).

6. Once urine begins to flow, continue to exert gentle pressure on the bladder and direct the stream into the kidney dish. If there is any resistance, do not continue and do not squeeze the bladder in an attempt to void urine.

7. When the flow discontinues, release the pressure.

8. Transfer the sample immediately into the appropriate sterile container.

From a litter tray

Samples collected from litter trays containing non-absorbent litter may be adequate for some purposes, e.g. specific gravity and glucose estimation, but are not suitable for most other purposes due to contamination.

One approach to collecting the sample is to place an empty litter tray in the kennel and wait; however, many cats refuse to use a litter tray if they are unable to bury what they have passed. There are a number of non-absorbable cat litters available that can be used to circumvent this problem.

If the litter tray method is used, the VN must be sure that it has been rinsed thoroughly after cleaning and that hypochlorites (bleaches) have not been used as these can alter the pH of the sample. The sample should be transferred as soon as it is voided into a sterile universal container.

Catheterisation (see Box 5.7 & 5.8)

Urinary catheterisation involves passing a catheter into the bladder via the urethra and is difficult in a conscious cat. Great care must be taken if the cat is not

---

BOX 5.7   MALE CATS: URETHRAL CATHETERISATION

1. Collect equipment (e.g. catheter, three-way tap, 10 ml syringe, lubricant, disposable gloves, sample container).
2. The assistant holds the patient in lateral recumbency and the hind limbs are drawn forward away from the penis.
3. Wash hands and wear gloves.
4. Gently cleanse the prepuce with surgical scrub and rinse.
5. Another assistant should open the external catheter package to enable operator to take the sterile inner pack.
6. Without jeopardising asepsis, the operator should estimate the length of catheter to be inserted.
7. Cut the end off the catheter package and cut a further 'feeder' section approximately 2.5 cm long.
8. Expose just the tip of the catheter and apply sterile lubricant.
9. Retract the prepuce to expose the penis and gently put traction on the penis in a caudal direction to help straighten the penile flexure.
10. Use the other hand to pass the catheter into the urethral opening. Remove the stylet (if present).
11. Continue feeding the catheter along the urethra gently (it should pass easily; if this is not the case, the penile flexure is probably not fully straightened, or it may be necessary to re-evaluate the size of the catheter). Initially the urethra angles towards the spine, then runs parallel to the spine.
12. Once the catheter is in the bladder, urine should begin to flow into the package.
13. Discard the first few millilitres of urine then collect 6–10 ml in a sterile syringe.

BOX 5.8   FEMALE CATS: URETHRAL CATHETERISATION

1. Collect equipment (as Box 5.8).
2. Assistant to restrain cat in lateral or ventral recumbency, extending the tail over the cat's back to stretch the skin over the genital region.
3. Wash hands and wear gloves.
4. Gently cleanse around the vulva with surgical scrub and rinse.
5. Another assistant opens external catheter package to enable operator to take sterile inner pack.
6. Estimate the length of catheter to be inserted (without jeopardising asepsis).
7. Expose just the tip of the catheter and apply sterile lubricant.
8. With one hand, pass the catheter into the urethral orifice via the vulva by angling the catheter ventrally and running its tip along the floor of the vulva and vagina, keeping it on the mid-line.
9. Continue gently, feeding the catheter along the urethra. It should pass easily into the bladder.
10. Once the catheter is in the bladder, urine should begin to flow into the package.
11. Discard the first few millilitres of urine then collect 6–10 ml in a sterile syringe.

sedated or anaesthetised as there is an increased risk of iatrogenic trauma. There is also a risk of introducing infection to the urethra and bladder and so you must ensure an aseptic and atraumatic technique.

Catheterisation is a useful method of collecting urine when a free flow sample cannot be obtained and, if good sterile technique has been used, the sample may be used for bacterial culture and sensitivity tests.

TECHNIQUE – GENERAL POINTS
1. Ensure all equipment is ready.
2. Typically, a conventional cat catheter or a Jackson's cat catheter is used for obtaining samples from the male and female feline patient. A standard catheter is preferred as it allows better maintenance of aseptic technique when placing the catheter (see Boxes 5.7 & 5.8). For long-term indwelling catheters it is best to use a urinary catheter made from silicone, to avoid irritation of the urethra.
3. General anaesthesia or sedation is usually required for urinary catheterisation of feline patients.
4. A lubricant such as KY-Jelly™ can be used, and will not damage any latex catheters (the lubricant can be sterilised in small containers for this use).
5. Clean around external genitalia if necessary to remove discharges and dirt.
6. The operator should wash their hands prior to starting and wear non-sterile gloves.
7. Care should be taken not to insert catheters too far because they can bend or kink or at worst turn back on themselves and knot.
8. Never twist or turn the catheter when it is placed in the urethra as this may cause trauma.

Cystocentesis

Cystocentesis involves passing a needle through the abdominal wall into the bladder to remove the urine. This method of collection is the preferred method for bacteriology as the sample is not contaminated. It may also be used to drain the bladder when there is an obstruction. This procedure is generally well tolerated in conscious cats but it involves penetration of the abdominal cavity and therefore under the RCVS Code of Conduct guidelines it can only be performed by a veterinary surgeon.

Handling and storage of samples

Following collection, sample pots should be labelled appropriately with time, date and patient details. Plain, sterile commercially available containers are most commonly used. Jam jars or other old food containers should not be used as they may be contaminated. Storage tubes containing boric acid should be used for urine culture to prevent the bacteria multiplying. These tubes have a red top, and contain white powder. They must be filled to the marked line to ensure that the sample contains the correct concentration of preservative. If there is insufficient urine to reach the mark, the boric acid in a single tube can be subdivided into several other tubes to achieve a correct ratio.

Urinalysis should be performed within 30 minutes of collection to prevent changes in pH, increases in bacterial numbers and degenerative changes. Samples for crystal analysis should not be refrigerated, as this will cause large numbers of crystals to form.

In-house urine analysis

Appearance

Before analysing the urine record its overall appearance. Normal urine in the cat is quite yellow (well-concentrated) and clear. Common abnormalities include paleness (less concentrated urine, i.e. low specific gravity), redness (haematuria or haemoglobinuria) and cloudiness (increased protein, crystal or cell content).

Specific gravity (see Box 5.9)

A refractometer is used to assess the specific gravity (SG) of urine, i.e. its density relative to distilled water. It is essential that the refractometer be calibrated before each SG reading to prevent false results. Place a drop of water onto the prism and check that the scale reads 1.000; if not, adjust the reading using the graduated collar on the refractometer. Refractometers are calibrated for use at room temperature, so it is important to ensure refrigerated samples are allowed to come to room temperature before testing.

BOX 5.9   TECHNIQUE: REFRACTOMETER

1. Wear gloves.
2. Invert urine sample to ensure thorough mixing.
3. Use a pipette to place two drops of sample onto the prism and replace the prism cover.
4. Hold the refractometer up to the light and read the SG of the sample.
5. Record the results.
6. Clean the prism using distilled water and dry.

The normal SG in the cat is >1.035. Low urine SG may be indicative of a number of systemic diseases (e.g. renal disease, diabetes mellitus) and further tests should be performed.

The urine SG reading on dipstick is not reliable and should not be used.

Urine chemistry using dipsticks (see Box 5.10)

Various commercially available biochemistry dipsticks are available which test a range of parameters of which the most useful are pH, protein, ketones, bilirubin, blood and glucose. Many of the sticks are designed for human use so some parameters, such as the white blood cell count, are inaccurate for the feline patient. In addition inaccurate results can occur with out of date strips, old urine samples or preserved samples. The urine must be in contact with the test pad for the recommended time to ensure accurate results. A recent meal will influence the pH of the sample (post-prandial alkaline tide).

Sediment examination (see Box 5.11)

Sediment is examined for the presence of cellular material (red and white blood cells, neoplastic, epithelial or inflammatory cells), microorganisms, urinary casts and crystals. In the feline patient normal urine does not contain a large amount of sediment. The presence of a large number of casts (hyaline, cellular, granular and waxy casts) may indi-

cate various disease processes including inflammation and renal disease. The presence of crystals in urine may or may not be of clinical significance; phosphate and struvite crystals can occur in healthy cats.

The urine sample needs to be centrifuged and the sediment examined under the microscope. Fresh samples must be used for this purpose as storage allows spontaneous formation of crystals and cell lysis to occur.

Urinary catheters

In addition to collection of urine for analysis, catheterisation of the bladder may be performed for a range of other procedures. For example, monitoring urine output, relieving urine retention, to empty the bladder before some surgical or radiographic procedures and to perform hydropropulsion to dislodge obstructions in the urethra.

The technique and general considerations for placement of a urinary catheter have been described in the previous section (p. 96).

BOX 5.11   TECHNIQUE: URINE SEDIMENT

1. Gather equipment – fresh urine sample, disposable gloves, centrifuge and centrifuge tubes, pipette, microscope slide and cover slip, microscope, appropriate stain.
2. Centrifuge all or some of the urine sample for 5 minutes at 2000 rpm or according to the instructions supplied with the centrifuge.
3. Gently remove most of the supernatant fluid with a pipette, leaving a few drops at the bottom. Discard the supernatant appropriately.
4. Resuspend the sample by flicking the bottom of the tube (with the lid on!).
5. Stains, such as Sedistain™ or methylene blue can be used, but may create artefacts.
6. Pipette a few drops of the sample onto a microscope slide and apply cover slip avoiding air bubbles.
7. Examine under low power and low illumination.

BOX 5.10   TECHNIQUE: URINE TEST STRIP

1. Gather equipment – fresh urine sample, test strips, pipettes or syringe, disposable gloves.
2. Wear gloves.
3. Ensure test strips are in date.
4. Invert urine sample to ensure thorough mixing.
5. Remove a stick from container and replace lid immediately.
6. Cover all test squares with urine (using a pipette or dipping the stick into the urine sample).
7. Note the time or set timer for required period.
8. Compare reaction colours with colour scale on the label. Read and record the results at the correct times.

Table 5.6 Sediment examination

Item	Source	Frequency in normal urine	Interpretation
Red blood cells	Urine samples may be contaminated with RBCs as a result of collection methods (e.g. cystocentesis)	<5 per high-powered field.	Large number of RBCs occur as a result of bleeding into the urogenital tract – e.g. due to cystitis, neoplasia or renal disease.
Epithelial cells	Renal tubule cells (small round cells), transitional epithelial cells (variable shape – usually 2–4 times size of a WBC) or squamous epithelial cells (large flattened cells with small nucleus).	Small numbers are sometimes seen.	Epithelial cells are shed from the urinary tract, but large numbers may indicate urinary tract infection or neoplasia.
Bacteria	Bacteria may be seen in old urine samples, and the sampling method may cause high numbers of bacteria to be seen (e.g. catheterisation).	Negative	High numbers of motile bacteria indicate bacterial urinary tract infection. Culture and sensitivity testing of a cystocentesis sample is indicated. A Gram-stain may provide immediate indication of bacterial morphology.
Crystals	Common in normal cats. Important to examine fresh urine (within 2 hours of collection) as crystals form as the sample cools.	Variable	Struvite and phosphate crystals can occur as a result of normal renal concentrating ability in cats therefore may be present in normal cat urine. Presence of crystals is not necessarily an indication of urolithiasis. Also note that crystals are sometimes not seen in cats with a urolith and that the type of crystals seen may not reflect the type of urolith if present. See Ch. 6, p. 147 for further information.
Casts	Accumulations of cells or other material within the renal tubule, that are then passed into the urine but maintain the shape of the tubule in which they formed May be hyaline, cellular, granular, waxy or fatty.	<1–2 hyaline or granular casts per low-power field	Large numbers of casts signify renal tubular disease.

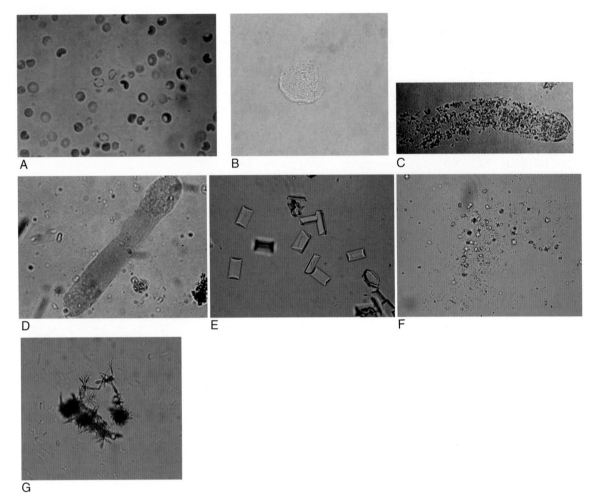

Figure 5.9 Sediment examination: A, red blood cells; B, epithelial cell; C, granular cast; D, hyaline cast; E, triple phosphate crystals; F, calcium oxalate crystals; G, ammonium urate crystals (courtesy of IDEXX Laboratories).

Repeated catheterisation is likely to increase the risk of infection and particular care and observation of these patients should be carried out. For the maintenance of indwelling catheters see Chapter 6 (p. 148).

Types of catheter

CONVENTIONAL CAT CATHETER
- Available in nylon.
- Single use.
- Smaller version of conventional dog catheters.
- Size range 3 and 4 FG.

JACKSON'S CAT CATHETER (see Fig. 5.10)
- Indwelling 'tom cat' catheters.
- Nylon with additional metal stylet and plastic flange to suture to the prepuce.
- Size range 3 and 4 FG.

SILICONE CAT CATHETER (see Fig. 5.11)
- Best used when needing a longer term indwelling catheter, as it reduces the chance of causing irritation and urethritis.
- Smaller version of conventional dog catheters.
- Size range 3 and 4 FG.
- Usually not used to 'unblock' the urethra as the catheters lack stiffness.

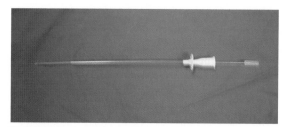

Figure 5.10 Jackson catheter.

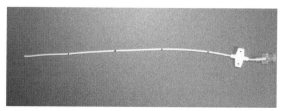

Figure 5.11 Silicone urinary catheter.

5.3 FAECAL SAMPLING

Introduction

Macroscopic examination of faeces, in conjunction with clinical signs shown by the cat, can provide some information about the intestines and help in the selection of further diagnostic testing (see Table 5.7). Abnormalities in the consistency, volume, colour and any sign of dyschezia may help to differentiate between a small or large intestinal problem.

Obtaining samples

Faecal samples are usually collected after they have been passed. Cats tend to bury their faeces, making it more difficult for samples to be obtained and samples collected from the garden can be contaminated. Washable (non-absorbent) cat litter can be used in litter trays so that faecal samples can be obtained by this method. Faeces can also be collected directly from the rectum although cats do not tolerate this procedure particularly well and may require sedation. It is

Table 5.7 Macroscopic examination of faeces – physical changes	
Physical changes in appearance	**Possible causes**
Consistency	Diarrhoea is seen in a wide range of disease processes, including diseases outside the intestinal tract (renal disease, thyroid disease etc) and diseases within the intestinal tract (for instance infectious diseases, inflammatory diseases or neoplastic diseases etc).
Volume	Increased in small intestinal disease – usually large volume of very watery faeces. Decreased in large intestinal disease, but usually the frequency of defaecation is increased.
Colour	Very pale faeces may be due to increased faecal fat content (steatorrhoea) or due to lack of bile pigment in biliary obstruction. Colour may also be affected by the food the cat eats.
Fresh blood	Fresh blood mixed through the faeces usually originates from the colon. Fresh blood on the surface of the faeces suggests that it originates from the distal colon or rectum.
Black, tarry faeces (melaena)	Digested blood usually due to haemorrhage in small intestine.
Mucus	Mucus in the faeces is often seen in large intestinal disorders, e.g. colitis.
Straining (tenesmus)	Usually indicates a large intestinal problem.
Parasites	Tapeworm segments and adult roundworms may be seen in faeces.
Thin or flattened shape	May indicate intestinal narrowing due to neoplastic lesions.

however useful to do this while a cat is under general anaesthetic for further investigation anyway.

Faecal samples should be examined as soon as possible to minimise changes (e.g. eggs hatching). Samples requiring storage should be refrigerated, or may be mixed with equal parts of 10% formalin, if bacterial culture is not required.

Faecal smears

Smears can be made to examine faeces for parasitic eggs and trophozoites, however, it is easy to miss eggs if only small numbers are present. Smears can also be stained and examined for undigested food material.

Preparation of a direct faecal smear

1. Collect all equipment (sample, microscope slides, spatula or loop, saline, appropriate stains if required, cover slips, microscope).
2. Wear gloves.
3. Place one to two drops of saline onto the middle of a microscope slide.
4. Using spatula or loop, collect a small amount of faeces and mix into the saline.
5. Add a drop of stain. (Iodine will stain starch granules dark blue/black, Sudan III will stain fat globules orange/red.)
6. Cover the sample with cover slip, avoiding air bubbles.
7. View under × 40 objective lens.

Faecal flotation

Faecal flotation is a more sensitive tool for detecting parasite eggs. There are various methods available. The use of a saturated sugar or salt solution is described here using the McMaster technique (see Box 5.12).

BOX 5.12 PREPARATION OF A FAECAL FLOTATION TO IDENTIFY PARASITIC EGGS AND OOCYSTS

1. Collect all equipment (sample, saturated sugar or salt solution, spatula, two beakers, microscope, Pasteur pipette).
2. Weigh 3 g of faeces and add to a beaker with 45 ml of saturated solution of sugar or salt water.
3. Mix the solution thoroughly with a spatula.
4. Pour the solution through a sieve or strainer into the second beaker.
5. Leave the solution to settle for 15 minutes at room temperature or centrifuge at 1500 rpm for 3 minutes.
6. Pipette off the supernatant for further examination and discard the rest of the solution.
7. Use a Pasteur pipette to withdraw a small amount of the supernatant.
8. Fill the counting chamber of a McMaster slide and apply the cover slip.
9. Allow to stand for a further five minutes.
10. View under low power (x10 objective lens). See Fig. 5.12.
11. Identify all eggs and oocysts and count all of the eggs seen over the grid.
12. The number per gram of faeces is calculated by multiplying the number of eggs within the chamber by 50.

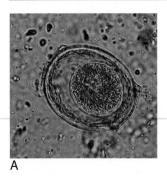
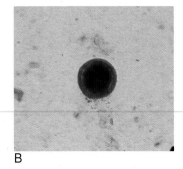
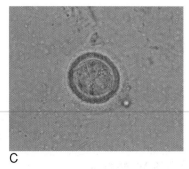

A   B   C

Figure 5.12 Faeces: Endoparasites: A, *Toxascaris leoninea*; B, *Toxocara cati*; C, *Dipylidium caninum* (courtesy of IDEXX Laboratories).

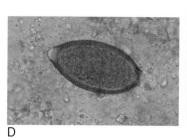
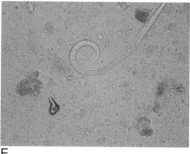
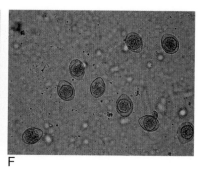

D   E   F

Figure 5.12—cont'd D, *Trichuris*; E, *Aelurostrongylus abstrusus*; F, coccidia (courtesy of IDEXX Laboratories).

5.4 SKIN SAMPLING

Introduction

Samples from the patient's skin and fur may be obtained to examine for the presence of dermatophytes, yeasts, bacterial infections and ectoparasites.

The method of collection will depend on the suspected infection and this will determine the test to be performed, for instance:

- Skin scrapings are used primarily to detect burrowing mites such as *Sarcoptes* and *Demodex*. Skin scrapings are usually carried out by veterinary surgeons.
- Coat brushings are performed to detect fleas, lice and *Cheyletiella* infestation.
- Hair plucks may be taken and submitted for fungal culture or examined for lice and *Cheyletiella* eggs, which are attached to the hair shaft.
- Clear adhesive tape may be used to collect fleas, lice and harvest mites and to demonstrate the presence of microbes such as *Malassezia*.
- Ear wax can be collected and examined for presence of *Otodectes cynotis*.

Obtaining samples

Coat brushing technique
1. Wear gloves.
2. Place the patient onto a large sheet of white paper.
3. Vigorously brush the coat with a brush (Mackenzie brush or sterile tooth brush can be used for this).
4. Collect the dislodged material and transfer some of it onto a microscope slide with some liquid paraffin.
5. Examine under the microscope.

Hair plucking technique
When collecting a hair sample it is important to ensure that the hairs are plucked rather than clipped. Plucking ensures that the entire length of the hair, from root to tip, is collected. Wear gloves to collect the sample and pluck the hairs from the periphery of any skin lesions.

SELF-INDUCED ALOPECIA
Examination of the tips of the plucked hairs under a microscope will distinguish between alopecia due to self-grooming and alopecia due to spontaneous hair loss. If the cat has been over-grooming the tips of the hairs will have jagged broken ends, whereas if hair loss is spontaneous the plucked hairs will have finely tapered, undamaged tips.

ECTOPARASITES (see Fig. 5.13)
Place the sample on a microscope slide, cover with a cover slip and examine the whole sample for evidence of lice, mites and parasite eggs. Liquid paraffin may be applied to the sample before examination.

DERMATOPHYTES (see Fig. 5.13)
There are a number of ways to check for the presence of ringworm:

- Microscopy: Place the sample onto a microscope slide. A drop of 'Quink' ink may be added to the sample to make visualisation of the spores easier. Put a cover slip on the sample and examine the hairs for spores under ×100 or ×400 magnification.
- Woods lamp: see p. 105.
- Fungal culture: Hair pluckings are collected and carefully inoculated using sterile forceps onto one of two media: Sabouraud's agar or dermatophyte test medium (Dermafyt™), which is available in

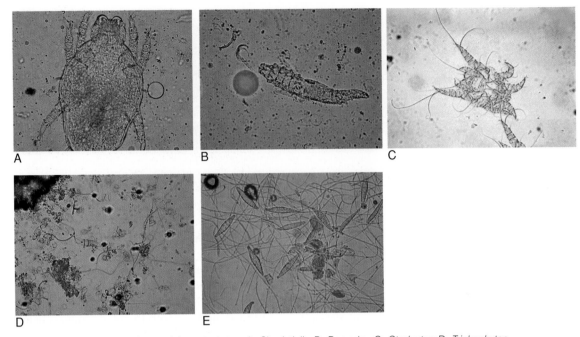

Figure 5.13 Skin ectoparasites and dermatophytes: A, *Cheyletiella*; B, *Demodex*; C, *Otodectes*; D, *Trichophyton mentagrophytes*; E, *Microsporum* (courtesy of IDEXX laboratories).

commercial fungal culture kits for use in practice. The unit containing the culture should be sealed with biohazard tape and kept at room temperature for 7–10 days. It should be checked daily for the appearance of a white colony and concurrent red coloration of the medium, which indicates the presence of a dermatophyte (although there is the possibility of contamination with a saprophyte fungus). If there is no growth after three weeks, the sample can be considered negative for ringworm.

Tape strip technique

1. Wear gloves.
2. Choose the area to be tested and if necessary, separate the hairs to allow access to the skin below.
3. Press a length of clear adhesive tape firmly onto the area then peel it off. Debris from the coat and skin will stick to the tape strip. The process can be repeated using the same tape strip if insufficient sample is collected at the first attempt.
4. Transfer the tape, sticky side down onto a microscope slide for examination under low power. If the sample is to be stained, e.g. when examining for *Malassezia*, stick the two ends of the tape strip to the ends of the glass side, leaving a loop of tape free in the central section. This will keep the tape strip from becoming tangled when it is dipped into the stain solutions.

5. Stain the sample, e.g. with Diff-Quik™ or methylene blue.
6. Unstick the tape and re-position so that the sample is over the slide.
7. Examine under high magnification, using oil immersion, for presence of yeasts and fungal hyphae.

Ear swab technique

1. Wear gloves.
2. Using a cotton bud, gently collect some of the ear wax from the external ear canal.
3. Transfer the wax onto a microscope slide by gently rolling the swab across the surface of the slide.
4. Mix the wax with 2–3 drops of liquid paraffin or KOH and break up any clumps using a sterile needle so that the sample is not too thick.
5. Apply cover slip and examine under microscope.

Preserving samples

As with most laboratory tests, it is usually better to examine the sample immediately, however, if this is not possible or if the sample is to be sent to an external laboratory for analysis it is important that the sample does not dry out. Potassium hydroxide or liquid paraffin may be used as the lubricant.

With the exception of air-dried smears, it is not advisable to send prepared microscope slides through the post, as the sample is likely to slip off the slide.

Samples from skin scrapes can be placed into a 5 or 20 ml sterile universal sample pot along with the blade and sent to the laboratory. Samples of ear wax can be stored by cutting the cotton bud and placing it into a universal sample pot.

Ultraviolet (Wood's lamp) examination technique

A Wood's lamp is an ultraviolet light that can be used to help detect certain strains of ringworm. Around 50% of *Microsporum canis* strains fluoresce an apple-green colour when examined under this light. The technique can produce both false negative and false positive results, so it should not be used as the sole diagnostic test for ringworm. It is most useful as a means to determine which hairs to use for culture.

1. Choose a room that can be effectively darkened.
2. Turn on the lamp and allow at least five minutes for it to warm up.
3. Wear gloves.
4. Wear eye protectors.
5. Turn off main light.
6. With the patient restrained, hold the lamp over the affected areas and examine the hair and skin for apple-green fluorescence.

5.5 BLOOD PRESSURE MEASUREMENT

Introduction

High blood pressure (hypertension) is a common problem in older cats, and is often associated with underlying disease processes such as chronic renal failure and hyperthyroidism. In these patients regular blood pressure measurements are indicated as a way of determining if treatment is required or to determine the success of treatment.

Direct measurement of arterial blood pressure by means of arterial catheterisation provides accurate and sensitive readings, however, this method generally requires sedation or anaesthesia for the placement of the catheters and must be performed by highly skilled trained staff. It also requires specialist equipment and so direct measurement is usually limited to specialist practices.

There are various ways in which indirect blood pressure measurement can be achieved in practice. The Doppler method provides the most satisfactory and reliable indirect method for use in conscious cats. It should be noted that this method is unlikely to produce a totally accurate result, but it will identify cats with a clinically significant problem, and is particularly useful to identify changes in blood pressure in an individual patient.

Blood pressure will increase markedly in a stressed animal, and this can be problematic when measuring a cat's blood pressure in a hospital environment. Stress to the feline patient should be minimised prior to and during blood pressure measurement by careful handling and ensuring that the room is quiet and calm. Cats are very likely to be stressed in the veterinary practice and this can lead to the release of adrenaline. The associated vasoconstriction caused by this can lead to misleadingly high blood pressure measurements

In patients with low blood pressure a reading may be difficult to obtain at all due to the difficulty of finding a peripheral arterial pulse.

Blood pressure measurement: Doppler technique (see Box 5.13)

A small inflatable cuff is wrapped around an extremity over an artery (see Table 5.8) and an ultrasound transducer probe is positioned over the artery, distal to the occluding cuff (see Fig. 5.14).

It is essential to use an appropriate size of the cuff to ensure accurate results. The width of the cuff should be approximately 40% of the circumference of the extremity to which it is being applied. An overly large cuff may result in an abnormally low blood pressure reading and conversely, a cuff that is too small can produce an overly high reading.

The cuffed area should be positioned at the same level as the heart. The cuff should not be applied too tightly and in fractious cats it can be helpful to further secure it with a piece of tape.

Diastolic blood pressure measurement is less easy to determine than the systolic pressure, as it can be

Table 5.8 Positions of blood pressure cuff		
Extremity	Position of cuff	Artery
Forelimb	Midway between elbow and carpus	Common digital
Hindlimb	Proximal to hock	Dorsal metatarsal
Tail	Base of the tail	Ventral coccygeal

BOX 5.13 TECHNIQUE: BLOOD PRESSURE MEASUREMENT

1. Allow the cat adequate time to become settled in its surroundings. If possible arrange for the owner to be present to restrain the cat as this will reduce stress.

2. Collect all equipment – Doppler monitor, ultrasound gel, appropriate sized cuff.

3. Clip the hair over the artery. Some authors prefer not to clip as this may stress the cat, but to work some ultrasound gel into the fur over the artery instead.

4. It is advisable to return the feline patient to its owners or kennel for a while at this stage so that it is less stressed at the time of measurement.

5. Position the cat on the table in a natural sitting position, which is comfortable for the cat.

6. Place ultrasound gel on the transducer and place it over the artery and listen for an audible pulse. Moving the probe against the fur produces a very loud noise, which will frighten the cat. If you are using headphones this will not be a problem, but if you are not using headphones keep the volume turned right down until the probe is in place against the leg. Don't press too hard with the probe, as this will collapse the artery, obliterating the pulse.

7. As soon as the pulse is heard, inflate the cuff until the pulse stops.

8. Deflate the cuff gradually.

9. Observe the pressure dial and note the point where an audible blood flow restarts (this denotes the systolic blood pressure).

10. Continue to deflate the cuff and note the point at which the signal changes in pitch (this denotes the diastolic blood pressure).

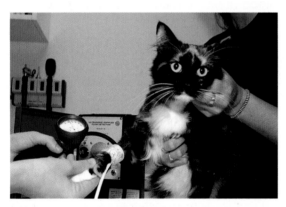

Figure 5.14 Blood pressure measurement in a cat. Reproduced with permission from V. Barrs

difficult to assess the change in flow sound. Most people simply obtain a systolic pressure when using the Doppler method.

It is best to discard the first blood pressure measurement as at that stage the cat is still likely to be stressed. Another 4–5 measurements should be taken and the lowest blood pressure should be noted as probably the most accurate. It is important to realise that indirect blood pressure measurements are not 100% reliable, but only give indications. Systolic blood pressures below 160 mmHg are normal, above 180 mmHg are too high. The area between 160–180 mmHg is a grey area, where repeating blood pressure measurement at a later date is indicated.

5.6 INTRAVENOUS CATHETERS

Introduction

Intravenous catheters are placed to provide continuous, secure, comfortable access to the circulation. Continuous venous access i.s required for the intravenous administration of fluids, and is particularly useful in critically ill patients requiring regular intravenous injections of drugs. All anaesthetised patients should have an intravenous catheter placed before induction of general anaesthesia, to provide venous access in the event of an emergency.

Sites of placement

Catheters may be placed either peripherally via the cephalic vein, lateral or medial saphenous vein or centrally via the external jugular vein or femoral vein (see Table 5.9). The choice of site depends on the purpose of the catheter. For example, central access is required for central venous pressure (CVP) monitoring and for administration of irritant compounds such as parenteral feeding solutions. Central catheters can also be used to collect blood samples and are useful if frequent

Table 5.9 Advantages and disadvantages of sites of catheter placement

Vein	Location	Advantages	Disadvantages
Central access			
Femoral	Medial aspect hind limb	Central venous access. Enables rapid infusion of large quantities of fluid. Well-tolerated. Less likely to become occluded or kinked than peripheral catheter. Can be left in place for longer periods.	Not used as frequently so fewer people able to perform the technique. Sedation maybe required during catheter placement. Meticulous care is required to avoid catheter contamination and phlebitis. Catheters are more expensive.
Jugular	Side of the neck	As for femoral catheter.	As for femoral catheter. May be easier to keep clean, but may be more difficult to place as the feline neck is quite short.
Peripheral access			
Cephalic	Cranial aspect of front limb	Easily accessible. Commonly performed technique therefore higher success rate of placement.	Prone to occlusion if the cat bends its elbow. Cat able to chew/lick catheter and tubing.
Lateral saphenous	Lateral aspect of lower hindlimb (between hock and stifle)	An alternative vein if other veins cannot be used.	Delicate vessel prone to damage by catheter and extravasation of fluid. Prone to soiling with urine/faeces.

blood sampling is required. In addition, the intended duration of use of the catheter and the demeanour of the patient should be considered. There is some debate about the length of time catheters should remain in place, however, as a general guide peripheral catheters should be removed after a maximum of three days and central lines after seven days. Ideally, the largest available vein should be used, but this may not be possible if it has been damaged by previous catheterisation.

Placement technique

Always collect and prepare all the equipment you need before starting:

1. Electric clippers or scissors.
2. Skin prep swabs (povidone-iodine or chlorhexidine).
3. Swab soaked in isopropyl alcohol.
4. Local anaesthetic ointment, e.g. EMLA™ cream (optional).
5. Intravenous catheter of appropriate size*.
6. T-connector or bung – fill with heparinised saline (3-way tap not recommended as they are too bulky in the feline patient).
7. 2 ml syringe with heparinised saline.
8. Warmed intravenous fluids if required.

*The size of catheter selected will depend on the size of the patient. As a general guide 22–24 gauge over the needle catheters are suitable for adult cats for peripheral use and 20–22 gauge through the needle catheters for jugular catheterisation. Smaller gauge catheters will be required for kittens and very small cats.

9. Administration set (normal or ideally paediatric).
10. Securing tape.
11. Bandaging materials.
12. Assistant.

The assistant should restrain the patient gently but firmly (refer to Chapter 4). The assistant can also distract the cat, by blowing on its nose or ear, or scratching the cat's head (if both hands are not involved in restraining the cat) just as the needle goes through the skin. This is often the most painful part of the procedure and a momentary distraction can help keep the cat still.

Many people advocate the application of a local anaesthetic cream such as EMLA™ to the catheterisation area to help reduce the pain on insertion (a thick layer should be applied under an occlusive dressing 45 minutes before catheterisation to allow the local anaesthetic effect to develop).

In animals in shock or dehydration, it may be advantageous to make a nick through the skin just above the vein to help visualise and catheterise the vein more easily. The skin is pulled away from the vein and a small cut is made in the skin using a number 11 surgical blade (see Fig. 5.15), or the bevel of a hypodermic needle. The catheter can then be inserted through the skin at this point.

The administration of certain sedatives can dramatically drop the blood pressure making catheterisation much more difficult. If possible catheterisation should be carried out before their administration.

Surgically prepare the site. Clip a large area over the anticipated catheter insertion point (scissors may be used if animal becomes stressed by the noise of the clippers). Use surgical scrub (iodine-povidone/chlorhexidine) to thoroughly cleanse the skin. Rinse off scrub solution with swab of isopropyl alcohol. Allow to air dry.

Good hygiene is essential during catheter placement and at all times when handling the catheter and administration lines and ports. Always wash hands with a surgical scrub solution.

The assistant can open the catheter packet just prior to starting to allow you to take the catheter without jeopardising asepsis.

Placement of peripheral catheter (right-handed technique)

1. Assistant raises the vein.
2. Remove the catheter from its protective plastic cover, taking care not to touch any part of the needle.
3. Using the left hand, immobilise the vein by stretching the skin between the thumb and fingers. Position the thumb so that it is just lateral to the vein (see Fig. 5.16A).
4. Select the venipuncture site: choose a position towards the distal end of the clipped region, where the vein is straight and long enough to accommodate the entire length of the catheter.
5. Holding the catheter in the right hand, insert the needle with the bevel facing upwards.
6. Advance the catheter one-third of the way into the vein. (Should feel a 'pop' and venous blood should appear in the hub – Fig. 5.16A.)
7. Stabilise the stylet hub with the left hand.
8. With the right hand, gently advance the catheter into the vein (Fig. 5.16B) and then remove the stylet.
9. If correctly positioned, blood should be flowing freely from the catheter hub.
10. The assistant stops raising the vein and moves thumb down to apply pressure over the skin covering the catheter to help reduce blood flow.
11. Attach the pre-filled T-connector/bung (Fig. 5.16C).
12. Secure catheter with tape (see p. 110).
13. Flush catheter with small quantity of heparinised saline.
14. Connect fluid supply if necessary.
15. Apply bandage over catheter and administration set to help prevent contamination, patient interference and accidental removal.
16. Apply Elizabethan collar if necessary.
17. Examine the site at least daily for evidence of infection or swelling.
18. Change catheter site every three days.
19. Look for signs of thrombophlebitis, subcutaneous administration, haemorrhage etc.

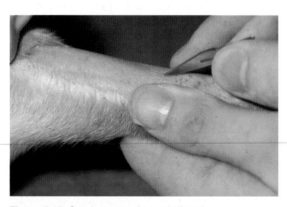

Figure 5.15 Cut-down onto the cephalic vein.

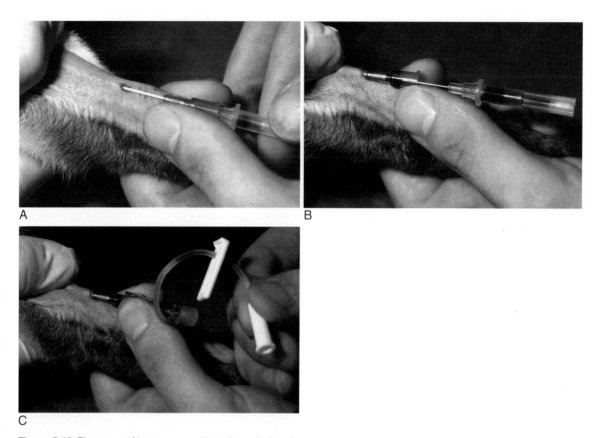

A   B

C

Figure 5.16 Placement of intravenous catheter in cephalic vein.

Placement of a jugular catheter (femoral catheter)

1. Assistant restrains the animal in lateral recumbency, extending head to enable access to the jugular (or extending the lower hind limb for the femoral vein).
2. A small sandbag placed under the neck will enhance visualisation and catheterisation of the jugular vein.
3. Clip the hair over the jugular (femoral) area to approximately 10 × 10 cm around the proposed catheter entry site.
4. Aseptically prepare the site using surgical soap.
5. Rinse soap suds off with isopropyl alcohol swab.
6. Raise the vein by applying pressure with the thumb to the jugular groove (inguinal area for femoral vein).
7. Holding the through the needle catheter firmly in one hand, insert through the skin in a caudal direction towards the thoracic inlet (in proximal direction towards the groin for femoral vein).

8. Stabilise the jugular vein (femoral vein) with the free hand and with one sharp movement, pass the catheter into the vein.
9. When blood appears in the hub and lumen of the catheter advance the catheter 1 cm further.
10. Holding the catheter in the right hand, thread the catheter into the vein by pushing it through the metal needle within the plastic sleeve.
11. Disconnect the plastic sleeve from the needle.
12. Take the metal needle out of the skin and place the protective plastic needle guard over the needle and snap closed.
13. Place injection cap on to catheter.
14. Flush catheter with heparinised saline.

For placement of a femoral catheter the cat needs to be placed in right lateral recumbency and the left hind limb needs to be held out of the way. The medial thigh needs to be prepared as for the jugular catheter. The technique for placement of the catheter is the

109

same as for the jugular catheter. After placement the plastic needle guard (containing the metal needle) is secured to the cranial aspect of the hind limb to avoid soiling by urine or faeces.

Securing the catheter

Many catheters fail not because of poor placement techniques but because they have been badly secured in place. Effective securing of the catheter is essential not only to prevent the patient from removing it but also to avoid damage to the vein.

A light-weight, easily removed (by the veterinary staff rather than the patient!) tape such as Micropore™ is preferable for use in cats. Elastoplast and zinc oxide stick well but are painful and difficult to remove.

The tape is passed around the limb, under the hub of the catheter initially, and then on its second rotation around the limb, over the catheter hub (see Fig. 5.17A). This provides a barrier between the hub and the skin and helps to anchor the catheter in place. It is important not to place the tape too tightly as this will interfere with the circulation and cause

marked swelling of the distal limb. T-connectors and administration lines should also be taped in place (see Fig. 5.17B) incorporating a loop of tubing in the system to help prevent removal of the catheter in the event of the tubing being pulled on. A light bandage is then placed over the whole system (see Fig. 5.17C).

Jugular and femoral catheters are usually sutured into place and further protected with padding and bandages. An Elizabethan collar may be necessary if the patient is seen to interfere with the bandages or lines in any way; however, they seem to cause distress in many feline patients and so if possible are best avoided.

Maintenance of catheters

Strict adherence to aseptic technique is essential to avoid development of nosocomial infections. Hands must be washed before handling the catheter, associated lines and connectors.

The VN needs to be aware of potential problems associated with catheter placement and the signs associated with each (see Table 5.10). It is essential that the

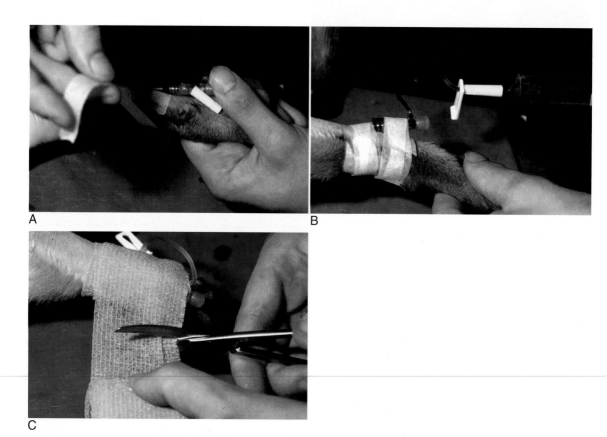

Figure 5.17 Securing an intravenous catheter.

Table 5.10 Common complications of catheter placement and their causes	
Problem	**Cause**
Extravasation (fluid accumulation in the subcutaneous space around the catheter site)	Damage to the vein during catheter placement. Catheter has become dislodged.
Local and systemic infection	Poor hygiene during placement. Poor management of the catheter and administration ports. Patient interference.
Distal paw oedema Thrombophlebitis	Securing tapes or bandages have been applied too tightly. Thrombus formation can occur on the outer surface of the catheter (fibrin coats the outside of the catheter which can lead to the formation of a thrombus), within the lumen of an unused catheter and on the vessel wall at the catheter insertion site. Regular flushing with heparinised saline will help to reduce the risk of thrombus formation.
Air embolism	Poor technique used to set up and connect fluid bags and administration lines and allowing inadvertent injection of air into the system. This may be potentially fatal and should be avoided at all cost.

catheter insertion site is examined daily for evidence of erythema, swelling, or discharge. The lymph nodes above and around the catheter site should also be palpated each day to assess for evidence of enlargement. A core body temperature should be obtained at least twice daily to detect early signs of pyrexia. If the catheter is not being used for a continuous infusion it must be flushed with heparinised saline 2–4 times daily to maintain a patent lumen.

If any of the above complications arise, the best solution is to remove the catheter and place a new catheter in another vein.

5.7 ENTERAL NUTRITION

Introduction

It is important that nutrition is maintained in the hospitalised feline patient. Malnutrition can impair the function of the immune system, slow down tissue repair, and can alter the metabolism of drugs. The veterinary nurse should be able to identify quickly which patients are not eating sufficient quantities and help decide on an appropriate feeding regime to suit the needs of the patient's demeanour and condition.

Nurses must not only be able identify which patients require nutritional support but must also be competent at maintaining the feeding equipment and tubes and be able to calculate the daily calorie requirements according to the patient's disease or condition (see Chapter 3).

Indications for assisted feeding

- Anorexia for more than three days.
- Conditions associated with inadequate food intake lasting longer than three days.
- More than 10% body weight loss.
- Physical limitations, e.g. oral ulceration, facial trauma etc.
- Following oral surgery – to allow tissues to heal and reduce pain caused by eating.
- Generalised loss of muscle mass.
- Generalised lethargy of more than three days in severely ill animals.

Methods of administering enteral nutrition

- Patient encouragement.
- Assisted oral feeding.
- Syringe feeding.
- Naso-oesophageal tube feeding.
- Oesophagostomy feeding.
- Gastrostomy tube feeding.
- Enterostomy tube feeding.

Encouragement, assisted oral and syringe feeding

Hospitalised feline patients unfamiliar with their surroundings are often stressed. With noisy dogs around and strange smells the hospitalised cat often refuses to eat. With gentle encouragement, and by talking and stoking the patient, they can often be encouraged to eat. For more information on encouraging cats to eat, and the use of appetite stimulants, see Chapter 3.

Naso-oesophageal tube feeding

A small (3.5–6 French gauge) feeding tube of polyurethane or silicone is placed via the nostril into the oesophagus. Naso-oesophageal tubes are preferred to nasogastric tubes in which the tube extends through the cardia into the stomach. Placement of a tube through the cardia commonly leads to gastric reflux, vomiting and oesophagitis. Advantages and disadvantages of naso-oesophageal tubes are listed in Table 5.11.

TUBE PLACEMENT

Tube placement is easy and is best done in a fully conscious cat so that placement of the tube in the trachea is less likely to occur. Firm restraint of the head is required when the tube is first introduced into the nose, but once the tube is correctly in place the cat should tolerate it well.

1. The handler restrains the cat in a natural upright position. It is useful to have the cat backing into the handler, so there is no possibility of it going backwards when you are inserting the naso-oesophageal tube.
2. Place a drop of a local anaesthetic solution into one nostril (Fig. 5.18A).
3. Pre-measure and mark the length of tube required to reach from the cat's nostril to the level of the ninth rib (Fig. 5.18B).
4. Place a small amount of sterile lubricant gel on the tip of the tube.
5. Once the local anaesthetic has had time to work, introduce the tip of the tube into the nostril. Firm restraint of the head is required at this stage:
   - Hold the cat's head with one hand.
   - Tilt the cat's head upwards.
   - Hold the tube in your other hand; grip the tube close to its tip and rest your hand against the cat's cheek for extra support and so that you can move your hand as the cat moves its head.

6. Gently run the tube along the floor of the nasal cavity aiming slightly towards the mid-line. Go rapidly at first since the cat will sneeze until the tip has reached the back of the throat.
7. Smoothly advance the tube until the mark is reached (Fig. 5.18C). At this point the cat should be comfortable with the tube, if it is coughing or sneezing excessively the tube may be in the trachea, so take it out and start again.
8. Check carefully to ensure that the tube is in the oesophagus.
   - Attach an empty syringe to the connector and draw back. If a vacuum is produced the tube is correctly placed but if the tube is in the trachea a small amount of air will be aspirated.
   - Slowly instill 2–3 ml of sterile water into the tube (Fig. 5.18D) and check for coughing, but beware that not all cats with cough when the tube is incorrectly positioned in the airways.
   - If in doubt take a lateral thoracic X-ray to check the position, or withdraw the tube and start again.
9. Once you are fully satisfied that the tube is correctly placed, attach butterfly tabs of tape and suture or glue the tube to the cat's head, in the mid-line above the eyes (Fig. 5.18E).
10. Fit an Elizabethan collar and tape the excess tubing to the outside of the collar (Fig. 5.18F) or use a light stockinette body bandage.

MANAGEMENT OF THE TUBE

1. Before each use check the measurement markers on the outside of the tube to ensure it has not become displaced. If in doubt, repeat the checks outlined previously to ensure that the tube is still in the oesophagus.
2. Flush the tube with 5–10 ml tepid water before and after each feed to reduce the risk of the tube becoming blocked.
3. Keep the intubated nostril clean and comfortable – emollient creams may be helpful.

COMPLICATIONS (see Table 5.11)
- Local irritation – nose bleeds and rhinitis.
- Misplacement of the tube into the trachea causing inhalation pneumonia – check tube position before each use!
- Vomiting, diarrhoea or occasionally reflux oesophagitis causing potential stricture formation.

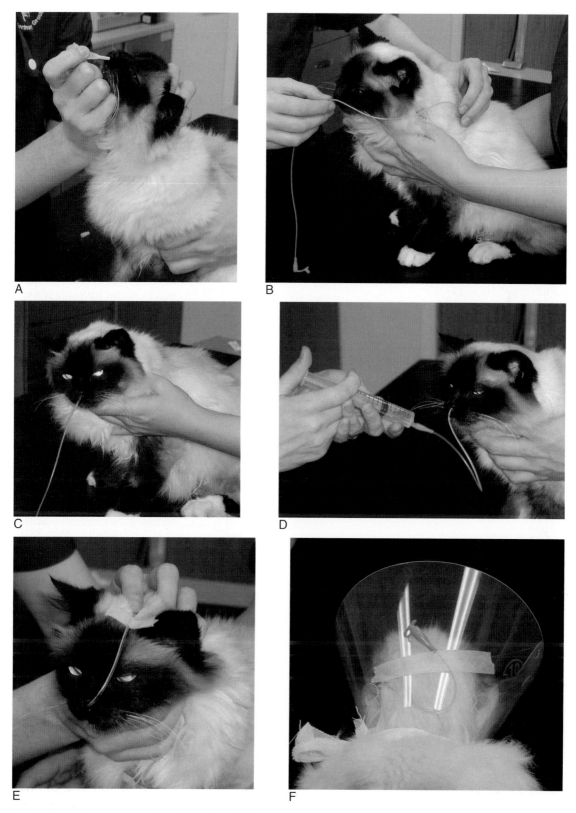

Figure 5.18 Placing a naso-oesophageal tube (see text).

- In general cats refuse to eat normally when they have a naso-oesophageal tube in place. They will go up to their food bowl, but back off as soon as the tube touches the food.

Oesophagostomy tube feeding

A larger (14–16 French gauge) feeding tube is placed into the oesophagus via an external skin incision on the lateral aspect of the patient's neck. Advantages and disadvantages of oesophagostomy tubes are listed in Table 5.12.

Gastrostomy tube feeding

Gastrostomy tubes are wide-bore tubes placed either during a surgical gastrostomy or percutaneously placed by endoscopic gastrostomy (PEG tubes). Advantages and disadvantages of gastrostomy tubes are listed in Table. 5.13.

USE AND MAINTENANCE OF FEEDING TUBES

Before each feed the tube position should be visually checked. If there is any doubt that the tube has been partially displaced its position must be checked by a veterinary surgeon before it is used again.

If the tube is correctly positioned 1–2 ml of sterile saline should be syringed through the feeding tube before administering any food. If the animal coughs or shows signs of distress the position of the tube should be re-checked. If the tube is fully or partially blocked do not attempt to pass more food through it until it has been unblocked (see later).

Liquid food may be administered via the feeding tube by repeated bolus administration split throughout the day. The maximum stomach capacity is 50–90 ml/kg (but is reduced following periods of inappetence). Up to 30–45 ml/kg of food can be given per feed.

Table 5.11 Advantages and disadvantages of naso-oesophageal feeding tubes

Advantages	Disadvantages
• Relatively easy to place • Quick and easy to remove – no sedation or general anaesthesia required.	• Only suitable for short-term use (up to one week). • The internal bore of the tube is very narrow so very few food types can be used without blocking the tube. • Should not be used in vomiting, unconscious, or dyspnoeic patients. • Should not be used in patients with nasal, pharyngeal or oral disease. • Easy for patient to dislodge the tube therefore Elizabethan collar required – causing distress in many feline patients.

Table 5.12 Advantages and disadvantages of oesophagostomy feeding tubes

Advantages	Disadvantages
• These tubes are suitable for short- to medium-term use. • Useful in patients with trauma or disease to the nasal or oral cavity. • Larger feeding tubes can be used therefore a wider range of foods can be administered. • Usually well-tolerated by the patient (may be able to go home with tube in place).	• Involves a surgical procedure for placement. • Requires general anaesthesia for placement. • Not suitable for use in vomiting patients. • Stoma site can become infected therefore daily cleansing of site required. • The tube cannot be used for the first 24 hours after placement (seal needs to form first to prevent leakage).

Table 5.13 Advantages and disadvantages of gastrostomy feeding tubes

Advantages	Disadvantages
• Good for long-term nutritional support (can be in place for several months). • Extremely well-tolerated by most patients. • Easy to administer foods • Wide tube therefore a wider variety of liquid foods can be given.	• Requires a general anaesthetic for placement – either during gastrotomy or by endoscopy. • Gastrostomy tubes should be left in place for a *minimum* of five days, so are not suitable for short-term use. • The tube cannot be used during the first 24 hours after placement (seal needs to form first to prevent leakage).

Initially, food should be introduced slowly by giving a third of the daily allowance over the first day divided into 4–6 feeds. For the first 24 hours, the food should be diluted by 50% to reduce the chance of diarrhoea. The food is ideally warmed to body temperature. Tubes must always be flushed with saline after feeding to prevent clogging the tube with food. A spigot or gate clamp should be placed over the end of a gastrostomy tube during placement, and it is essential that the nurse remembers to replace the bung after using the tube. The VN should observe the patient with a feeding tube closely and evaluate their response to the administration of food. The veterinary surgeon in charge should be notified if there is any evidence of vomiting, regurgitation, bloating or diarrhoea. The patient's body weight should be checked daily and recorded. In the event of inhalation of food, feeding should be stopped and the tube removed.

The nurse should check the tube entry site daily. Dressings and bandages are required for gastrostomy and oesophagostomy tubes.

For calculations of caloric requirements see Chapter 3.

Tube obstruction

This is more likely to occur with narrow bore tubes, or when using a wide bore tube to feed semi-liquid food.

- Avoiding obstructions.
  - Flush the tube with 5–10 ml of tepid water before and after each use.
  - If drugs are administered through the tube use liquid formulations and flush with water before and after each dose. Any other formulation will encourage clump formation, which may block the tube.
- Clearing obstructions.
  - Instill warm water into the tube and alternately apply gentle pressure and suction.

- Instill carbonated water into the tube and leave it for about 1 hour before applying gentle suction; if this fails then try Coca-Cola in place of the carbonated water.
- Introduce a flexible wire or endoscopy biopsy forceps into the tube to dislodge the obstruction.

5.8 WOUND MANAGEMENT

Introduction

The veterinary nurse's aim during wound management is to ensure that the wound heals as rapidly as possible. Correct wound management, including appropriate use of dressing materials, can help to achieve this, by ensuring the optimal wound healing conditions. There are four main factors to consider in the management of wounds:

- The type of wound (classification).
- Initial treatment and care of wounds.
- Continued management of the wound with appropriate dressing materials.
- Long-term management – signs of wound breakdown and delayed healing.

Classification of wounds

Clean
A clean wound describes a surgical wound made under aseptic conditions. There has been no break into a contaminated area (e.g. gastrointestinal tract).

Clean-contaminated
A clean-contaminated wound describes a surgical wound, made under aseptic theatre conditions, but

where there has been an incision into a contaminated area such as the gastrointestinal tract.

Contaminated

Some kind of contaminant has entered the wound. Surgical wounds with a major break in asepsis (for example where spillage from a contaminated area such as the gastrointestinal tract has occurred) are classified in this way, as are most fresh traumatic wounds, e.g. recent animal bites and wounds from road traffic accidents.

Dirty

Dirty wounds are wounds in which an active infection has become established. They can develop either from a surgical wound that extends into an area where infection is present or as a progression from a contaminated wound. If debris and bacteria are left in the wound for more than 6–8 hours the bacteria will start to multiply, and establish an active infection. The contaminated wound has now become a dirty wound and requires a different approach to management.

Initial treatment of wounds

It is essential that all wounds are thoroughly flushed and cleaned as soon as possible after the initial injury to remove contaminants and reduce the risk of the wound becoming infected. Ideally, wound cleaning should occur in the first 6 hours following injury although this is not always possible.

Healing will not occur until debris and infection is removed and cleaning and decontamination of the wound is the most effective way of reducing long-term bacterial contamination. Wound cleansing should be carried out in a clean/sterile environment (e.g. theatre or theatre prep-room).

Cleaning the wound
- It is advisable to swab wounds over 8 hours old for bacterial culture and sensitivity.
- Apply a water-soluble lubricating gel to the wound so that clipped fur sticks to the gel and is easier to remove from the wound during lavage.
- Remove hair from around the wound. Use scissors with the blade coated with lubricating gel for clipping the hair around the wound edges, so that the clipped hair sticks to the scissors rather than falling into the wound.
- Lavage the entire wound with copious quantities of *warmed*, sterile, isotonic saline.

- In very contaminated wounds, *warm* tap water may be used initially to remove gross dirt. Prolonged used of tap water is not recommended due to its low osmolality, which will damage the exposed tissues.

Wound lavage

Sterile saline should be used to thoroughly lavage the wound. The pressure with which the lavage fluid is applied is important. High pressures may force debris and bacteria further into the wound, while low pressures have been shown to provide ineffective lavage. Aerosol pumps, attached to drip bags are commercially available however, a 20 or 30-ml syringe and 19-gauge hypodermic needle also provides the ideal lavage pressure.

Continued wound management

Dressing materials

There is a plethora of dressing materials in use in veterinary practice and there are many commercially available products, which claim to provide the optimum conditions for wounds at different stages of their healing. As new products become available, and new research is carried out, advice changes as to which is the optimum management regime for each wound type. It is currently suggested that the products to use are best selected taking into consideration the exudation levels in the wound (see Table 5.14). No single product, or regime, will be applicable to all wound types.

Signs of wound breakdown and delayed healing

A number of systemic and environmental factors can impair healing and it is essential that the nurse is able to recognise the clinical signs of wound breakdown and delayed healing.

- Inflammation.
- Erythema.
- Separation of the wound edges.
- Patient interference.
- Discharge.
- Pyrexia.
- Malodour.
- Change in patient's demeanour.

Table 5.14 Dressing materials commonly used in veterinary practice during management of open wounds

Stage of healing	Dressing material	Action and advantages	Disadvantages
Inflammatory – with exudate	Dry-to-dry – a dry sterile surgical gauze swab is applied to the wound surface and removed each day.	Each time the dressing is removed, a layer of necrotic material and debris is removed.	Should never be used on granulating wounds – on removal a certain amount of the healthy, healing cells are disrupted and removed. The removal of these dressings is often painful for the patient thus necessitating repeated sedation.
	Wet-to-dry – these work in a similar way to dry to dry. The gauze swab is first soaked in sterile saline before being applied to the wound.	The wetness of the dressing reduces the viscosity of wound exudates so that they may be absorbed more easily. The fluid then evaporates and the dressing becomes dry by the time it is removed thus pulling away the unwanted materials.	As above, but these dressings have added disadvantages because the moist environment is more conducive to bacterial growth and the tissues surrounding the wound may become macerated if the dressing is too wet. Use of cold wetting solutions sometimes causes discomfort to the animal.
	Calcium alginate – e.g. Kaltostat™, AlgiSite™, Sorbsan.™ These 'sheets' of dressing should be moistened with saline and cut to the shape of the wound.	The dressings stimulate macrophages to debride the wound and also absorb exudates. The sheet forms a gel when absorbing exudates, which cleans the wound. These dressings are haemostatic and encourage epithelialisation and granulation. They can continue to be used in the granulation phase of healing.	Continued use can be expensive. Must be cut to the size of the wound; overlap onto uninjured tissues tends to cause maceration of the healthy tissue.
	Hydrophillic dressings – e.g. Allevyn™	The hydrophilic structure of the dressing allows controlled absorption of exudate of up to ten times its own weight. It has a non-adherent layer, which facilitates quick, less painful dressing changes than with the dry- and wet-to-dry dressings. There are a variety of shapes available some of which can be used to 'plug' deep cavity wounds. Can be left in place for up to five days.	Continued use can be expensive.

Table 5.14 Dressing materials commonly used in veterinary practice during management of open wounds—cont'd			
Stage of healing	Dressing material	Action and advantages	Disadvantages
Repair stage	Hydrocolloid – e.g. hydrogels such as Intrasite™ and Biodress™ are interactive moist dressing materials.	Their use has been shown to accelerate wound healing by providing an optimum wound temperature, promoting cell migration from the edges of the wound andencouraging cell mitosis.growth. They are able to remove excess exudates and toxic components whilst giving protection from secondary infection. They are easy to remove and do not cause trauma or pain at dressing changes.	These dressings are contraindicated in the presence of infection or incomplete debridement – exudates remain trapped on the wound surface and this may encourage bacterial These dressings are expensive for long-term use

Care of dressings and owner advice

- Prevent self-trauma – apply Elizabethan collar if necessary.
- Check bandages regularly.
- Keep the bandage dry.
- Keep the feline patient inside whilst the bandage is in place.

Inform owners of the signs of wound breakdown (identified above) and advise them to return to the clinic if they are worried.

Wound drains

Drains (see Table 5.15) can be used to remove fluids and/or gas from wounds or body cavities. They are positioned during a surgical procedure and remove substances by either passive or active drainage.

Passive drains work by overflow, gravity and capillary action. Most of the fluid is removed by passing over the surface of the drain. Efficiency depends on the size and surface area of the drain and the way that they are positioned in respect of the wound. The outflow end (distal end) of the tube must be positioned lower than the wound to promote removal of fluids by gravitation.

Care of surgical wound drains

When nursing patients with wound drains, you should always be aware of, and check for, complications and deal with them appropriately:

- Wound breakdown – especially when drains exit through the primary incision.
- Ascending infection – from distal end of tube into the wound.
- Blocked drains.
- Local tissue irritation.
- Interference by the patient.

It is essential that you carry out effective hygiene procedures for these animals. Cleaning the drain daily, removing soiled bandages, cleaning the surrounding skin and changing bedding materials frequently will do much to prevent complications occurring in the first place.

- Drains should be placed aseptically at the time of initial surgery to the area.
- The drain should enter and leave the skin at a site a small distance away from the wound.
- Ensure the drain is sutured securely to the skin.
- Clip hair around the drain exit site.
- About 5 cm of the drain should protrude from the skin surface.

Table 5.15 Types of drain

Type of drain	Description and use
Penrose drain	A flattened soft latex rubber tube, which is available in a variety of widths (0.5–2.5 cm). Fluid exits primarily along the outside of the tube although some will pass via the inner lumen. Gauze tape can placed within the lumen increasing the capillary action – this is called a cigarette drain.
Tube drain	Made of polythene, silicone or rubber, this is a more rigid tube than the Penrose drain. It may be used as a passive or active drain and can be fenestrated to improve efficiency and prevent obstruction. However, it can collapse with active suction and the rigidity of the material may cause local tissue irritation.
Sump drain	A tube drain constructed with two or more lumens. The inner lumen acts as a vent for access, reducing the likelihood of the drain blocking. The outer lumen drains the fluid. With these drains, there may be an increased risk of contamination from the environment.
Sump–Penrose drain	Combination of Sump and Penrose to make a triple lumen drain. The outer fenestrated Penrose drain helps to prevent tissue adhering to the sump drain. These drains remain functional for long periods of time without becoming blocked. Patency can be further maintained by flushing the tube.
Corrugated tube	These are ribbed malleable strips of PVC or rubber. Drainage occurs entirely over the surface of the drain, as there is no internal lumen.
Compressible plastic containers	These are simple, cheap devices. They are squeezable bottles, which are squeezed initially and then by the action of expansion, create suction on the wound, allowing continuous drainage. They are light and can be taped to the patient providing up to 24 hours of suction.

- Apply white soft paraffin around exit site to prevent skin excoriation.
- Cover with sterile dressings to prevent contamination and to absorb exudates.
- Change bandage frequently and check the wound and drain.
- Prevent self-trauma using Elizabethan collar.

Suture technique for minor wounds

It is important that the nurse who sutures basic wounds is thoroughly trained in this procedure and that he or she is aware of the legal implications of performing minor surgery under The Veterinary Surgeons Act 1966. The choice of suture material will depend on the area being repaired and the length of time the suture will be required to help hold the healing skin to repair. As a general guide, monofilament, non-absorbable sutures should be used in skin to prevent wicking of fluid containing bacteria.

Taper-cut needles are ideal for skin as the cutting tip pierces the skin easily whilst the round body of the shank of the needle minimises tissue trauma as the needle passes through the tissues.

Simple interrupted sutures are relatively easy and quick to place and providing good technique is applied, give good appositional support to the wound. It is important to minimise tension on the wound and therefore the placement of sutures is crucial to allow wound healing to occur. Sutures should be placed about 5 mm from the wound edge at intervals of 5 mm. Sutures should not be too tight but sufficiently taught to ensure the wound edges are slightly everted. Knot tying is equally important in the suture technique as incorrectly or poorly tied knots can come apart and lead to dehiscence of the wound. An instrument tied square knot should be used.

The needle is inserted through the tissue on one side of the wound and passed through to the opposite side. The suture material is knotted using a square knot ensuring that the knot itself is offset so it does not sit over the wound edge.

5.9   CHEST DRAINS

Chest drains may be placed to remove air or fluids from the thoracic cavity. Removal of air or fluid is achieved by either continuous suction or by intermittent drainage. In some situations such as a traumatic pneumothorax, evacuation of air via a chest drain is required. In most practices intermittent drainage using syringes and a three-way tap will be used. When aspirating from tubes, it must be done gently to prevent aspiration of lung tissue.

Continuous closed suction is indicated when there is a lot of air or fluid accumulation for example, in the case of a tension pneumothorax, high volume pleural effusion or following a thoracotomy. There are various systems available for continuous drainage, all based on underwater bottle systems. The end of the thoracotomy tube is attached to a bottle semi-filled with an antiseptic solution. This acts to collect fluid, provide a one-way water seal and provide negative suction. These devices should be placed at least one meter below the patient and maintain a suction pressure of 5–10 cm of water. Heimlich valves should not be used in cats as their small thoracic size generates insufficient expiratory pressure for effective drainage.

A chest drain will need constant management. The VN must be aware of the potential problems associated with chest drains and adhere to strict hygiene methods to prevent iatrogenic problems and asepsis. The wound needs to be checked daily for signs of irritation, infection or wound breakdown. The wound needs to be cleaned, the soiled bandages replaced and the surrounding bedding changed frequently. It is important to make sure the patient cannot get to the tube as this may cause either problems with infection or potentially a fatal air leakage into the chest (pneumothorax) if the patient manages to chew through the drain. The drain needs to be closed at all times for this reason.

The presence of a drain within the thorax induces an effusion of 2–3 ml/kg in 24 hours and because of this the drain should be removed as soon as possible. It is also important to realise that chest drains in the cat are very uncomfortable. This is another reason to remove the drain as soon as possible. Pain management is essential to ensure the patient remains as comfortable as possible.

NURSING COMMON DISEASES

CHAPTER 6

Annette Litster, BVSc PhD FACVSc(Feline Medicine)
Jacquie Rand, BVSc DVSc DipACVIM

6.1 RESPIRATORY DISEASE

Upper respiratory disorders

The upper respiratory tract comprises the nose, mouth, throat and sinuses. A wide range of disorders may affect these areas, including:

- Upper respiratory viral infections (calicivirus and herpesvirus).
- *Bordetella bronchiseptica.*
- Chronic bacterial rhinitis and sinusitis.
- Fungal rhinitis – especially *Cryptococcus neoformans.*
- Neoplasia – especially lymphosarcoma and squamous cell carcinoma.
- Foreign bodies.

Cats affected by upper respiratory tract disease tend to develop obstruction of normal airflow and often present with nasal discharge. Secondary bacterial infections are common, whatever the primary cause of the disease, and contribute significantly to the clinical signs seen. The most common upper respiratory infections are described in more detail below, but the nursing requirements for cats with upper respiratory disease of any cause tend to be similar.

Feline viral upper respiratory tract disease

The most common causes of upper respiratory tract disease in cats are viral infections:

- Feline herpesvirus-1 (FHV, also known as rhinotracheitis virus).
- Feline calicivirus (FCV).

Both viruses cause sneezing, pyrexia and depression. FHV can also cause keratitis (inflammation of the cornea), and FCV infection is often associated with oral ulceration.

Clinical signs are worse if young kittens become infected when maternal antibody levels wane or if the husbandry is poor, for example if there is overcrowding, poor nutrition, poor ventilation or poor hygiene. Other factors such as stress or concurrent diseases will worsen the clinical signs.

Both FHV and FCV are shed in ocular, nasal and oral secretions for 1–3 weeks after acute infection. Virus is shed in droplets formed by sneezing, and can spread over only about 1.2 m, so close proximity is required for direct spread of infection. Fomites (inanimate objects that may harbour infectious agents, especially human clothing, cages and food bowls) are also important, particularly in FCV transmission because this virus is relatively stable outside the host. Both viruses are susceptible to most disinfectants including alcohol, quaternary ammonium compounds, and bleach.

Feline herpesvirus (FHV; feline rhinotracheitis virus)

PATHOGENESIS

The incubation period is 2–17 days. Clinical signs generally resolve within 10–20 days, but on recovery from acute disease cats develop a prolonged (months to years) carrier state during which virus can be shed in the saliva. Virus is shed intermittently, for 1–10 days at a time, often following periods of stress, e.g. boarding in a cattery or veterinary hospital, visits to cat shows, treatment with immunosuppressive doses of steroids, or during lactation. Clinical signs may or may not be apparent during episodes of viral shedding.

FHV survives outside the host for less than 24 hours, and is very susceptible to drying out.

CLINICAL SIGNS OF FHV

The earliest sign is usually paroxysmal sneezing (many sneezes within the space of a few seconds). This is followed by development of severe ocular and nasal discharge, which is initially serous and progresses to mucopurulence. Dried discharges cause crusting, which may lead to nasal obstruction, and young kittens' eyelids may become sealed closed.

Cats often develop anorexia, depression, pyrexia and dehydration. Keratitis may occur in the acute phase of the disease, or as chronic sequelae to infection, and may progress to corneal ulceration. FHV can also cause a persistent or recurrent rhinitis and sinusitis because of damage to the nasal epithelium and subsequent osteolysis. These cats present with recurrent sneezing, and a mucopurulent nasal discharge, which is only temporarily responsive to antibiotics.

Kittens are typically presented with clinical signs at about 5–6 weeks of age. This is about a week after peak lactation for the queen, which may induce her to shed virus and spread the infection to the litter. Clinical signs usually resolve in 1–4 weeks. Abortion or foetal absorption may occur in pregnant cats if there is a severe FHV problem within a breeding cattery. Adult cats may also be affected following exposure to the virus.

Feline calicivirus (FCV)
PATHOGENESIS

The incubation of FCV is 2–10 days, and clinical signs can vary from mild to severe depending on the viral subtype and the immune status of the cat. Following acute infection there is usually a prolonged carrier state lasting for months to years, during which virus is shed constantly. FCV survives outside the host for 8–10 days.

CLINICAL SIGNS OF FCV

Clinical signs are often milder than FHV. Early signs include lethargy, anorexia and pyrexia. There is often only mild serous ocular/nasal discharge, and sneezing may occur but is not paroxysmal. Tongue ulcers, if they occur, are characteristic of FCV. In severe cases ulcers may also be found on the hard palate, lips, footpads and/or nares. These range from small vesicles to large ulcers. In rare cases FCV can cause pneumonia and this may be fatal.

FCV infection is often associated with a persistent mild unilateral or bilateral conjunctivitis with a serous or red-stained discharge. Chronic gingivitis and periodontal disease are also often reported in some carriers.

Bordetella bronchiseptica

B. bronchiseptica is a bacterial infection that can affect both cats and dogs. In cats it is most commonly implicated as a secondary pathogen, but in some cases it can act as a primary pathogen. Cats from rescue centres and overcrowded multi-cat households are more

BOX 6.1   KEY POINT: FHV AND FCV

Once infected with FHV or FCV, most cats will become carriers for years, shedding FCV constantly or FHV intermittently.

likely to be affected. Mild upper respiratory signs such as sneezing and oculonasal discharge are common, but coughing and submandibular lymphadenopathy may also occur. Bronchopneumonia may be seen in kittens less than 10 weeks old.

Transmission occurs via intimate contact between cats, by aerosol or intranasal routes of infection. There have been occasional reports of spread of Bordetella bronchiseptica between dogs and cats.

The organism does not survive long outside the host and is readily killed by many common disinfectants. However, in a heavily contaminated environment survival may be long enough to allow indirect transmission.

Treatment is with an appropriate antibiotic and good nursing care.

Nursing the cat with upper respiratory tract disease

As a general rule, cats with *viral* upper respiratory tract disease (URTI) should be treated as out-patients, unless they are dehydrated, to minimise hospital contamination. Barrier nursing techniques should be used (see Chapter 4). Dehydration is common when discharges are severe, and should be corrected with fluid therapy.

Crusted discharges should be cleaned from the eyes and nose. Airway humidification will make the discharges less viscous and will help clear the respiratory tract. This can be achieved by using a vaporiser or nebuliser, or by taking the cat into the bathroom at shower time.

Nutrition is important in the management of this condition, and hand feeding with strong smelling foods (sardines or fried chicken) may be needed initially to tempt the cat to eat (see Chapter 3). Appetite stimulants may be helpful. If anorexia is prolonged (>4 days) and the cat objects to assisted feeding, an oesophagostomy or percutaneous, endoscopically placed gastrostomy (PEG) tube should be placed under general anaesthesia. Naso-oesophageal tubes are less appropriate because of the presence of nasal and sinus obstruction.

Good nutrition is an essential requirement for a good immune response, and when anorexia persists longer than 1–2 days, vitamin supplementation is indicated.

If there is a mucopurulent nasal discharge or other evidence of a secondary bacterial infection, broad-spectrum antibiotics should be prescribed. Intranasal topical decongestants or oral decongestants may be helpful in the short term but should not be used for more than a few days.

Lower respiratory tract disease

The lower respiratory tract comprises the trachea, the bronchial tree, the lungs and the pleura. Common clinical signs associated with lower respiratory diseases are dyspnoea and coughing.

Allergic bronchitis/feline asthma/chronic bronchitis

This is the most common cause of chronic coughing in cats. In allergic bronchitis/asthma, the coughing is due to an immune-mediated hypersensitivity reaction to inhaled allergens such as pollens, house dust, cat litter dust, and cigarette smoke. This hypersensitivity reaction causes inflammation and reversible airway obstruction, which results from bronchoconstriction, excessive mucus secretion and inflammation and oedema of the bronchial tree. Exhalation is more impaired than inhalation because the lower airways are affected. The allergic component is not found in all cats with bronchial disease, but the signs in chronic bronchitis can be just as severe.

CLINICAL SIGNS

Usually middle-aged to older cats are presented and coughing is the most frequent sign. Many cats are presented with wheezes and occasionally crackles on auscultation. There may be episodes of dyspnoea, which can be severe enough to cause open mouth breathing and cyanosis.

NURSING TREATMENT OF THE BRONCHITIC CAT

Once the diagnosis is made, the first step is to determine if the clinical signs are intermittent or if they occur daily. If clinical signs occur daily, the next step is to decide if they are mild, moderate or severe.

1. **Mild clinical signs** – These do not affect the daily life of the cat.

BOX 6.2 KEY POINT: FELINE ASTHMA

Feline asthma is a diagnosis of exclusion, so other causes of chronic coughing must be thoroughly investigated before asthma is diagnosed.

2. **Moderate clinical signs** – These sometimes affect the cat's quality of life, e.g. it may tire easily, or wake up at night coughing.
3. **Severe clinical signs** – In these cats, there is a continual problem, which clearly limits the cat's ability to lead a normal life.

Human, and perhaps feline, bronchitic airways show evidence of chronic ongoing inflammation whether or not the patient is symptomatic. As a result, for cats with daily clinical signs, treatment strategies are most successful if they are directed towards decreasing the underlying inflammatory component of the disease. Inhaled corticosteroids are now available that do not cause systemic side effects, and this treatment has greatly enhanced our ability to successfully treat cats with inflammatory bronchial disease (see Chapter 4).

Cats presented with acute asthma are initially treated with supplemental oxygen, and if available, with inhaled corticosteroids and bronchodilators which produce rapid alleviation of signs with minimal stress to the cat. If inhaled therapy is not possible then intravenous anti-inflammatories and bronchodilators are required, and must be administered using minimal restraint and concurrent oxygen supplementation. The general principles of nursing dyspnoeic cats must be adhered to (see Chapter 7).

Pleural effusions

A pleural effusion is an accumulation of free fluid within the pleural space, i.e. between the lungs and the thoracic wall. Pleural effusions are a common cause of severe dyspnoea in cats. They may arise as a consequence of a number of conditions.

Cats with pleural effusion from any cause have reduced pulmonary capacity and are at severe risk of hypoxia. When managing these cats the first priorities are to maintain adequate oxygenation and to drain at least some fluid from the thorax in order to allow improved lung function. Needle thoracocentesis should be performed as soon as possible, and before any other diagnostic tests are undertaken, if the cat is dyspnoeic. When drainage is performed, it is essential to collect and store samples of the accumulated fluid. Samples should be handled aseptically and stored in appropriate containers: heparinised tube (for protein analysis), EDTA tube (for cytology) and plain tube (for bacterial culture). Results of analysis will allow the fluid to be categorised, which may provide valuable information as to the likely cause of the effusion. The fluid may be categorised as a transudate, modified transudate, or effusion. Effusions can be further subdivided into chylous, purulent or haemorrhagic effusions. Ultrasound examination of the chest may be performed once the cat is stabilized, and before more fluid is drained from the chest.

Pyothorax

PATHOGENESIS AND CLINICAL SIGNS

Cats with a pyothorax present with dyspnoea, anorexia, depression and often a fever. Anaerobes are involved more frequently than aerobes, and mixed infections may occur. *Bacteroides* and *Fusobacterium* are the most common anaerobes cultured, and *Pasteurella multocida* is the most frequent aerobe. These organisms are usually commensals in the cat's oral cavity. The source of infection is often not identified in pyothorax, but there are a number of possibilities. These include haematogenous spread, e.g. from a recent cat fight abscess and direct extension from adjacent tissues via penetrating injuries/foreign body, e.g. a puncture wound from a cat fight or a grass awn.

NURSING THE CAT WITH PYOTHORAX

The mainstays of pyothorax management are thoracic drainage and appropriate antibiotic therapy. Initially, drainage may be performed using a butterfly needle and syringe. Once the cat is stable, insert a chest drain and flush with sterile saline twice daily. The chest drain is removed when the drainage fluid is clear and there are no bacteria.

Chylothorax

PATHOGENESIS AND CLINICAL SIGNS

Chylothorax is an accumulation of milky fluid, which contains high concentrations of lipids. Most are idiopathic (cause unknown) and result from obstruction to the flow of lymph in the thoracic duct associated with lymphangiectasia. Of the known causes, the most common are thoracic neoplasia and obstruction of lymph flow into the venous circulation as a result of congestive heart failure. Other potential causes include jugular thrombosis, which may occur secondary to

jugular catheterisation. Traumatic rupture of the thoracic duct is now thought to be an uncommon cause of chylothorax.

Cats are presented with dyspnoea and sometimes cyanosis, and milky white fluid can be aspirated from the pleural space. Coughing is sometimes associated with chylothorax. Additional signs may include depression, anorexia, weight loss and pale mucous membranes. Chyle has a characteristic milky appearance and may be pink if there is haemorrhage. A cream layer forms when it is left to stand or centrifuged and chyle becomes clear with the addition of ether.

NURSING THE CAT WITH CHYLOTHORAX

As with all effusions, the immediate priority is to drain the effusion by thoracocentesis. Investigations to look for any underlying problems, such as cardiac failure or thoracic neoplasia should be undertaken. An indwelling chest drain may be required for ongoing management, especially in idiopathic cases. The main goal of ongoing medical management is to provide the nutritional and metabolic needs of the patient until the effusion resolves.

BOX 6.3   KEY POINT: CHYLOTHORAX

In idiopathic cases aspiration of chyle via surgically inserted chest drains usually needs to be maintained for months, so owners of the cat with chylothorax should be warned that treatment may be prolonged to ensure their commitment.

6.2   CARDIAC DISEASE

Types of heart disease

Congenital heart disease

Congenital cardiac disease is relatively rare in cats compared to dogs. Kittens or young cats with congenital heart disease usually have cardiac murmurs and may also have signs of congestive heart failure. If the heart disease is severe, kittens are often stunted in their growth.

Acquired heart disease

Acquired heart disease may affect the heart muscle (cardiomyopathy) or the heart valves. Cardiomyopathies are the most common group of acquired heart diseases in cats, while primary valvular disease is relatively uncommon.

Echocardiography is essential to diagnose the different types of heart disease.

Cardiomyopathies

HYPERTROPHIC CARDIOMYOPATHY (HCM)

This disease most commonly affects middle-aged to older cats, but it can be found in kittens as young as 5–6 months of age. The heart muscle of the left ventricle is thickened and as a result the left ventricle will not fill well during the relaxation phase (diastole). The volume of blood filling the heart chambers is less than normal and the cardiac output is reduced. Blood which cannot enter the left ventricle accumulates in the left atrium and in the pulmonary circulation, causing congestive heart failure. Neuroendocrine responses to the reduced cardiac output also play an important part in the volume overload that exists in cats with cardiac failure.

RESTRICTIVE CARDIOMYOPATHY

Endocardial and myocardial fibrosis are thought to play a major role in the pathogenesis of this condition. The heart muscle becomes stiffer as a result and is therefore less able to relax and contract. This type of heart muscle disease is associated with left atrial enlargement and occasionally focal thickening of the left ventricular septum and free wall. A definitive diagnosis of restrictive cardiomyopathy can only be reached on the basis of cardiac biopsies obtained at post mortem examination.

DILATED CARDIOMYOPATHY (DCM)

This condition is most commonly due to dietary taurine deficiency, and is now extremely rare because of widespread pet food supplementation with taurine. However some cats do develop DCM despite being fed a diet with adequate taurine, and it is thought that these cats may have a genetic predisposition to the disease.

In DCM all cardiac chambers are dilated. In this condition the heart chambers are filling well, but the contractility of the heart is markedly reduced, causing reduced cardiac output and heart failure.

Pericardial effusion

Pericardial effusion is the accumulation of fluid in the space between the heart wall and the pericardium (pericardial sac). When the stretching capabilities of the pericardial sac are exceeded, the resultant high intra-pericardial pressure can collapse the right side of the heart and restrict cardiac filling (tamponade). Cardiomyopathy and feline infectious peritonitis are the most common causes of pericardial effusion in cats.

Cardiomegaly with a globoid cardiac shadow is seen on chest radiographs.

Bacterial endocarditis

This is a rare condition in cats, and the aortic and/or mitral valves are usually affected. Cats usually present with signs of congestive heart failure and often sepsis (fever, lethargy, a high white cell count with increased neutrophils, and bacteraemia). *Streptococcus, Bartonella henselae* and Gram-positive cocci may be identified when blood is cultured. The diagnosis is made on cardiac ultrasound and blood culture. The prognosis is poor to grave.

Clinical signs of cardiac failure in the cat

Cats with cardiac failure usually present relatively late in the disease process because they tend not to show premonitory signs (see Box 6.4). Initially they may be sleeping more, but often owners attribute this to the weather or ageing. Because of this, there is usually not a history of exercise intolerance or dyspnoea.

In the early stages, the only indication of cardiac disease may be the presence of a heart murmur. However, not all cats with heart murmurs have cardiac disease (stress, old age, anaemia, hyperthyroidism and hypertension can all cause murmurs to develop) and not all cats with cardiac disease have a murmur.

As cardiac disease progresses, the heart attempts to compensate for the decrease in function by increasing the heart rate. At that stage, the femoral pulse will usually be weaker than normal and the capillary refill time may be prolonged (normal should be less than 2 seconds). The owner may notice a reduction in activity.

The underlying heart disease usually continues to progress and heart failure will eventually develop. The cat will become more lethargic, start breathing faster, lose weight and have a reduced appetite. During the later stages, there will be fluid build-up either within the lungs (pulmonary oedema) or in the pleural space (pleural effusion) and the cat will have severe breathing difficulties.

It is important to realise that the early stages are often missed, and that cats with chronic heart failure frequently present in severe respiratory distress or even collapse.

Monitoring the cat with cardiac failure

Cats in cardiac failure need to be closely and frequently monitored because the condition is often dynamic and affected cats are often close to decompensation. The clinical examination should focus on the following areas:

- **General examination** – In particular, the cat should be observed for attitude, posture, body condition and anxiety level.
- **Respiration** – The respiratory rate should be counted and the cat observed carefully for any signs of dyspnoea. Dyspnoea should be classified as inspiratory or expiratory and as restrictive (fast and shallow, due to reduced lung compliance, for instance due to pleural effusion) or obstructive (slow and deep, due to airway narrowing).
- **Mucous membrane colour and refill** – Refill time should be less than 2 seconds and membrane colour should be monitored for any changes (Fig. 6.1).
- **Arterial pulses** – The femoral arteries should be palpated on the medial thighs. Both sides should be compared for strength, regularity and rate.

BOX 6.4   KEY POINT: CONGESTIVE HEART FAILURE

> Because cats disguise the early signs of cardiac disease, they usually present in an advanced stage of congestive heart failure.

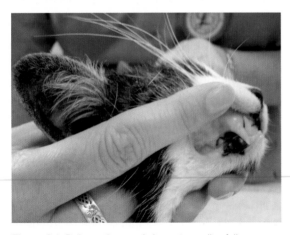

Figure 6.1 Pallor and cyanosis in acute cardiac failure. Reproduced with permission from J. Beatty.

Nursing the cat with cardiac failure

Cats with congestive heart failure have reduced lung capacity because of the presence of pulmonary oedema or pleural effusion. They are usually dyspnoeic, and the general principles outlined in Chapter 7 must be adhered to. Initial emergency management may involve:

- **Cage rest** – essential to reduce respiratory oxygen requirement.
- **Oxygen** – essential for the cat in acute decompensated heart failure, because the reduced lung capacity (either due to pulmonary oedema or pleural effusion) will cause hypoxia.
- **Diuretics** – used to reduce the volume overload in cats with heart failure, and will help reduce the workload of the heart. These drugs are given by the intravenous route in emergencies.
- **Vasodilators** – act directly on the blood vessels to cause vasodilation, thus reducing cardiac work. Vasodilating drugs may be applied topically to a shaved patch of skin in a well-vascularised area such as the groin or axilla.
- **Positive inotropic drugs** – aid the cardiac muscle in contracting effectively. These drugs are especially useful in cases where the heart contractility is markedly reduced, such as in DCM.
- **Anti-dysrhythmic drugs** – may be necessary if there are life-threatening dysrhythmias.

Once the signs of heart failure have resolved, other drugs can be added to help reduce the workload and increase the effectiveness of the heart muscle function:

- **ACE-inhibitors** – ACE-inhibitors counteract the neuroendocrine response induced by the heart failure. These drugs work by reducing the retention of sodium and water, which will reduce the volume overload and the workload of the heart.
- **Beta-blockers** – These drugs slow the heart and reduce systolic blood pressure to decrease cardiac afterload. Their use is controversial and they should not be used if the cat has signs of heart failure.
- **Calcium channel blockers** – Calcium channel blockers reduce systolic blood pressure and facilitate relaxation of the heart muscle. Again their use is controversial, and they should not be used when the cat is in heart failure.
- **Aspirin** – Aspirin prevents the relatively sticky feline platelets from adhering to each other, and may be used to reduce the risk of formation of new thrombi (see later).

Feline aortic thromboembolism (FATE)

FATE is very serious, often fatal, and is usually a complication of cardiomyopathy. Cardiac chamber dilation results in turbulent blood flow, which allows blood clotting (thrombus formation) to occur. The primary thrombus is usually formed in the left atrium, but fragments of the clot (thromboemboli) may break off and enter the peripheral circulation via the left ventricle and aorta. These thromboemboli then become wedged, most commonly in the terminal aorta, preventing flow of blood to the hind limb(s). Thromboemboli may also lodge anywhere else in the body, for instance in the renal circulation causing acute renal failure.

As a result of the thromboembolism, the tissues distal to the blocked artery lose their blood supply. In FATE the lack of blood supply to the hind limbs causes an acute onset of paresis/paralysis with hard, painful muscles, and pallor of the footpads or claws that bleed minimally, if at all, when cut.

Often these cats also have concurrent signs of heart failure. Treatment should be supportive to manage the heart failure and try to improve the circulation to the affected limb(s). This condition is extremely painful and pain relief is essential.

Heat can be applied for 10–15 minutes to increase circulation to an area that is cool to the touch. Heat will also help to relieve pain and warm up the limb before exercising or stretching. The recommended method is moist heat. A warm wet rolled hand towel is applied to the area with a larger thick dry towel placed over it to keep the heat in.

Joint mobilisation and massage are also useful techniques for treating poor circulation in the limbs of cats with FATE. Joint mobilisation is a passive movement, either with an oscillatory motion or a sustained stretch slow enough that the cat may stop the motion if it is uncomfortable. Gentle massage has been shown to be beneficial in reducing stress, enhancing blood circulation, reducing swelling and enhancing relaxation. Massage may also relieve pain induced by muscle spasm and reduce adhesions caused by scar tissue. Ten to fifteen minutes of gentle limb massage should be performed frequently each day, paying careful attention to and being guided by the cat's response to this form of therapy.

Complications following sudden reperfusion of the limb are common and often life-threatening. If the cat survives the initial episode recurrences are common and FATE has a guarded to poor prognosis.

Hypertension

Hypertension in cats is usually associated with a primary medical condition such as renal failure or hyperthyroidism. Hypertension itself may cause secondary cardiac failure from increased afterload (the pressure the heart must pump against to circulate the blood through the arterial system). Hypertension is also associated with increased end-organ damage such as renal failure or damage to the central nervous system.

The most common presenting clinical sign of hypertension is the acute onset of blindness resulting from retinal haemorrhage and retinal detachment. Systolic arterial blood pressure can be measured in conscious cats using a Doppler ultrasound blood pressure monitor (see Chapter 5).

When hypertension is diagnosed it is important to treat any underlying disease and to treat the hypertension itself. The blood pressure needs to be checked on a regular basis to make sure the medication is effective, but does not cause hypotension. In the initial stages the medication often needs to be adjusted and occasionally multiple drugs are necessary to control the blood pressure.

6.3 ENDOCRINE DISEASE

Diabetes mellitus

Diabetes mellitus is caused by an absolute or relative lack of insulin, a hormone which has an essential role in regulation of blood glucose concentration. Insulin is produced by the pancreas and its function is to allow the cells of the body to absorb glucose, amino acids, and fat from the blood. Insulin insufficiency decreases utilisation of glucose, amino acids and fat, and increases tissue breakdown.

Diabetes mellitus causes:

- Hyperglycaemia as a result of:
  - reduced uptake and utilisation of glucose;
  - increased production of glucose through gluconeogenesis and glycolysis.
- Lipidaemia as a result of:
  - increased lipolysis and release of free fatty acids;
  - decreased uptake of triglycerides into adipose tissue.

Classification of diabetes
TYPE 1 AND TYPE 2

- **Type 1 diabetes:** This occurs in middle-aged dogs, and is equivalent to the 'juvenile' or insulin-dependent form in humans. It is caused by immune-mediated destruction of pancreatic β-cells. There is an absolute lack of insulin with this form of diabetes. This appears to be very rare in cats.

- **Type 2 diabetes:** This is the most frequent form found in cats, and was previously called 'adult onset' or non-insulin-dependent diabetes mellitus (NIDDM). It is due to a gradual decline in β-cell function combined with increased peripheral resistance to the effects of insulin. The most consistent histological finding is amyloid deposition in the pancreatic islets. Islet amyloid is derived from the hormone amylin or islet amyloid polypeptide, which is secreted with insulin from β-cells. Affected cats are also frequently obese (see Fig. 6.2) which leads to additional insulin resistance.

OTHER SPECIFIC TYPES OF DIABETES

Other specific types of diabetes occur if the pancreas is destroyed by another disease process, e.g. pancreatic adenocarcinoma or pancreatitis, or if there is a high concentration of hormones which antagonise insulin action i.e. cortisol, adrenaline, growth hormone, progesterone or glucagon. This may be iatrogenic, from administration of progestogens or long-acting steroids, or may arise spontaneously if the cat has hyperadrenocorticism or acromegaly (a growth hormone producing tumour). Other specific types of diabetes account for approximately 10–20% of feline cases.

Pancreatitis is also a common histological finding in diabetic cats, but whether it is a cause or a result of diabetes is unclear. In most cases the inflammation does not seem sufficiently severe to cause diabetes by itself, but its presence may contribute to β-cell loss.

Diagnosis of diabetes mellitus

The diagnosis is usually based on a combination of signalment, clinical signs, physical examination and results of laboratory tests.

SIGNALMENT
- Age – Affected cats are usually over 5 years old.
- The majority of affected cats are male.

CLINICAL SIGNS
- Polyuria and polydipsia (PU/PD).
- Polyphagia (increased food intake).
- Weight loss.

PHYSICAL EXAMINATION

Diabetic cats are usually normal body weight or obese (Fig. 6.2), but become emaciated in the later stages of the disease. Hepatomegaly may be found on abdominal palpation, abdominal radiographs or abdominal ultrasound.

In long-standing cases where control of blood glucose has been poor, there may be signs of diabetic neuropathy. This is a condition affecting the peripheral nerves and usually results in an inability to raise the hock joints off the ground (plantigrade stance – see Fig. 6.3). The condition often resolves over weeks to months once the blood glucose is controlled by insulin therapy.

LABORATORY TESTS

Blood glucose concentration is increased in diabetes, and once the renal threshold for glucose is exceeded

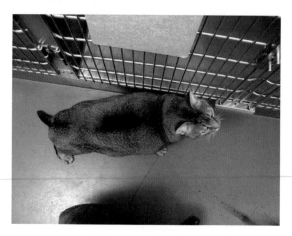

Figure 6.2 Overweight, inactive cats are predisposed to the development of Type 2 diabetes mellitus.

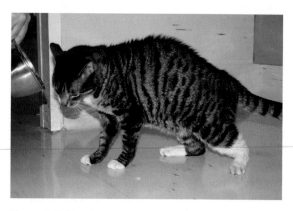

Figure 6.3 Chronic diabetes mellitus may result in diabetic neuropathy, presenting with a plantigrade stance.

this results in glucosuria (glucose in the urine). The presence of glucose in the urine produces an osmotic diuresis, which is the cause of the polydipsia and polyuria. In severe cases, there may also be ketonuria associated with diabetic ketoacidosis. In cats, blood glucose concentration may also be increased as a result of 'stress'. This may be the stress of being in the hospital, but also the stress of concurrent other diseases. Struggling, which may occur during blood sampling or physical examination, is a potent cause of stress hyperglycaemia. Stress causes the release of hormones such as adrenalin and cortisol, which counteract the effects of insulin, causing a significant increase in blood glucose. If this stress hyperglycaemia causes blood glucose concentration to exceed the renal threshold for glucose, it will also cause 'overspill' of glucose into the urine. For this reason it is not possible to differentiate feline diabetes mellitus from stress, based only on the presence of hyperglycaemia and glucosuria. However, persistent hyperglycemia for more than 5 hours is most likely the result of diabetes mellitus, especially if glucose concentration is greater than 16 mmol/l.

Increased serum fructosamine concentration is a marker for diabetes in cats. It is formed by irreversible binding of glucose to serum proteins. The rate at which fructosamine is formed depends on the amount of glucose in the blood, but the rate at which it is cleared from the blood is constant. Fructosamine concentration starts to increase after two days of hyperglycaemia, and serum concentration gives a good indication of the mean blood glucose level over the preceding 10–14 days. Normal serum fructosamine levels are less than 407 μmol/l in cats.

Management of uncomplicated diabetes

The aims of therapy for the diabetic cat are diabetic remission or resolution of PU/PD, normalisation of body weight, and maintenance of blood glucose concentration between 7–15 mmol/l throughout a 24-hour cycle.

Cats with uncomplicated diabetes do not have a history of illness or depression, and are not severely ketotic. They are usually presented for evaluation of PU/PD, inappropriate urination and/or weight loss, or their diabetes may be identified during a routine health screen. In these cases management usually relies on normalisation of body weight, regulation of food intake and regular injections of insulin to control the blood glucose. A proportion of cats will not be diabetic after 2–3 months of diabetic management.

DIET AND WEIGHT CONTROL

If the cat is obese, a weight loss program (see Chapter 3) should be commenced, as obesity increases insulin resistance. The rate of weight loss should be conservative – approximately 1–2% per week, as more rapid weight loss may result in hepatic lipidosis and liver failure.

A low carbohydrate, high protein diet is the best choice for diabetic cats, as it reduces fluctuations in blood glucose compared to a more traditional feline diet, which is higher in carbohydrates. If the cat is a 'grazer', it is best to allow it to continue this pattern of feeding. If the cat is more used to being fed twice daily, it is best to time the meals with the insulin injections.

If the cat is underweight and/or ill, treatment with insulin should be started and the cat fed ad libitum. A low carbohydrate, high protein diet is still ideal, but it is most important these cats eat regularly, so a diet that the individual cat finds palatable should be used.

Insulin treatment

Most diabetic cats cannot be stabilised by dietary manipulation alone, and will require additional treatment with insulin injections. While some cats can be adequately stabilised using once daily insulin, the majority of cats will be better controlled if they are injected twice a day. This means that the owner needs to be very committed to the long-term treatment of their cat, and must have a lifestyle that enables them to do this.

There are several types of insulin on the market, which differ in duration of action from very short-acting types of insulin (such as the soluble insulins) to longer acting insulin (such as lente and PZI). The other difference between insulin types is the source, for instance bovine, porcine, human or synthetic insulin. Glargine is a human insulin that is currently showing much promise in the treatment of diabetic cats. It has a long duration of action and achieves a high remission rate in diabetic cats.

Most owners will initially be reluctant to inject their cat, but once they have been carefully taught how to give the injection they usually soon become very confident (see Box 6.5). It often falls to the veterinary nurse to teach the owners how to inject their cat and patience is vital at this point. Owners will also need encouragement and support along the way once they have mastered the technique, and this is another important role for the veterinary nurse.

The starting dose of insulin will be low and is gradually increased over time until the appropriate dose for the individual cat is found. It is important the owner knows that regulation may take a while and

BOX 6.5 TEACHING THE OWNER OF A DIABETIC CAT TO USE INSULIN

- Storage: insulins must be kept in the fridge and it is important to have the bottle out of the fridge for as short a period as possible. Pharmaceutical companies recommend discarding any unused insulin after one month. This is because each time a needle is introduced into the bottle there is a risk of bacterial contamination which would inactivate the insulin. However, with careful attention to cleanliness, most insulins can be used for several months.

- Mixing of insulin: gently roll the bottle to mix the solution before use if a suspension is being used. Vigorous shaking must be avoided as it will cause damage to the insulin molecules.

- Teach the owner how to fill the syringe to the required level, ensuring there are no air bubbles trapped in the syringe which will reduce the actual volume of insulin supplied. Make sure the right syringes are dispensed as there are syringes that are calibrated for insulin containing 40 units/ml and 100 units/ml. If the syringe is inadvertently changed from a 100 U/ml syringe to 40 U/ml syringe, serious overdosing can occur. Similarly, changing from a 0.5 ml to a 1 ml 100 U/ml syringe can lead to an overdose, because the gradations represent different volumes.

- Teach the owner how to give a subcutaneous injection by demonstrating and explaining the technique first, and then allowing the owner to practice using sterile saline.

- Nervous owners often find it helpful to inject their cat while the cat is eating, so that the cat is distracted.

that ongoing monitoring is essential. Monitoring of the cat's clinical signs (especially water drunk, urine production, appetite, weight, general demeanour) is a useful way to assess whether an adequate amount of insulin is being given, but serial blood glucose measurement and fructosamine measurement will also be required in all cases. The owner can be a great help in keeping a diary of the clinical signs:

- Water drunk should be measured over 48 hours each week, as increasing water intake may be a sign of poor diabetic control. Similarly, any changes in food intake or appetite should be noted.
- Owners can also be provided with urine dipsticks to allow home urine testing, ideally at least once each week. Depending on the insulin used, there may be a trace of glucose in the overnight urine. However, there should never be ketones in the urine and if ketonuria occurs, the cat should be examined immediately by a veterinarian. If the urine dipstick is persistently negative for glucose the cat needs to be checked by a veterinarian to make sure hypoglycaemia is not an issue.
- If accurate measurement of weight can be performed at home, weekly weight records are useful. Any continuing or sudden weight loss should be investigated. Paediatric weighing scales may be purchased for this purpose.

Cats are not well-controlled if there is a return of PU/PD, weight loss, weakness or ataxia, or if there is

ketonuria or consistent absence of urine glucose (see also Box 6.6). In these cases the owner needs to bring the cat back to the surgery for further evaluation. Since diabetic remission is relatively common, owners should be advised to watch especially for signs of insulin overdose, such as negative urine glucose on an overnight sample or weakness/ataxia.

Serial measurements of blood glucose concentration (glucose curves) are necessary for fine regulation of diabetes. When blood glucose curves are performed at the surgery, it is important that the VN takes the minimum necessary volume of blood each time, as frequent (every 2–4 hours but sometimes hourly) blood sampling will be required. One drop of blood is sufficient for use in hand-held glucometers. The blood glucose curve will provide information about the efficacy and duration of action of the insulin being used, in that individual cat. The veterinary surgeon can then use this information to adjust the dose of insulin, the frequency of injection, and/or the type of insulin used.

Management of diabetic ketoacidosis

Affected cats are presented as 'unwell', usually with a history of depression, anorexia, and vomiting. On clinical examination they are dehydrated, and laboratory workup reveals severe ketoacidosis with glycosuria and ketonuria. In these cats the absence of insulin, sometimes in combination with other increases in metabolic demands (e.g. concurrent illness or dehydration), has triggered a switch from metabolising

BOX 6.6   TROUBLESHOOTING CHECKLIST FOR POOR DIABETIC CONTROL

- Is there improper administration of insulin, e.g. poor injection technique by an inadequately trained owner?
- Is there inadequate mixing of the insulin in the vial if a suspension is being used?
- Is outdated or heat damaged insulin being used?
- Is there inaccurate assessment of blood or urine glucose levels? This commonly occurs with urine dipsticks.
- Is there any possibility of insulin resistance? This may occur due to the administration of drugs such as corticosteroids or progestogens, or with growth hormone producing tumours.
- Is insulin being over- or underdosed as a result of an inadvertent change in type of insulin or insulin syringe?

glucose and protein, to using free fatty acids, which are oxidised to ketones. This produces some short-term benefits because ketones are utilised for energy instead of glucose. However, the accumulation of large amounts of ketones produces acidosis, CNS depression, vomiting, and osmotic diuresis and resultant dehydration. This is exacerbated by the osmotic diuresis that already exists because of glycosuria.

The veterinary team should always look for the precipitating factor, especially pancreatitis as the underlying diabetes has probably existed in uncomplicated form for some time. Haematology, biochemistry, and urinalysis should be performed to provide a minimum database.

In the ketoacidotic patient, intravenous fluid therapy is very important to improve hydration and control electrolyte imbalances. Insulin therapy is started, initially with short-acting soluble insulin, given intravenously or intramuscularly every hour, or supplied by a continuous infusion. Once dehydration has resolved and the cat has good peripheral circulation, treatment with a longer acting insulin can be started.

Complications in the treatment of the diabetic cat
HYPOGLYCAEMIA

Giving too much insulin will cause hypoglycaemia, which is potentially fatal, and is of much more concern than the presence of hyperglycaemia. In cats, the signs of hypoglycaemia are sometimes vague, with just an increase in lethargy, so it is particularly important to educate the owner to be aware of this risk. However, more severe signs include an ataxic 'drunken' gait, dilated pupils, trembling, and occasionally seizures or coma. If hypoglycaemia is suspected, the owner should treat their cat with an oral solution of glucose designed for use in human diabetic patients, or rub honey into the gums, and contact the practice for advice as soon as possible. Urine samples that are

consistently negative for glucose should alert the veterinary surgeon that the cat may be receiving too much insulin and is at risk of hypoglycaemia.

DIABETIC REMISSION

Diabetic remission occurs if the cat's insulin-producing cells recover sufficiently to produce adequate amounts of insulin. Increasing peripheral sensitivity to insulin by weight reduction in obese cats also aids this process. Remission of diabetes takes at least 2 weeks to occur, and so a period of 1–4 weeks between insulin dose increases is recommended. If diabetic remission occurs, the cat may relapse weeks, months or years later, so the owner should be vigilant in monitoring water intake and urine glucose. Early reinstitution of insulin therapy can achieve a second and third remission.

In some cats, good control of diabetes may result in a decreased requirement for insulin, while in other cases the insulin requirement may increase after several months of therapy as further loss of insulin-producing cells occurs.

THE SOMOGYI OVERSWING EFFECT

The Somogyi overswing effect results from the administration of excessive doses of insulin. This leads to clinical or subclinical hypoglycaemia, which results in a compensatory stress hormone response. These hormones increase blood glucose, thus protecting the brain from hypoglycaemia. Blood glucose measurements will be high in these cases, which can lead to a decision to increase the insulin dose. This is in fact the opposite of what is required, and increasing the insulin dose will cause a worsening of the hypoglycaemia and a more marked Somogyi overswing. It will also decrease the duration of insulin action, and lead to apparent insulin resistance.

Hyperthyroidism

Hyperthyroidism is a disease of old cats, and the average age at presentation is 12–13 years. It is extremely rare for cats under 8 years to be hyperthyroid. In the majority (approximately 98%) of cases the condition is due to benign hyperplastic nodules within the thyroid gland(s) and both left and right sides are affected in around 70% of cases (Fig. 6.4).

Excessive thyroid hormone has multisystemic effects, because thyroxine regulates metabolic processes in most tissues.

Clinical signs

Clinical signs are slowly progressive, and veterinary attention is often delayed until signs are advanced, because most affected cats remain active with a good appetite.

There is a history of weight loss in over 90% of cats, which results from an increase in metabolic rate. Irritability, hyperactivity and polyphagia occur in about 80% of cases. The increased appetite compensates inadequately for the increase in metabolic rate. Some cats have gastrointestinal signs, such as vomiting and diarrhoea. Some cats will have an increase in thirst and urine production. Cats with thyroid disease may have high blood pressure, and this generally resolves after treatment.

In a small proportion (about 10%) of cases the hyperthyroid cat presents as lethargic and anorexic. This form is known as 'apathetic hyperthyroidism'.

Some of the physiological effects of hyperthyroidism will tend to mask concurrent chronic renal failure, and there is the potential for underlying renal disease to be 'unmasked' when the hyperthyroidism is controlled.

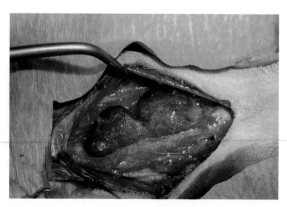

Figure 6.4 Enlarged adenomatous thyroid gland. Reproduced with permission from V. Barrs.

Diagnosis

Hyperthyroidism is often suspected on the basis of clinical signs and physical examination. The thyroid gland is often palpably enlarged and serum total thyroxine (T4) concentration is above the reference range.

Occasionally serum total thyroxine level is within the normal range, and further tests (such as serum free T4, or a T3-suppression test) are necessary to diagnose the disease.

Treatment

There are three treatment options:

- Chronic administration of an anti-thyroid drug.
- Surgical thyroidectomy.
- Radioactive iodine (I^{131}) administration.

The method of choice depends on the general health status of the cat, the age of the cat, and the availability of therapy.

MEDICAL THERAPY OF HYPERTHYROIDISM

Cats that are treated medically have little requirement for nursing care as these patients are treated on an outpatient basis.

Anti-thyroid drugs block the synthesis of active thyroxine, but do not destroy adenomatous thyroid tissue. Hyperthyroidism will recur within 1–3 days if the drug is discontinued.

Around 15–20% of cats experience some adverse effects to anti-thyroid drugs. Owners should be warned to report any signs of ill health immediately. Anorexia, vomiting and lethargy are the commonest problems. Other less frequent problems include blood cell disorders and severe pruritus, and in these cases treatment must be stopped and an alternative treatment should be started.

Once treatment with an anti-thyroid drug has been started, repeat monitoring of the thyroid concentration is necessary to establish the correct dose of the drug.

BOX 6.7   KEY POINT: HYPERTHYROIDISM

> Medical treatment for hyperthyroidism will continue for the remainder of the cat's life, so owners must be committed to long-term therapy.

SURGICAL TREATMENT

Surgical resection of the adenomatous thyroid gland(s) is often the treatment of choice for cats with no other major medical problems.

Surgery is not indicated in cats with pre-existing kidney disease. Surgical candidates are stabilised with anti-thyroid drugs prior to surgery to reduce their anaesthesia risk. When monitoring anaesthesia it is important to be aware of the possibility for cardiac dysrhythmias and also the risk of hypothermia as these cats are usually underweight.

Postoperative care is usually straightforward, unless the parathyroid gland or its blood supply has been damaged during the surgery. In these cases life-threatening hypocalcaemia can occur, requiring emergency treatment and nursing care.

RADIOACTIVE IODINE (I¹³¹)
This treatment involves a single dose of I^{131} given orally, subcutaneously or intravenously. Almost all cats treated by this method become euthyroid within 3 months, and most within 2 weeks. This is a very safe, effective and permanent treatment for hyperthyroidism, but it involves handling radioactive iodine and nursing a cat that is emitting radioactivity in the days to weeks after treatment. For this reason, the cat must be hospitalised in approved facilities after treatment until its surface radioactivity has dropped to a safe level. Faeces and urine are radioactive, and must be disposed of in an approved manner.

Approved facilities and specially trained staff are required for I^{131} treatment, which in practice usually means referral to a specialist centre. Cats must also be in a stable medical condition, so they can safely be managed with minimal handling for a period of days to weeks after treatment. This treatment is expensive, but provides a permanent cure, so can be cost-effective in the long term.

6.4 GASTROINTESTINAL DISEASE

Gastrointestinal disorders are common in cats and may cause signs such as vomiting or regurgitation, diarrhoea and weight loss.

Regurgitation

Regurgitation is the term used to describe the passive elimination of undigested food from the oesophagus. It can be distinguished from true vomiting (active elimination of food and fluid from the stomach) based on the absence of premonitory signs; a relatively short time elapsing since eating; and the material brought up being undigested and in a tubular shape. By contrast, vomiting is preceded by retching or signs of distress; a more prolonged period since eating; and the material that is brought up may be partially digested, perhaps with bile staining, and will be acidic when tested with a pH strip. However, in cats it can sometimes be difficult to differentiate regurgitation from vomiting because the signs overlap, for example, in megoesophagus regurgitation can occur hours after eating.

Regurgitation is an uncommon problem in cats and it results from conditions affecting the oesophagus, the most common of which are oesophagitis, oesophageal strictures and foreign bodies, although oesophageal tumours and congenital oesophageal abnormalities can also occur.

Causes
- **Oesophagitis** – Reflux of gastric juices into the oesophagus can cause severe focal oesophagitis and commonly occurs during general anaesthesia, especially if the cat has been tilted with the head below the rest of the body or if the chest/abdomen has been compressed after placement of an endotracheal tube, e.g. to determine if the tube is correctly placed. Post-anaesthetic oesophageal strictures can be very difficult to manage, so all care should be taken to avoid gastric reflux during general anaesthesia. Dosing of tablets and capsules that contain irritant drugs (e.g. tetracyclines) can also cause local oesophagitis. Tablets and capsules commonly lodge in the oesophagus for a period of time after being swallowed and can cause focal irritation and subsequent inflammation which can eventually lead to stricture formation. It is therefore good practice to syringe a few millilitres of water into the cat's mouth after dosing any tablets or capsules in order to encourage immediate transit into the stomach. VNs should adopt this practice, and should educate owners to do the same when they are dosing their cat at home.
- **Oesophageal stricture** – An oesophageal stricture is a focal narrowing of the oesophagus which develops as a consequence of oesophageal scarring at a site of chronic oesophageal inflammation (oesophagitis).
- **Foreign bodies** – Cats commonly ingest fragments of bone or string (with fish hook or needle still attached).

Clinical signs
Cats that have a foreign body trapped in their oesophagus will start showing clinical signs almost immediately.

They will have a reduced appetite, difficulty in swallowing, and regurgitation.

If the problem is secondary to inflammation of the oesophagus there may be some signs of hypersalivation, discomfort and regurgitation at the time, but oesophageal strictures due to scar contraction usually take 2–3 weeks to develop. Cats will have a decreased appetite during this time. Depending on the size of the stricture lumen, some cats may still be able to cope with liquidised food and water.

Diagnosis

The diagnosis is suspected on the basis of history and clinical signs and is confirmed by endoscopy or contrast radiography. Occasionally a string foreign body may be caught around the base of the tongue and may be seen when inspecting the mouth.

Treatment

The treatment of an oesophageal stricture involves gradual dilation of the stricture under general anaesthesia using progressively larger tubes or specialised inflatable catheters. It often requires several treatments to completely break down the stricture and is more successful if treatment is instigated soon after the initiating event. A gastrostomy tube may then be placed to manage nutrition and to give the oesophagus time to heal.

Oesophageal foreign bodies may be removed endoscopically or surgically.

Vomiting

Vomiting is a common sign associated with gastric and intestinal disorders in the cat, but it can also be a sign of a primary disease outside the gastrointestinal tract, such as chronic renal failure or hyperthyroidism. It is important to consider these metabolic causes of vomiting before concentrating only on gastrointestinal causes. It is also important to note that in cats intestinal disease often causes vomiting rather than diarrhoea.

Causes

The most common causes of vomiting associated with primary gastrointestinal disease are inflammatory conditions, such as food intolerance, food allergy and idiopathic inflammatory bowel disease (IBD), and also the accumulation of hair in the stomach, especially in long-haired cats.

Intestinal neoplasia and intestinal obstruction (e.g. due to a foreign body or an intussusception) are also important causes of vomiting.

FOOD INTOLERANCE AND FOOD ALLERGY

Food intolerance is an abnormal response to an ingested food or food additive, e.g. the inability of many cats to digest lactose in milk, due to lack of the enzyme lactase. Food intolerance does not have an immunologic basis, whereas a genuine food allergy (hypersensitivity) is an adverse reaction to a food or food additive, with a proven immunologic basis. Food intolerance and food allergy are very common causes of gastrointestinal signs in cats (see Box 6.8).

BOX 6.8   KEY POINT: CHRONIC VOMITING

A common cause of chronic vomiting in an otherwise well cat is food allergy/intolerance, usually to a dietary protein source that the cat has eaten repeatedly. Food allergy/intolerance is highly diet responsive once a suitable diet is found, which usually contains a protein source that the cat has not encountered before.

IDIOPATHIC INFLAMMATORY BOWEL DISEASE

This is a common condition in cats that can cause vomiting, diarrhoea and/or weight loss. It is believed to be due to an immune-mediated reaction. There is an accumulation of inflammatory cells within the bowel mucosa, causing tissue destruction, and impaired digestion and absorption of food. The cause, or trigger, of the reaction is unknown and thought to be multifactorial.

INTESTINAL NEOPLASIA

Lymphoma, lymphosarcoma and adenocarcinoma are the most common tumours in the feline intestine. Benign tumours are rare.

Clinical signs

Vomiting may be acute (signs last for less than 10 days) or the problem may be chronic (persists longer than 10 days). In chronic cases the problem may have been present for years, may be waxing/waning or gradually worsening. In some cases the vomiting episodes are accompanied by inappetence, and affected cats may be underweight. In cases of food allergy or idiopathic inflammatory bowel disease diarrhoea may also be a symptom.

The consumption of grass or houseplant leaves may be an indication of underlying nausea.

Diagnosis

If the problem is acute in onset and the cat is clinically stable, it is usually appropriate to try symptomatic treatment before undertaking diagnostic tests to find an underlying problem.

Many healthy cats will vomit around once a month to rid their stomach of hair, accumulated by constant grooming and this may be considered within the normal range. If vomiting is more frequent further tests are necessary to investigate the underlying cause of the problem. A dietary trial is often an appropriate option if the cat appears healthy in all other respects, and food intolerance/allergy is suspected. If the problem is food intolerance/allergy, once a suitable single-protein source diet is fed, vomiting will cease. Most cats respond to a sole diet of chicken or raw beef, and once vomiting has ceased, a more balanced diet may be gradually introduced, being careful to discontinue any new choice that provokes vomiting, and return for a few days to the 'safe' diet. The choice of further tests is based on the history, signalment and physical examination of the cat. Investigations usually involve blood tests, abdominal radiography or ultrasonography and in some cases gastrointestinal biopsies, either obtained surgically or via endoscopy.

Treatment

ACUTE VOMITING

1. Withhold food for 24 hours, and only allow water to drink. The cat may need to be confined to the house during this period to prevent hunting and scavenging behaviour. The period of fasting should not be prolonged (unless there is a medical indication) as this may exacerbate the gut problems.
2. If drinking water produces vomiting, i.v. or s.c. fluids will be required (for calculation of fluid requirements see p. 83).
3. After fasting the cat for 24 hours, small quantities of single, high quality protein food such as chicken or raw beef can be offered.
4. Gradually re-introduce the cat's normal diet after several days without vomiting.

CHRONIC VOMITING

1. Identify and treat the underlying cause. This may involve long-term feeding of a hypoallergenic diet, or may require surgical or medical management of the underlying problem.
2. Support the patient with i.v. fluid therapy when needed.

Diarrhoea

Diarrhoea is a common problem in cats with gastrointestinal disease. Acute diarrhoea (signs last for less than 4 weeks) is commonly caused by dietary indiscretion, stress, or any rapid change of diet, and often resolves without treatment, or following feeding of a simplified diet. Chronic diarrhoea can be more problematic and requires more detailed investigation into the underlying cause. It is sometimes helpful to try to categorise the diarrhoea as 'small bowel' (enteritis) or 'large bowel' (colitis), according to the appearance of the stools, their volume and frequency (see later). However, many cats with chronic diarrhoea have conditions which affect both small and large bowel, and so the distinction is often difficult to make, and less helpful than it would be in a dog with chronic diarrhoea.

Causes

DIETARY

Abrupt dietary change is a frequent cause of acute diarrhoea in young kittens, and occurs because there is insufficient time for intestinal brush border enzyme activity and pancreatic secretions to adjust to major changes in the nutrient content of the diet. In this case the problem is categorised as a temporary maldigestion syndrome rather than as a food allergy. Genuine dietary intolerance and food allergy occasionally cause acute diarrhoea, but more usually cause chronic vomiting.

BACTERIAL ENTERITIS

- *Campylobacter jejuni:* This organism can be isolated from the faeces of around 10% of normal cats, but it can cause diarrhoea in cats, dogs and humans. It is an opportunistic pathogen, and mainly causes signs in young cats with intercurrent GI disease, for example *Salmonella* or *Giardia*. In adult cats, the organism is usually asymptomatic, but in some cats may cause chronic or intermittent large bowel diarrhoea and anorexia/vomiting for periods of between 2 weeks to several months. It is associated with poor sanitation and crowded housing and infection is usually via contaminated food and water. The organism is shed for 1–4 months after infection and may be spread to humans.
- *Salmonella:* Infection is usually associated with poor husbandry, and is asymptomatic in many cats (*Salmonella* can be isolated from the faeces of up to

14% of normal cats). If it does cause signs of disease, about 50% of symptomatic cats have gastroenteritis, while other affected cats present with abortion, stillbirth, neonatal death, or septicaemia. The disease is usually found in young cats (<1 year old), malnourished cats, cats under stress (e.g. associated with surgery, hospitalisation, or concurrent illness), and cats treated with glucocorticoids or chemotherapy. Diagnosis is made by positive microbial culture in the faeces of cats with gastroenteritis, or by culture from the blood or internal organs in septicaemia.

PROTOZOAN ENTERITIS

- **Isospora** is the commonest gastrointestinal coccidian infection in cats. Two species infect cats – *I. felis* and *I. rivolta*. Infection of both the definitive host (cat) and the intermediate host (mice and other mammals) is by ingestion of sporulated oocysts. Cats may also become infected when hunting by the ingestion of tissue cysts in the intermediate host.

  I. felis infections are usually asymptomatic, and not pathogenic in healthy weaned kittens. Clinical signs usually appear only if the kitten is very young (<1 month old), there are a large number of oocysts ingested, or the cat is immunosuppressed e.g. due to overcrowding, transport, re-homing or intercurrent infection.

  I. rivolta infection is usually a cattery problem, causing diarrhoea and weight loss in queens after each litter, and in kittens from infected queens. Infection is confirmed by detection of distinctive oocysts on microscopic examination of the faeces, but *I. rivolta* oocysts are often absent from the faeces of infected cats, so diagnosis can be problematic in some cases.

- **Giardia** is a motile protozoan, which can infect a wide range of host species, including cats, dogs and humans. Infection is usually through drinking contaminated water. *Giardia* has a direct life-cycle, i.e. there is no intermediate host involvement. The parasite colonizes the small intestine of the infected host and infective oocysts are then intermittently shed into the faeces. Cysts can survive outside the host for weeks to months in cool, moist conditions. *Giardia* infection is often asymptomatic, but may cause acute or chronic diarrhoea (continuous or intermittent), with soft to watery faeces, often with mucus. Diagnosis is by microscopy of multiple zinc sulphate centrifugal flotations. The oocysts are shed intermittently so examination of a single sample is only diagnostic in 70% of cases rising to 90% success rate on examination of three successive faecal samples. Motile parasites (trophozoites) may be seen in fresh smears of diarrhoeic faeces, but are not a source of infection, since they are destroyed by gastric acid. Direct faecal smears have a <20% detection rate if only one sample is examined, and a 43% detection rate if three smears are assessed.

NEMATODE INFECTIONS

Roundworm (*Toxocara cati*, *Toxascaris leonina*), hookworm (*Ancylostoma tubaeforma*, *Ancylostoma braziliense*) and tapeworm infections (*Dipylidium caninum*, *Taenia taeniaeformis*) are rare causes of diarrhoea in adult cats. Clinically apparent roundworm and hookworm infections mostly occur in kittens kept in poor conditions and are controlled by regular administration of anthelminthics and good husbandry.

Clinical signs

Clinical signs of diarrhoea are rapidly evident to owners of cats that use litter trays, but may go unnoticed in cats that have access to the outdoors and are efficient at self-grooming. Careful questioning of the owner is therefore required, and in some cases it is helpful to confine the cat indoors for a period to allow the faeces to be examined.

In considering the likely cause(s) of the diarrhoea and determining further diagnostic tests, it can be helpful to try to distinguish whether the problem is located in the small bowel or the large bowel, although as previously mentioned many cats with chronic diarrhoea will have mixed signs.

Small bowel diarrhoea is characterised by:

- Increased volume.
- Moderate increase in frequency (2–3 stools per day) with no significant increase in urgency – diarrhoea is usually passed outdoors, or in the litter tray.
- Absence of fresh blood and mucus.
- Absence of straining.
- Weight loss.
- There may sometimes be vomiting accompanying the diarrhoea.

Large bowel diarrhoea is characterised by:

- Increased frequency but little overall increase in volume (more than three small stools passed per day).
- Increased urgency – faeces may be passed in inappropriate places around the house.

- Straining to defaecate, sometimes accompanied by vomiting.
- Presence of fresh blood and mucus. In some cases straining to defaecate produces only small volumes of mucoid material with no appreciable faecal content.
- Absence of weight loss.

Diagnostic tests

In cases of acute self-limiting diarrhoea, no diagnostic tests are necessary. If the diarrhoea becomes chronic and/or the cat becomes debilitated further tests are indicated.

Multiple faecal samples should be submitted for full analysis (direct microscopy, special stains, faecal flotation and bacterial culture for enteric pathogens) as this will hopefully identify any infectious (and potentially zoonotic) cause. However, further diagnostic tests may be necessary: blood tests are often unremarkable and diagnostic imaging (radiography, ultrasonography) and gut biopsies (surgical or endoscopically) may be required.

Treatment

SYMPTOMATIC THERAPY FOR ACUTE DIARRHOEA

Dietary management: Bowel rest is helpful in the short term (24 hours) since food is abrasive, and may cause mucosal cell loss. However more prolonged food restriction may be harmful because the gastrointestinal mucosal cells take a significant proportion of their nutrition directly from the bowel contents rather than from the blood stream.

- If the cat is vomiting, withhold all food for 24 hours.
- If the cat is not vomiting, feed small meals, frequently i.e. 4–6 times daily initially, providing only around 30% of the required calories in the first 24 hours. A suitable diet will be an easily digested diet, containing high quality protein and relatively low proportions of fat and carbohydrate, for instance lean cooked meat. In contrast to dogs, rice and other starches are poorly tolerated in cats and can cause or exacerbate diarrhoea if fed to excess.
- Once the stool is normal, *gradually* reintroduce the cat's normal food. Cats that suffer from repeated episodes of acute diarrhoea may benefit from long-term use of a hypoallergenic diet (using a 'novel' protein, i.e. a protein the cat has not been fed before).

Fluid therapy: This is very important if the cat is dehydrated. A balanced electrolyte solution containing lactate (e.g. Hartmann's solution) is a good choice as bicarbonate is lost in diarrhoea, causing metabolic acidosis. Lactate is metabolised in the liver to bicarbonate, so helps to redress this loss.

THERAPY FOR CHRONIC DIARRHOEA

The cat should receive supportive care in terms of diet and fluid therapy as necessary. The most important part of the management is identification and treatment of the underlying cause.

If the diarrhoea is caused by an organism with zoonotic potential, the owner should be warned of the risks to human health. If an infectious cause has been identified strict hygiene measures must be applied when treating the patient in the hospital.

BOX 6.9   KEY POINT: TREATMENT OF DIARRHOEA

Acute diarrhoea may initially be treated symptomatically without a definitive diagnosis. Chronic diarrhoea should not be treated symptomatically and diagnostic tests *must* be done.

Constipation/obstipation

Constipation is a common problem in cats, and is defined as difficult or infrequent passage of faeces. Obstipation refers to intractable constipation due to irreversible loss of colonic function, and it results in dilation of the colon, which is usually referred to as 'megacolon'.

Causes

Constipation is usually a problem of middle-aged to older cats and there are a number of causes:

- **Dehydration** – The feline colon absorbs water from the bowel contents very efficiently, and chronic dehydration may lead to constipation due to excessive drying of the stool e.g. in older cats with chronic renal failure.
- **Obstruction** – This is usually due to a narrow pelvis or abnormal pelvic bone growth. This may be due to dietary calcium deficiency in kittens (nutritional secondary hyperparathyroidism) or more commonly is caused by malalignment and bony callous formation associated with healed pelvic fractures.

- **Nerve dysfunction** of aged cats causing colon hypo-motility. This is a common cause of obstipation in older cats, especially Burmese.
- **Foreign body**, e.g. hair, bones. Accumulated hair is a common cause of constipation in longhaired cats and can be prevented by regular grooming or even full body clipping if necessary. Hair also accumulates in cats that groom excessively, which is usually associated with skin irritation.
- **Painful defecation** – Anal sacculitis, anal stricture or fractured pelvis may cause pain when attempting to defaecate (occasionally cats will actually cry out when passing faeces). This will inhibit some cats from attempting to defaecate, and the owner must be observant to notice that motions have not been passed recently.
- **GI tumours** are a rare cause of constipation in the cat.

Clinical signs

Cats are often presented with a history of straining to pass a small volume of dry faeces. Occasionally, there is some blood or mucus because of irritation of the colonic mucosa. This should be differentiated from straining to pass urine (stranguria), and many owners will confuse the two signs, so careful questioning is required as stranguria may be a medical emergency.

Occasionally there is a history of vomiting, and constipated cats are often lethargic, inappetent, and have an unkempt coat. The cat may adopt a hunched/crouched posture due to abdominal pain.

Diagnosis

Usually the history, signalment and clinical signs point towards a defaecation problem and hard, non-compressible faecal masses are detected on abdominal palpation. Abdominal radiography is helpful in assessing the extent of the problem (see Fig. 6.5), especially with regard to the size of the colon and pelvic canal. This may be sufficient to make the diagnosis, but in some cases further tests will be necessary to identify the underlying cause of the problem.

Treatment

Treating the underlying problem at an early stage wherever possible is important to avoid permanent damage to the colon, resulting in obstipation and megacolon. Symptomatic treatment of the constipation is also required:

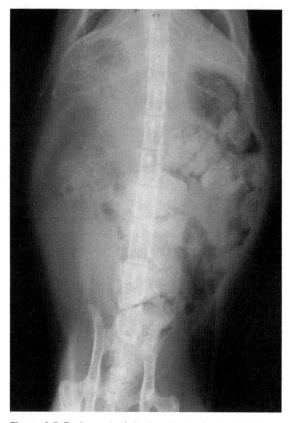

Figure 6.5 Radiograph of obstipated cat, showing colon impacted with faeces.

1. **Restore fluid and electrolyte balance:** This is essential if dehydration is a contributory factor, and is essential in all cases before an enema is given. Most enemas have the effect of drawing fluid into the bowel from the circulation and will exacerbate any fluid and electrolyte abnormalities, which may be potentially fatal.
2. **Remove faeces:** The method depends on the severity of the constipation, but is usually initially via an enema (commercially available pediatric enema [microenema], hand-warm water or laxative). If this is performed under general anaesthesia, an endotracheal tube must be placed in case vomiting occurs as a result of stimulation of the colon. Enema solutions that are high in phosphates must be avoided as they are highly toxic to cats. Manual evacuation is usually required in severe cases.

If the underlying cause can be treated at an early stage, the problem may be cured. However, in many cases the underlying cause cannot be found, or cannot be corrected, or is not identified until the colonic damage has become chronic and irreversible. In these cases there are several treatment options, and many cats will benefit from long-term use of a combination of medical treatments. In severe cases, surgery will be required.

MEDICAL MANAGEMENT

- Increase oral fluid intake: Feed canned rather than dry food, and offer tasty fluids such as dilute fish or beef broth to drink.
- Oral laxatives:
  - Increase dietary fibre by the addition of fibre such as psyllium, canned pumpkin or creamed corn to the diet.
  - Petroleum wax is a lubricant laxative and can be helpful in mild cases. If it is given in liquid form (e.g. liquid paraffin), it must be mixed with food, because if it is dosed by syringe there is a risk of aspiration, resulting in severe irritant damage to the lungs.
  - Lactulose: This is a syrup containing poorly absorbed polysaccharides which act as an osmotic laxative.
- Periodic microenemas.

SURGICAL MANAGEMENT

- Pelvic re-configuration – orthopaedic surgery to widen the pelvic canal in cats with post-pelvic fracture narrowing.
- Subtotal or total colectomy (removal of the colon). This is used in severe, recurring constipation and megacolon which are refractory to medical treatment, or sometimes when owners are unable to administer treatment, leading to frequent reoccurrence of signs.

BOX 6.10   KEY POINT: CHRONIC CONSTIPATION

Chronic constipation is often a lifelong problem that requires the owners to observe the cat carefully and maintain a regular management regime.

Pancreatitis

Inflammation of the pancreas is increasingly recognised as an important disorder in cats. In the majority of cases there is chronic, low-grade inflammation (chronic pancreatitis) but acute pancreatitis, more commonly seen in dogs, can also occur.

Pathogenesis

Chronic pancreatitis in cats is often associated with cholangitis and inflammatory bowel disease. The exact cause is not known. It is thought that bacteria may ascend from the gut into the common bile duct and pancreatic duct, causing inflammation and an exaggerated immune response.

Clinical signs

Anorexia, lethargy and dehydration are the most common presenting signs in cats, unlike the classic signs of vomiting and abdominal pain that are exhibited in dogs. In chronic pancreatitis, the signs may be very subtle, and tend to be intermittent in nature.

Diagnostic tests

Confirmation of the diagnosis is difficult. The clinical signs are very non-specific and further tests will be necessary to make a presumptive diagnosis. Unfortunately there are currently no reliable, non-invasive tests that confirm the diagnosis. Serum amylase and lipase are not useful in the diagnosis of feline pancreatitis. Trypsin-like immunoreactivity (TLI) and pancreatic lipase immunoreactivity (PLI) may be helpful in some, but not all, cases. Abdominal ultrasound is useful if changes in the pancreas are seen, but in some cases there will be no gross changes, and when lesions are seen it can be difficult to differentiate chronic from acute changes.

A pancreatic biopsy is necessary to confirm the diagnosis. An exploratory laparotomy may be considered too invasive in mildly affected cases. Severely affected cats, for whom definitive diagnosis would be more valuable, are often metabolically unstable, and surgery is associated with more risks of adverse effects. A presumptive diagnosis is therefore often made.

Treatment

The main treatment is supportive care. Aggressive fluid therapy is the cornerstone of treatment during acute episodes of inflammation, not only to correct the dehydration, but also to provide circulatory support. Food should be withheld for 1–2 days if vomiting is present, to reduce pancreatic secretions, followed by a gradual return to full feeding using a highly palatable and highly digestible, low-fat diet.

BOX 6.11   KEY POINTS: PANCREATITIS

- Feline pancreatitis is difficult to diagnose and may be missed if a careful diagnostic workup is not performed.
- The pathogeneses of pancreatitis, inflammatory liver disease and inflammatory bowel disease may be linked in cats.

In cats that are not vomiting, and especially those that have not eaten for more than 3 days, food should not be withheld, and if the cat is inappetent, placement of a feeding tube should be considered. Subclinical cobalamin (vitamin B_{12}) deficiency may be a complication of chronic pancreatitis and this can be addressed by supplementary injections.

6.5   LIVER DISEASE

The liver serves a number of vital functions, including:

- **Digestion:** The liver secretes bile, which plays an important role in fat digestion and absorption. Bile emulsifies large fat particles from the food, so that enzymes from the pancreas can break them down; it also aids in transport and absorption of the end products of fat digestion.
- **Detoxification:** Liver cells (hepatocytes) detoxify metabolic by-products and also act as gatekeeper to prevent toxins from the GI tract entering the circulation. Bile is a vehicle for excretion of waste products from the blood, especially bilirubin, which is an end product of haemoglobin destruction, and cholesterol, which is synthesized by the hepatocytes.
- **Clotting factors:** The liver produces clotting factors, which have vital roles in the complex process of blood coagulation.
- **Energy metabolism:** The liver plays an important part in the maintenance of blood glucose concentrations, by storing excess glucose as glycogen, and releasing it as glucose when required. It is also an important source of glucose formed via a process called gluconeogenesis.

Inflammatory liver disease

Pathogenesis

The cause of feline inflammatory liver disease is unknown, but it is suspected that biliary and pancreatic reflux, and loss of immune tolerance to normal gut and liver antigens may be involved in the pathogenesis.

There are two forms of disease:

1. **Neutrophilic cholangitis.**

   – *Acute phase:* There is an infiltration of neutrophils into the bile duct areas and hepatic tissues. Bacteria such as *E. coli* (from the GI tract) are sometimes cultured in the bile in the acute phase. Bacterial infection ascending the bile duct from the duodenum is a possible cause.
   – *Chronic phase:* In the chronic phase, there is an infiltration of lymphocytes, plasma cells and some neutrophils into the bile duct areas and hepatic tissue. This may represent a more advanced stage of the same process that causes acute neutrophilic cholangitis, and it may progress to cause liver fibrosis.

2. **Lymphocytic cholangitis.** In lymphocytic cholangitis, the bile duct areas and surrounding hepatic tissues are infiltrated by small lymphocytes. Also, bile duct inflammation and fibrosis are often seen in this condition. This disease may wax and wane over several years.

Clinical signs

Cats with inflammatory liver disease are presented with anorexia, weight loss and lethargy. In chronic cases these signs may be intermittent. Occasional vomiting may be reported, and on clinical examination, jaundice (see Fig. 6.6), an enlarged liver and/or fever may be found. In severe, chronic cases there may also be ascites.

Diagnosis

Serum biochemistry shows elevated liver enzymes and bilirubin, and there are often significant increases in fasting and post-prandial bile acids. There may be increased numbers of neutrophils on haematology, especially in acute neutrophilic cholangitis. While these findings are indicative of inflammatory liver disease, they do not show which form of disease is present, and a liver biopsy is required to reach a definitive diagnosis.

Treatment

It is important to give the cat supportive care. This should include i.v. fluid therapy and nutritional support appropriate for the individual cat.

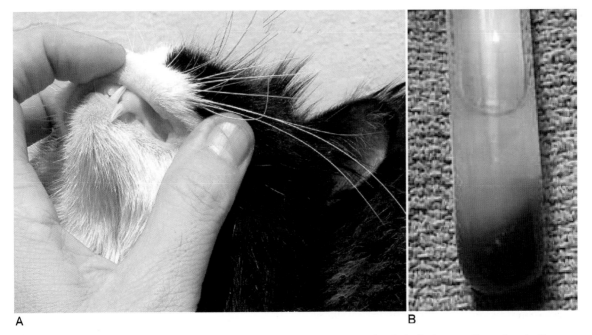

Figure 6.6 (A) Cat with jaundice. (B) Blood sample from the same cat, showing icteric (yellow) serum. Reproduced with permission from A. Gough.

Once the underlying disease process has been diagnosed, specific treatment can be started. Treatment for acute neutrophilic cholangitis centres on long courses (3 months or longer) of broad-spectrum antibiotics, whereas chronic neutrophilic cholangitis and lymphocytic cholangitis are treated with immuno-modulating drugs, as well as continued supportive care.

Cats with chronic liver disease may also develop a secondary blood clotting problem, because the liver has an important role in manufacturing blood clotting factors. These cats may benefit from additional vitamin K therapy. Ursodeoxycholic acid is a drug with multiple functions including reduction of toxic serum bile acid concentration, and it is used to treat hepatopathies. S-adenosyl methionine (s-AME) is an anti-oxidant, which may be helpful in promoting liver repair.

Nutritionally balanced diets are ideal for the cat with inflammatory liver disease. In cats with severe liver dysfunction the dietary protein levels need to be restricted.

Idiopathic hepatic lipidosis

Hepatic lipidosis is a potentially fatal condition, which can affect overweight cats that have a period of reduced food intake for any reason. Affected cats require aggressive intensive care and assisted feeding, but even so, a significant number of affected cats do not survive. Hepatic lipidosis can be avoided by keeping cats within the normal bodyweight range and by ensuring that obese cats are maintained at good levels of nutrition through periods of ill health.

Pathogenesis

Inadequate caloric intake causes the body to mobilise fat as an alternative energy source and as a result, triglycerides accumulate in the liver cells, overwhelming normal liver function.

Hepatic lipidosis occurs mostly in middle-aged cats, and there is a history of previous obesity in nearly all cats. It can be caused by feeding obese cats a severely calorie-restricted or highly unpalatable diet or where environmental factors lead to reduced food intake, for example the addition of a dominant, aggressive cat to the household. Anorexia secondary to other illness or other causes may also be the trigger for hepatic lipidosis.

Clinical signs

These cats are usually completely anorexic and rapidly become lethargic and depressed. Vomiting may also be reported. On physical examination, jaundice (see Fig. 6.6) and dehydration may be found.

BOX 6.12 KEY POINT: HEPATIC LIPIDOSIS

> Obese cats that lose weight acutely for any reason are at risk of developing hepatic lipidosis.

Diagnosis

Serum biochemistry usually reveals elevated serum bilirubin, alkaline phosphatase (ALP), alanine transferase (ALT) and aspartate transferase (AST). Hypokalaemia is found in 30% of cats, due to lack of intake and increased losses through vomiting. On haematology there is a non-regenerative anaemia in approximately 30% of cats. Abnormal coagulation tests occur in about 50% of cats.

A fine needle aspirate sample from the liver will show large lipid vacuoles in all the hepatic cells, but a liver biopsy is required for definitive diagnosis. Anaesthesia and surgery should be approached with care because of the hepatic failure and possible coagulopathy, and in some cases treatment will be initiated based on a presumptive diagnosis.

Treatment

It is of prime importance to start nutritional support as soon as possible, while searching for any underlying disease that may have caused the initial anorexia. If such a cause can be identified, it also needs to be treated.

Long-term nutritional support will be required, and is best given via a gastrostomy or oesophagostomy tube. Appetite stimulants should be avoided, as some of these are hepatotoxic.

A nutritionally balanced, energy dense feline diet should be fed, ensuring that adequate levels of carnitine and taurine are supplied, as these two amino acids are particularly important for fat metabolism and recovery from hepatic lipidosis. Liquidised canned diets are most appropriate for use via wide-bore feeding tubes. Specialist liquid diets are available for use with narrow-bore feeding tubes, but their caloric content tends to be relatively low, requiring large volumes to be supplied each day. Feline milk powder can be added to these liquid diets to increase the calorie density of the food. Vitamin supplementation (especially the B vitamins and vitamin K) is done by injection.

Feeding needs to be continued until the cat starts eating independently, which may take many weeks or months. Long-term care and a dedicated owner will be required to achieve full recovery.

If the cat is still obese after recovery, a conservative weight management plan should be commenced to prevent the recurrence of hepatic lipidosis.

Portosystemic shunts

A portosystemic shunt (PSS) is an abnormality of the blood supply to the liver, which allows blood to bypass the hepatocytes. In most cases it is a congenital abnormality caused by failure of the foetal blood circulation to convert to its adult form, but it can also be caused by acquired hepatic circulatory problems in adult cats.

Pathogenesis

In this condition, blood from the GI-tract (GIT) passes directly into the systemic circulation, bypassing the liver, and therefore avoiding detoxification.

Substances produced by microbes in the GIT, such as ammonia, mercaptans, and short chain fatty acids, are normally removed by the liver. In PSS, these substances are not removed, and accumulate to relatively high levels in the blood, especially after a meal, causing toxic effects in the brain, and resulting in hepatic encephalopathy.

There are also increased concentrations of bile acids in the serum, because of disruption of the normal recirculation of bile acids between the liver and the GI tract.

Clinical signs

Cats with congenital PSS are usually < 2 years old at diagnosis. They usually show stunted growth, and are presented for salivation, periods of bizarre behaviour and depression. Excessive salivation is the most common sign of PSS in cats. Intermittent neurological signs also predominate, such as abnormal mentation, aggression, depression, restlessness, dementia, blank staring, and head pressing (Fig. 6.7). More severe cases may display ataxia, blindness, and seizures.

Rarely, cats display GIT signs such as vomiting and/or diarrhoea, and about a quarter of all male kittens with PSS are cryptorchid (only one descended testicle). Affected cats also often have striking, copper coloured irides, but it is important to remember that in some cats, and especially some breeds, this is a normal finding, so it is not pathognomonic for the condition.

Diagnosis

Diagnosis is made by a combination of appropriate history, clinical signs and laboratory tests.

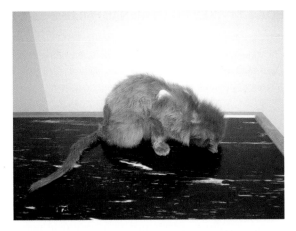

Figure 6.7 Head pressing and ataxia in a cat with portosystemic shunt (PSS). Reproduced with permission from V. Barrs.

Liver enzymes are often normal in affected cats, but liver function tests, such as fasting and postprandial serum bile acid tests, will be abnormal. Blood ammonia levels are also elevated, but are difficult to measure in practice, since blood must be analysed very rapidly after collection.

BOX 6.13 KEY POINT: PORTOSYSTEMIC SHUNTS

> Drooling is the most common clinical sign in cats with portosystemic shunts.

The urine may contain ammonium biurate crystals, and in more chronic cases these crystals may have formed into bladder stones.

Ultrasound examination of the liver and portal vasculature is usually diagnostic, but in some cases contrast radiography (portovenography) is necessary to find the shunting vessel(s).

Treatment

Treatment for a congenital PSS may be surgical or medical depending on the anatomy of the shunt. In cases of acquired PSS, surgery is not an option.

Surgical correction involves identification and (partial) ligation of the abnormal blood vessel. If this can be achieved, and if the normal blood vessels to the liver are well-developed, this can result in a complete resolution of clinical signs. Medical therapy is aimed at reducing the clinical signs of hepatic encephalopathy by reducing the accumulation of toxins. This includes:

- A low protein diet to reduce the amount of nitrogenous waste products, and to reduce the amount of substrate available for microbial growth.
- Oral antibiotics to reduce the numbers of GI microbes.
- Oral lactulose syrup to reduce ammonia absorption by reducing colonic transit time and reducing colonic pH. Diarrhoea is a side effect of this drug and the dose needs to be titrated to suit the individual.

6.6 URINARY TRACT DISEASE

Renal disease

The kidneys are made up of many microscopic units called nephrons, consisting of glomeruli, which filter blood, and renal tubules, which regulate the serum concentration of electrolytes and other substances. The kidneys also play a vital role in controlling blood pressure, via the renal angiotensin-aldosterone system, and in the production of red blood cells, via the production of erythropoietin.

Chronic renal failure (CRF)

Chronic renal failure (CRF) is associated with slow, progressive, irreversible deterioration of kidney function. There are a number of conditions, which can cause CRF in cats, but in the majority of cases the exact cause of CRF remains unknown. Age, genetics, environment and the impact of disease may all be important in its development. In recent years, more attention has been directed towards high blood pressure, low blood potassium concentration, and dental disease as possible contributing factors.

Although CRF can occur at any age, it is usually a disease of older cats. With advances in medical care, and improvements in feline diets, cats are now living much longer. Chronic renal failure is one of the leading causes of illness and death in older cats, but with early detection, and proper diet and hydration, it is possible for affected cats to remain clinically well and active for years.

Because the very early signs of chronic renal failure are subtle, the disease may only be recognised when it is advanced, and more dramatic signs are noticed. The clinical signs include weight loss, drinking more than usual (polydipsia – PD) or drinking from unusual places (Fig. 6.8), passing more urine than normal

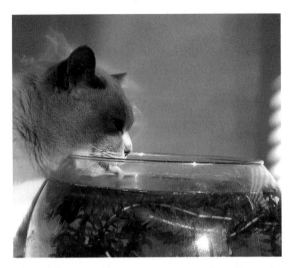

Figure 6.8 One of the most common signs of chronic renal failure is excessive water intake (polydipsia), and affected cats may drink from unusual places.

(polyuria – PU), loss of appetite or fussiness with food, and vomiting.

The earliest sign of renal failure is decreased urine specific gravity (dilution of the urine to a specific gravity of less than 1.035), caused by the inability of the kidney to conserve water. However, because of the tremendous reserve capacity of the kidneys, even this first clinical sign occurs relatively late in the course of disease. By the time urine specific gravity is reduced, the kidneys have already lost 65% of their functioning mass. Serum creatinine becomes elevated when 75% of the functional renal mass is lost, and serum phosphate levels rise when 85% is lost. Anaemia usually accompanies end stage CRF. The reasons for the anaemia are a reduced production of new red blood cells because of a lack of erythropoietin (a hormone synthesised by the kidney, responsible for stimulation of the red cell production in the bone marrow) and an increased destruction of red blood cells because of uraemic damage. Reduced food intake, leading to a negative protein and energy balance, contributes to the problem.

Once the diagnosis is made, the progression of disease can be followed by regular measurement of urine specific gravity, serum creatinine, electrolytes, phosphate, packed cell volume, blood pressure and body weight.

MANAGEMENT OF CHRONIC RENAL FAILURE

There are a number of management strategies that can be used to prolong life and ensure quality of life:

BOX 6.14   KEY POINT: RENAL FAILURE

If urine specific gravity is 1.035 or more, the kidneys are able to concentrate urine effectively and renal failure can be ruled out of the differential diagnosis.

- **Prescription renal diets** – Diets low in protein and phosphate alleviate some of the clinical signs of kidney failure and are available as both dry and canned foods. These diets provide the ideal nutritional balance for cats with chronic renal failure, and are also supplemented with additional potassium, water-soluble vitamins and poly-unsaturated fatty acids. Feeding a balanced 'renal' diet is one of the most important aspects of the management of CRF. However, some cats are unwilling to change their eating habits and care is required when attempting to change the diet. The most important thing is that the cat with CRF eats regularly so that weight loss is minimised.

- **Fluid therapy** – In advanced cases, initial treatment with intravenous fluids will be required to manage dehydration. In the longer term, continued fluid supplementation, via intermittent use of subcutaneous fluids and by encouraging increased oral fluid intake, will also be valuable. Plenty of fresh water should also be easily available, and canned foods may be preferable to dry foods if the cat will eat them, to facilitate water intake. The use of water fountains will encourage some cats to drink, as they often prefer running water, and some cats may be tempted to keep up their fluid intake by being offered a dilute low-salt broth made from meat, fish or chicken.

- **Potassium supplementation** – Large amounts of potassium are lost in the urine in renal failure, leading to weakness and possible deterioration in kidney function. In severe cases, there is ventroflexion of the head and neck, poor muscle tone, inability to jump and markedly reduced physical activity. Oral potassium supplementation is helpful, using potassium gluconate (available as tablets, powder, or a liquid supplement), or potassium citrate tablets.

- **Phosphate binders** – Blood phosphate levels are often high in cats with CRF, and this may lead to nausea and bone loss. The ideal way to control hyperphosphataemia is by the use of phosphate restricted 'renal' diets. However, if the cat will not eat the recommended diet, or if dietary phosphate restriction is not sufficient to manage the hyper-phosphataemia, additional orally administered phosphate binding agents may be required. These are inert substances, which bind to phosphate ions within the GI tract and prevent their absorption into the blood circulation. A palatable phosphate binding powder (Ipakitine™: Vetoquinol) is available in the UK. Alternatively, aluminium hydroxide tablets or liquids can be used with food. Blood tests will be required to monitor the effect of treatment, and to find the correct dose of phosphate binder for the individual cat.

- **Treatment for high blood pressure** – CRF may lead to high blood pressure, and this should be monitored (see p. 105). If the blood pressure is high, this should be treated and the effects of treatment monitored by repeated blood pressure measurements. Occasionally, high doses of drugs or multiple drugs are necessary to control the blood pressure.
- **Treatment for anaemia** – Anaemia is a common complication of CRF. Poor nutrition and iron deficiency should be addressed in the first instance. Androgens have been suggested as a means of treating CRF-induced anaemia, but response is often poor. In severe cases, the use of recombinant human erythropoietin (rHuEPO) can be highly effective, although some cats will gradually become resistant to its effects because of the development of anti-rHuEPO antibodies. The only other treatment option is repeated blood transfusion.
- **Water-soluble vitamin supplements** – These are required to make up for increased losses in the urine in CRF.
- **Anti-vomiting medications** – These may be prescribed if the cat is anorexic because of nausea, or has chronic vomiting from CRF.
- **Vitamin D** – This can be useful in cats that develop secondary hyperparathyroidism as a result of the chronic renal failure.

Autosomal dominant polycystic kidney disease (ADPKD)

Polycystic kidney disease is a genetically inherited disease, which causes fluid-filled cysts in the kidneys, and sometimes the liver. These cysts progressively enlarge and compress and damage normal renal tissue. Persians, Chinchillas and exotic short-haired cats are most commonly affected, but it can occur in other breeds too.

The condition is caused by a dominant gene and a gene test is now available to identify affected cats. Cats that are positive for the disease should not be used for breeding.

Affected cats may have the disease for years before renal failure develops and should be closely monitored for the development of clinical signs such as PU/PD and weight loss. Once clinical signs develop, affected cats are treated as for chronic renal failure (see previously).

Pyelonephritis

Pyelonephritis is a bacterial infection of the kidney tissue, usually caused by bacteria that are resident in the gut such as *E. coli*.

Cats often have a 2–4 week history of fluctuating inappetence, depression, PU/PD and weight loss, and there may be fever and dehydration. In acute cases, the kidneys can be painful, and haematology reveals the typical signs of a bacterial infection (an increased neutrophil count). There are bacteria and white blood cells, often in the form of casts, on examination of a centrifuged urine sediment.

Urine should be collected by cystocentesis and cultured, so that the correct choice of antibiotics can be confirmed. Long courses (4–8 weeks) of antibiotics are required, and urine should be cultured after the course to verify the elimination of infection. In the early stages of treatment, cats may need intravenous fluid support, and if there is permanent damage to the kidneys, medical management will also be required as described previously for renal failure.

Glomerulonephritis

Glomerulonephritis results from damage to the glomeruli by large molecules (immune complexes) produced by the immune system. The source of the immune complexes is often unknown, but may be associated with infection elsewhere in the body, neoplasia or with an immune reaction to certain drugs. These immune complexes stimulate an inflammatory reaction in the glomeruli, and renal filtering capacity is significantly reduced. Damage to the glomerular membrane results in loss of large amounts of protein in the urine (proteinuria).

Clinical signs in affected cats are usually related to low blood albumin concentration (hypoalbuminaemia), as a result of leakage of albumin through the damaged glomeruli. These cats will develop oedema (subcutaneous or ascites) when the albumin levels drop too low. There are also non-specific signs of chronic ill health such as weight loss, inappetence or anorexia and lethargy. In more advanced cases of disease, the kidney tubules are affected, resulting in more common signs of chronic renal failure, such PU/PD.

On laboratory tests, blood albumin concentration is low and urine protein concentration is high. The diagnosis is confirmed on renal biopsy.

Management focuses on treating the primary cause of the glomerulonephritis and slowing the loss of protein through the urine. Suitable diets contain only enough protein to maintain bodyweight and stabilise the blood albumin concentration, and have low levels of salt in order to reduce fluid retention (i.e. renal diets). Angiotensin converting enzyme (ACE) inhibitors are helpful in reducing the levels of proteinuria. If disease is advanced, with reduced urine specific gravity and elevated serum creatinine, additional management as for chronic renal failure is required (see p. 145).

Acute renal failure

Acute renal failure (ARF) in the cat most commonly arises as a complication of urethral obstruction. Other forms of ARF are relatively rare and usually caused by toxins that affect the kidneys (see Chapter 7), acute infections or problems with the blood supply to the kidneys (e.g. thromboembolic disease, p. 127).

In acute renal failure the kidneys produce reduced amounts of urine, if any at all, and toxic metabolites such as urea accumulate quickly in the serum. There are signs of severe metabolic acidosis, such as a rapid respiratory rate, and there is a rapid, potentially fatal increase in serum potassium concentration (hyperkalaemia). The kidneys may be enlarged on abdominal palpation.

Aims of treatment are to reverse the underlying cause where possible, and to stabilise fluid, acid–base and electrolyte balance until there is time for renal lesions to undergo healing. Because urine output is reduced or absent, fluid therapy must be administered with great care. Urine output and bodyweight should be closely monitored to avoid fluid overload and fluid accumulation in the lungs. Diuretics such as mannitol or frusemide may be used to promote urine production, and are most effective if given close to the time of renal injury. Serial monitoring of serum electrolyte and creatinine concentrations is essential for management of critically ill cats with acute renal failure. Close monitoring of acid–base balance is also helpful if it is available.

Lower urinary tract disease

There are a number of conditions which affect the feline lower urinary tract and the clinical signs shown by the cat will tend to be similar whatever the underlying cause.

Common signs include:

- Increased frequency of urination (pollakiuria).
- Straining to pass small amounts of urine (dysuria).
- Inability to pass any urine (stranguria).
- Blood in the urine (haematuria).

Owners notice the cat attempting to urinate more often than usual and perhaps in unusual places, such as bathtubs and shower recesses.

Male cats may be presented with complete urethral blockage, often as a result of the presence of a plug lodged in the long narrow urethra. The bladder is firm, distended and painful, and abdominal palpation must be gentle to avoid bladder rupture.

By contrast, in non-obstructed males and in females, the bladder is often small and contracted on abdominal palpation, because of spasm and frequent emptying. Bladder blockage is extremely rare in female cats, because of the wider diameter of the female urethra.

Owners should be advised to be alert for signs of lower urinary tract disease, as male cats, especially, must be assessed and treated promptly. Encouraging increased water intake is important for all cats with lower urinary tract disease. Prescription diets to encourage production of more dilute urine and to regulate urine pH are also a common aid to help prevent recurrence of the problem, especially if urinary calculi are involved.

Idiopathic feline lower urinary tract disease (iFLUTD)

Idiopathic FLUTD (also known as chronic interstitial cystitis) is a common, but poorly understood, disease in feline practice, and while numerous theories have been developed to explain the underlying cause, the condition remains idiopathic.

Cats usually present with recurring episodes of lower urinary tract signs. The episodes tend to be short-lived (usually 1–5 days duration) and eventually resolve spontaneously without treatment, but they tend to recur. The frequency, duration and severity of the episodes vary considerably from cat to cat.

Encouraging affected cats to take in increased amounts of water ensures continuous production of larger volumes of more dilute urine. This can be very helpful in reducing the severity of their clinical signs.

BOX 6.15   KEY POINT: FLUTD

Chronic interstitial cystitis in cats is idiopathic and signs are self-limiting. Since no therapeutic regime has been proven effective, the condition will often resolve and then relapse no matter what treatment is used.

Urolithiasis

Occasionally cats develop urinary calculi (uroliths), and these cats will present with lower urinary tract signs. Calculi are usually composed of struvite (magnesium ammonium phosphate) or calcium oxalate. Alkaline urine (high pH) and increased levels of urinary magnesium and phosphate can predispose to the development of struvite calculi, whereas acid urine (low pH) and high urinary calcium levels predispose to calcium oxalate calculi. It is thought that the widespread addition of acidifying agents to commercially available feline diets has resulted in a relative decrease in the frequency of struvite calculi and an increase in the proportion of calcium oxalate calculi in recent years. Struvite calculi can be dissolved by the use of urinary acidifiers and dietary reduction of magnesium and phosphate intake, but calcium oxalate calculi cannot be dissolved medically.

Both struvite and calcium oxalate calculi can form in the bladder and have the potential to lodge in the urethra. Calculi in the kidneys (nephroliths) and ureters (ureteroliths) are more likely to be composed of calcium oxalate, making their elimination much more difficult. Some indication of the nature of the calculus may be gained from urinalysis. Microscopic examination of urine sediment usually (although not always) reveals mineral crystals, each type with a characteristic shape (see Chapter 5, Fig. 5.9 and Table 5.6). However it is important to realise that the type of crystal seen on sediment examination may not be the same as the main component of the calculus. Urinary pH may also be a clue to the type of calculus present.

Bacterial infection is an uncommon cause of urolithiasis in cats, but is more likely to occur if the urine is more dilute than usual.

Urethral obstruction

EMERGENCY TREATMENT OF THE MALE CAT WITH URETHRAL BLOCKAGE

A male cat with complete or partial urethral obstruction should be treated as a medical emergency, because potentially fatal electrolyte and acid–base irregularities will occur within hours of obstruction.

Additionally, if the bladder enlarges to an abnormal size, the network of nerve fibres that stimulate normal bladder contraction during urination can be damaged, causing permanent loss of function.

Relief of urethral obstruction requires heavy sedation or general anaesthesia, to limit the potential for causing further damage to the urethra. This must be delayed until the fluid and electrolyte status of the cat has been addressed. Immediate bladder decompression by cystocentesis will relieve the pressure and alleviate the immediate crisis.

- **Fluid therapy:** Urethral obstruction produces a combination of dehydration, metabolic acidosis and hyperkalaemia as a result of acute obstructive renal failure. Fluid and electrolyte balance must be restored by intravenous fluid therapy (see p. 82) before undertaking general anaesthesia and relief of the urethral blockage. A solution of 2.5% dextrose in 0.45% NaCl is usually appropriate initially, to restore normal hydration status and decrease serum potassium concentration by expanding blood volume. Severe hyperkalaemia is a potentially fatal complication of acute renal failure. Serial blood electrolyte concentrations should also be measured initially every 1–2 hours. If measurement of serum potassium concentration is not possible, some indication of severe hyperkalaemia may be ascertained by regular cardiac auscultation and/or ECGs, as the heart rate will slow down, and irregularities of rhythm may occur, but this is an unreliable method of monitoring for hyperkalaemia. Once the urethral obstruction has been relieved, potassium-containing fluids, such as Hartmann's solution or Plasmalyte, with additional potassium supplementation, should be administered, because serum potassium levels can fall rapidly, during the inevitable period of post-obstructive diuresis.
- **Relief of urethral obstruction:** As soon as it is safe to anaesthetise the cat the process of unblocking the urethra by the passage of a urinary catheter can be undertaken by the veterinary surgeon. Once in place, the urinary catheter can be used to flush the bladder with sterile saline. A soft catheter is then usually placed and sutured into position and is kept in place for 24–48 hours to provide a patent urethra. There is often haematuria at first, but this should clear within 24–48 hours. The indwelling catheter is usually removed within 24–48 hours. In some cats, the urinary catheter will need to be replaced because of re-obstruction, or left in place longer, if the problem is a recurrence of a very recent episode. In male

cats where urethral blockage is recurrent, a perineal urethrostomy may be considered. This surgical procedure removes the narrow distal part of the urethra and joins the wider proximal urethra to the perineal surface to form a urinary opening. This procedure should only be used as a last resort, as it prevents the risk of urethral obstruction, but may predispose the cat to ascending bacterial urinary tract infections and does not address the underlying cause of the LUTD.

MAINTENANCE OF INDWELLING URINARY CATHETERS
(see Fig. 6.10)
Indwelling urinary catheters pose the risk of causing ascending urinary tract infections. To reduce the risk closed urine collection systems should be used when the cat has an indwelling catheter. The collection system usually consists of a fluid giving set attached to the urinary catheter at one end, with the other end attached to an empty fluid bag (see Fig 6.9). The tubing of the collection system should be taped to the cat's tail to prevent the weight of the system from dragging on the prepuce. If the cat gets distressed or if the cat moving around twists the collection system it is an option to remove the collection system. The catheter can be left open or a bung can be placed on the end of the catheter, which needs to be removed several times daily to allow evacuation of urine.

The time the catheter is left in place should be kept to a minimum. It is advocated not to use routine antibiotics to prevent infection as this is thought to contribute to a resistant bacterial population. Instead, the tip of the catheter should be cultured after removal, so the appropriate antibiotic can be used if anything is cultured. The nurse must observe the patient closely for development of pyrexia, discomfort, pyuria and other signs of UTI and it may be prudent to examine the urine sediment daily when an indwelling catheter is in place.

Before handling the urinary catheter and collecting system it is important to wash hands and to wear disposable gloves. The urine drainage bag is positioned lower than the level of the patient's bladder (see Fig. 6.9) to facilitate free urine flow. It is important to check the line and catheters on a regular basis to make sure they remain fully patent.

The patient needs to wear an Elizabethan collar to avoid damage to the urinary catheter and collection system.

Urinary incontinence

The most common causes of urinary incontinence in cats are pelvic nerve damage following a road traffic

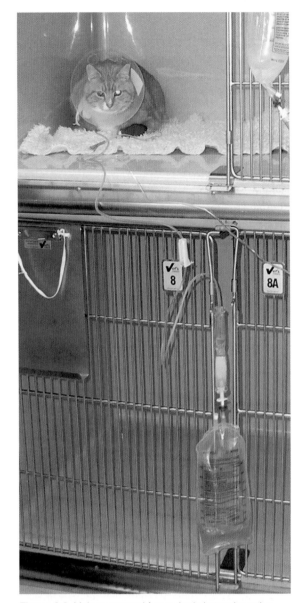

Figure 6.9 Male cat treated for urethral obstruction using urethral catheterisation and a closed urine drainage system.

accident, or local nerve plexus damage resulting from overstretching of the bladder in male cats.

The most common presentation is of a cat with a large, firm bladder, which sometimes dribbles urine because of overflow (overflow incontinence).

TREATMENT OF OVERFLOW INCONTINENCE
The most important factor in promoting healing of an overstretched bladder wall is to keep the bladder constantly decompressed. The best way to do this initially is by placement of a urethral catheter (see previously),

although it is not advisable to maintain this treatment for more than 3–5 days, because of the risk of bacterial urinary tract infection. Urine sediment should be regularly examined for the presence of bacteria and if infection occurs, antibiotic choice should be confirmed by culture and sensitivity of urine. Once the closed drainage system is removed, the bladder must be kept empty by regular manual bladder expression or cystocentesis every 6–8 hours. As the bladder starts to recover, the cat may be able to urinate independently following gentle bladder palpation, and at this stage, medical treatment may be helpful. Drugs that relax the external urethral sphincter assist urination.

HOME MANAGEMENT OF THE CAT WITH URINARY INCONTINENCE

The prognosis for return to urinary continence in most cats is quite good, especially if there has only been bladder wall damage, rather than spinal damage, however return of bladder function often takes several weeks. Occasionally cats do not regain continence, and if they are to be maintained as household pets, they will require regular bladder expression at home, 2–3 times daily. Owners of these cats need to be educated to gently palpate and express the bladder, and must be prepared to maintain this management in the long term. It is often helpful to combine regular bladder expression with medical therapy as described above. Care should be taken that urine is carefully cleaned from the perineal area after bladder expression, so that urine scald does not occur. Clipping the perineal area regularly and the application of an emollient barrier cream may aid in keeping the area clean.

BOX 6.16   KEY POINT: BLADDER PALPATION

Bladder palpation in cats with urethral blockages or overflow incontinence must be *gentle* to avoid bladder rupture.

6.7   INFECTIOUS DISEASES

Infectious diseases are an important cause of illness, and even death, in pet cats. Some infections have already been described in this chapter, for example, the upper respiratory tract infections (see p. 121), but some of the other most significant feline infectious diseases are described here.

Feline leukaemia virus (FeLV)

FeLV is a retrovirus, one of a family of RNA viruses which can enter a host cell and use the enzyme 'reverse transcriptase' to make a DNA copy of themselves (a provirus), which then inserts into the host cell's DNA. Once integrated into the host cell's DNA the provirus does not harm the cell, but it is able to produce new RNA viruses, which then escape from the cell by budding through the cell membrane.

Once FeLV becomes established it sets up a permanent infection, which may suppress the immune system, or cause cancer of the blood cells or lymph nodes. The virus can replicate within many tissues including bone marrow, the salivary glands and respiratory surfaces.

Transmission of FeLV

Viraemic cats continuously shed virus in their saliva, respiratory secretions and urine. Transmission of infection is by direct contact between cats, and saliva is the most important vehicle for spread. Mutual grooming, shared food and water bowls, bite wounds and prolonged, close contact between cats are the most common routes of transmission (Fig. 6.10). Spread via urine, faeces and fleas are much less likely. Iatrogenic transmission can also occur via contaminated needles, surgical and dental instruments or blood transfusions.

Most adult cats that become infected with FeLV are able to mount an effective immune response and eliminate the virus before it becomes permanently established. Kittens (<4 months old) are much more susceptible to infection, and are more likely to develop

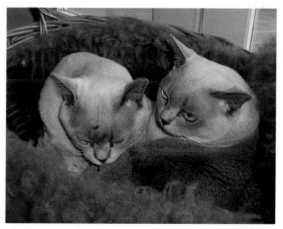

Figure 6.10 Feline leukaemia virus is usually diagnosed in young cats, and is spread by prolonged, close contact.

a permanent infection following exposure to the virus. Most infected cats are between 1 and 6 years of age and will have acquired the infection as kittens. If a queen with FeLV becomes pregnant she can spread the virus to her kittens in utero or via the milk, and kittens infected at this very early stage have a high death rate.

FeLV is a fragile virus, and spread via fomites is uncommon. The virus can survive for 1–3 days in moist environments, but it is inactivated in minutes in a dry environment. Common disinfectants, detergents and alcohol are all effective against FeLV.

Pathogenesis

Following infection, FeLV has a specific pattern of replication. There is initial viral replication in the local lymph nodes, followed by release of virus into the circulation, and spread of virus to all tissues. Once the virus enters the bone marrow, it establishes a permanent infection and the cat then becomes persistently viraemic, that is, there is continual production of new virus, which is released into the circulation. Persistently viraemic cats are a source of infection to other cats, and will eventually become ill from the effects of the virus.

Diagnosis

Diagnostic tests for FeLV are based on detection of viral antigen in the blood (or saliva), which may be present as early as a few days after infection. The ELISA and RIM tests, which are commonly used for in-house screening, can detect free viral antigen in whole blood, plasma, serum, tears or saliva. False-positive and false-negative results can occur using these tests, and the most reliable results will be obtained by using plasma or serum, rather than whole blood, saliva or tears. Kittens can be tested at any age, and maternal immunity or vaccination for FeLV does not interfere with FeLV diagnostic tests. Positive in-house tests should *always* be verified by an external laboratory, especially if the cat appears to be healthy, that is, if a positive result has been found on a routine screening test. If a positive result is confirmed in a healthy cat, the test should be repeated after 12 weeks to ensure that the cat is genuinely persistently viraemic.

Clinical signs

Persistent FeLV infection presents as four main syndromes, which may occur alone, or together:

1. Immunosuppression, presenting with various secondary infections. This accounts for about two-thirds of FeLV-related disease.

2. Neoplastic proliferation of blood cells or bone marrow cells, leading to leukaemia or lymphoma.
3. Degeneration of blood stem cells in the bone marrow leading to anaemia, or reduction in white blood cells.
4. Reproductive disorders including infertility, endometritis, foetal resorption, abortions, and fading kittens, which usually die in the first 2 weeks of life.

Treatment

The most important aspect of treatment is supportive care and management of the secondary problems that arise as a result of the virus. There are no specific anti-viral drugs that will eradicate the virus, although use of agents such as interferons and azidothymidine (AZT) may have some effect in limiting viral multiplication.

When considering whether to treat their FeLV-positive cat, owners must be aware that there is no cure for FeLV, and must also consider the risk the viraemic cat poses to other cats.

Prevention

As with any viral disease, it is best to prevent the infection. There are several ways in which this can be achieved:

- Prevent contact with infected cats.
  - In a single cat household, the cat must remain inside at all times, so that there is no possibility of contact with infected cats.
  - In multiple cat households and catteries, a program of testing all cats and removing or isolating infected cats should be instituted. Cages, food/water bowls, and litter boxes of negative cats must be disinfected regularly, and a barrier system adopted to keep negative cats, suspect cats, and positive cats separate. Follow-up testing must be performed on all positive cats to identify transiently infected or false-positive cats, which can then be separated from the persistently viraemic cats. After two consecutive negative tests, at 3–4 month intervals, a cat may be re-introduced into the cattery. Persistently viraemic cats must be euthanased, or re-homed and kept as indoor cats in a household in which there are no other cats. New owners should be warned of their poor prognosis. All new cats entering a multi-cat household must test negative before they are

introduced. It is important that contact with cats outside the household or cattery should be avoided.

- Vaccination has a role in preventing infection (see Chapter 2), but it is important to remember that no vaccine is 100% effective, and with FeLV, infection usually occurs at a young age and may occur prior to vaccination. As with any viral disease, it is best to prevent the infection.

BOX 6.17   KEY POINT: FeLV

Cats that are persistently positive for FeLV antigens have a very poor prognosis and over 80% succumb to the disease within 3 years.

Feline immunodeficiency virus (FIV)

Like FeLV, FIV is a retrovirus, so it uses the enzyme 'reverse transcriptase' to make a DNA copy of its viral RNA, which is then inserted into the host DNA. FIV is similar to the human immunodeficiency virus (HIV), but is only transmissible between cats.

FIV causes gradual suppression of the infected cat's immune system, eventually leading to chronic ill health, fever, weight loss, anorexia, secondary infections, and enlarged lymph nodes.

An important feature of FIV infection is that the disease is slow to progress, and there is a prolonged latent period before the onset of clinical signs. This asymptomatic period can last for a number of years and in many cases, infected cats remain healthy into old age and never exhibit clinical signs attributable to their FIV infection.

Transmission

FIV is transmitted in the saliva, mostly via biting, so adult cats with free access to the outdoors are at risk. Intact males are at the highest risk. It is unusual for the virus to be transmitted by social contact between co-habiting cats, so it is uncommon for the virus to spread in stable groups of cats that do not fight with each other. Vertical transmission of the virus (queen to kittens) has been achieved *experimentally* but FIV is not spread by sexual contact, close physical contact or by fomites.

Pathogenesis

There are four phases of infection:

1. **Acute stage** – This early stage of infection may last from several days to a few weeks. Clinical signs are often very subtle and are likely to go unnoticed but there may be general enlargement of the lymph nodes and perhaps a mild fever.
2. **Asymptomatic phase** – This phase may last for months to years. The cat is positive for FIV on serological testing, but remains clinically healthy. Many cats remain in this phase and do not progress to the next phase.
3. **Immunodeficient or AIDS-related complex phase** – In this stage there are persistent or intermittent chronic problems such as lower urinary tract disease, oral disease, chronic allergic bronchitis, miliary dermatitis, eosinophilic granuloma complex, chronic abscesses, sinusitis, uveitis, weight loss or diarrhoea.
4. **Terminal phase** – In the final stages of infection cats may become emaciated and develop terminal illness such as malignant neoplasia or renal failure.

Clinical signs

Common clinical signs in the immunodeficient phase of infection are:

- **Persistent generalised enlargement of the lymph nodes.**
- **Inflammation of the oral cavity** including gingivitis, stomatitis and periodontal disease.
- **Chronic upper respiratory tract** disease such as rhinitis (FHV, FCV or *Chlamydophila* infection may be involved) or chronic conjunctivitis.
- **Chronic infections of skin** (see Fig. 6.11), such as bacterial pyodermas, generalised demodectic or notoedric mange or chronic abscesses.
- **Chronic infections of the external ear** such as purulent otitis externa.
- **Chronic enteritis** and wasting associated with chronic small bowel diarrhoea and sometimes vomiting.
- **Opportunistic infections** such as *Toxoplasma gondii*, FCV, FHV, *Mycoplasma felis* infections or generalised demodectic or notoedric mange.
- **Central nervous system (CNS) signs** are less commonly seen, but may involve behavioural changes, seizures, uneven pupil size and muscle twitching.
- **Miscellaneous signs.** These include anorexia, weight loss, fever, recurrent cystitis, uveitis/glaucoma and neoplasia (most commonly lymphoma).

Diagnosis

An in-house ELISA or RIM test can be used to detect antibodies to FIV in a blood sample. Because FIV infection is permanent, the presence of antibody to FIV implies infection, however some false-negative results may occur. Most cats develop antibodies

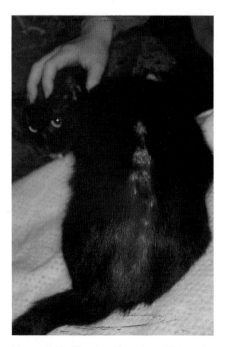

Figure 6.11 Chronic miliary dermatitis may be a presenting sign of the immunodeficient phase of FIV infection. Reproduced with permission from Cathy Curtis.

around 2–4 weeks post-infection, but occasionally it may take over 12 months. Some cats may not produce antibodies against the virus, especially in the terminal phase of infection. False-positive results are uncommon, but can occur. Positive in-house tests should always be confirmed by testing at an external laboratory, especially if the cat appears to be healthy. Kittens born from FIV-positive queens may receive FIV antibodies via the milk and will test positive on blood tests for FIV antibodies. These kittens are not infected with FIV, but their FIV-positive status on blood tests may continue until they are up to 6 months of age. For this reason, it is best to delay testing kittens for the presence of FIV antibodies in the blood until they are over 6 months old. Because FIV is usually transmitted by territorial fighting, infection of young kittens is rare.

On haematology, there may be a non-regenerative anaemia with reduced lymphocytes and neutrophils, and serum biochemistry may reveal high levels of globulins.

Treatment

As with FeLV, the main aim of treatment is to prevent secondary problems where possible by keeping the FIV-positive cat in good health through good nutrition,

deworming, vaccination where appropriate and regular dental care. If secondary problems occur, they must be identified early in their course, and must be treated whenever possible.

Some antiviral immunomodulatory drugs have been used in cats with FIV and have proven beneficial in some cats with chronic stomatitis. However, their effect is often limited, especially because cats are often diagnosed with FIV in the later stages of the disease, whereas these drugs are most effective if used early in the course of disease.

The long-term prognosis for cats with FIV seems to depend to some extent on the geographical area, as different strains of FIV are prevalent in different countries and there are clinical and prognostic differences between different strains. Prognosis worsens once the cat shows signs of immunodeficiency.

Prevention

All male cats should be castrated, and access to the outdoors should be reduced or eliminated. All incoming cats should be tested for FIV before being allowed to mix with others, in case initial territorial fighting occurs.

BOX 6.18 KEY POINT: FIV

Cats may remain healthy in the asymptomatic phase of FIV infection for years or even lifelong, but are infectious to other cats during this period. Ideally, they should be kept as totally indoor pets to prevent territorial fighting.

Feline infectious peritonitis (FIP)

FIP is caused by feline coronavirus (FCoV). There are many different strains of FCoV, most of which do not cause disease or cause mild diarrhoea. In some infected cats a mutation of FCoV occurs, producing a highly pathogenic form of the virus (FIPV) that can evade the cat's immune system and cause FIP. Most cats will eliminate FCoV, but in some, possibly those with less efficient cell-mediated immunity, the disease can progress to FIP.

Transmission

The main source of infection is FCoV viral shedding by healthy carrier cats. Most cats shed virus intermittently after infection and then eliminate FCoV altogether, but some become chronic FCoV shedders. Cats that have eliminated FCoV do not develop long-term protective immunity against future infection. Chronic shedders become a source of infection, re-infecting other cats in the household.

Transmission occurs via contact with virus-containing faeces or saliva, by mutual grooming, and through close contact. Shared litter trays and food bowls are the major source of transmission. Sneezed droplet transmission is also a possibility. FCoV is a relatively fragile virus, but in dry conditions has been shown to survive for up to seven weeks outside the cat, so fomite transmission is also possible. FCoV is readily inactivated by most disinfectants or by a 1:32 solution of bleach.

Pathogenesis
Cats of all ages can be infected with FCoV, but kittens and young cats are at highest risk of developing FIP. Genetic factors, stress, poor husbandry and nutrition, and exposure to chronically shedding carrier cats are all important in the pathogenesis of FIPV.

Once a non-pathogenic FCoV has mutated into the pathogenic FIPV it is carried throughout the body in macrophages, and is therefore transported to those organs that are rich in macrophages, such as the liver, spleen, lymph nodes and blood vessels.

The infected macrophages then trigger an immune-mediated inflammation of the blood vessels (vasculitis). The disease can present in a wide variety of ways and can be broadly categorised into two forms, the 'wet' or effusive form, and the 'dry' or non-effusive form.

The effusive form of FIP involves accumulation of protein-rich effusions in the body cavities (Fig. 6.12). Peritoneal effusion is the most common manifestation, but thoracic and pericardial effusions can also occur.

The non-effusive form of FIP involves granulomatous inflammation of any body organ. Clinical signs depend on the organs involved but neurological or ocular signs are common. Enlarged nodular kidneys (Fig. 6.12) may also be detected on abdominal palpation.

Clinical signs
Young cats (<2 years old) are most at risk of developing FIP, but elderly cats are also susceptible, probably because their immune system becomes less effective with increasing age.

Cats may present with a wide range of clinical signs, most commonly fever, anorexia, weight loss and malaise. There may be an abdominal effusion or a pleural effusion with straw-coloured, proteinaceous fluid. Neurological and ocular signs are more common in the non-effusive form of the disease.

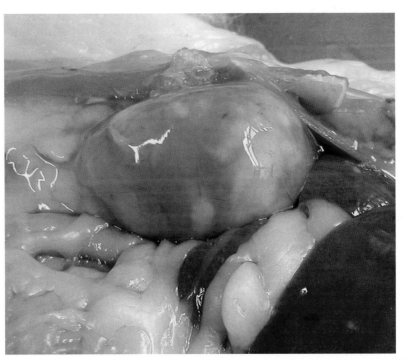

Figure 6.12 Straw-coloured peritoneal fluid and nodular kidney on necropsy in a cat with the 'wet form' of feline infectious peritonitis.

Diagnosis

Confirming the diagnosis of FIP can be difficult, especially in the non-effusive form of the disease. Presumptive diagnosis is based on a combination of age, clinical signs, biochemical and haematological changes, and fluid analysis (in the effusive form).

Histopathological examination of biopsy samples is required to confirm the diagnosis.

Coronavirus antibody titres are not useful for diagnosis of FIP. Many cats have been exposed to the non-pathogenic forms of the virus and will test positive, and a few cats with FIP will test negative, especially in the terminal stages of the disease.

Treatment

FIP is almost always fatal once clinical signs have begun. If the cat's appetite is good, then immunosuppressive doses of corticosteroids (e.g. prednisolone) and broad-spectrum antibiotics are worth considering, but their use is currently controversial.

If clinical signs are restricted to the eyes, topical steroids may be used to treat the uveitis.

Prevention

With regard to prevention of infection, there are three main points to remember:

1. Whether the cat develops FIP depends on how competent the immune system is. A well-fed, healthy cat kept in clean, well-managed surroundings has the best chance of resisting infection with FIPV.
2. Feline coronavirus is carried in the faeces of infected cats, and can be present in infectious quantities on litter trays, dishes, bedding, etc. for up to 3 weeks after they have been contaminated.
3. Most household disinfectants and detergents destroy FCoV.

PREVENTION OF FIPV-INFECTION IN THE CATTERY
- **Reduce faecal contamination.** Have 1 litter tray per 1–2 cats and change them at least once daily. Litter trays should be disinfected, and the area around them should be vacuumed. Longhaired cats may need to have their hindquarters clipped.
- **Reduce overcrowding.** No more than eight cats should be kept in an ordinary household, and catteries should not keep more than 20 cats unless special facilities are provided. Cats should be kept in stable groups of 3–4.
- **Good nutrition.** Homemade diets should be avoided, and good quality canned and dry foods

should be provided. Veterinary advice may be sought on the nutritional needs of cats at different ages and stages of reproduction.
- **Kittens.** A kitten room may be prepared and used for the last 1–2 weeks of the pregnancy. Litter trays and food and water bowls should be dedicated to this room, and washed in a 1:32 bleach solution. If queens that have produced kittens that have subsequently died of FIPV infection are to be used, the kittens should be removed from the queen at 5–6 weeks of age. These queens should be kept separate from all other cats. However, because it is likely that genetics plays an important role in susceptibility to FIP it may be more appropriate not to continue to breed from queens and stud cats that have previously produced kittens that have developed FIP.
- **Avoid stressing known antibody-positive cats.** This includes avoidance of elective surgery, rehoming, pregnancy, showing, and treatment with drugs that may suppress the immune system. Where stressors are unavoidable, for example re-homing and neutering, they should be delayed until the kitten is well-developed, and should not be carried out concurrently.
- **Vaccination.** The currently available FIPV vaccine provides only limited protection from infection. New vaccines are currently being developed.

BOX 6.19   KEY POINT: FIP

A positive feline coronavirus antibody titre only proves exposure to coronavirus, which is very common in cats and cannot be used to make a definitive diagnosis of FIP.

Toxoplasmosis

Toxoplasma gondii is an intracellular protozoan parasite whose definitive hosts are cats and other Felidae. There are two phases of the life cycle – the enteroepithelial (gastrointestinal) phase, and the extra-intestinal (tissue) phase.

When cats are infected by ingestion of an infected intermediate host or infective oocysts in cat faeces, the enteroepithelial life cycle begins, resulting in the shedding of oocysts into the faeces. The enteroepithelial phase only occurs in cats, and is common in kittens and young cats. It often causes no clinical signs. Because of the immune response of the gut to infection, cats usually only shed oocysts once for a short period during their life.

The extra-intestinal phase is far less common but potentially far more clinically severe. It occurs in many hosts, including cats and humans, and is of particular concern because of the risk of abortion and foetal damage if a woman becomes infected for the first time while pregnant (see later). Infection is usually the result of eating meat from infected intermediate hosts. There may be acute generalised disease, usually presenting as fever, dyspnoea and hepatitis in cats less than 1 year of age. Alternatively, chronic focal disease, often involving the CNS and/or the eyes, may occur in cats of any age. An asymptomatic carrier state exists, and infection may be reactivated by concurrent illness or suppression of the immune system, for example, following corticosteroid use.

Clinical signs

The extra-intestinal (tissue) phase has two main clinical presentations:

1. **Acute generalised toxoplasmosis** – This usually affects kittens and cats less than one year of age. Common presenting signs include fever, anorexia, and lethargy. Active pulmonary infection may result in tachypnoea or dyspnoea, and active hepatic infection is usually associated with increased liver enzymes. Neurological signs are seen with active infection of the brain and/or spinal cord, and the signs depend on location of infection.

2. **Localised toxoplasmosis** – This is more often found in older cats and is probably associated with reactivation of a latent infection. Clinical signs are usually referable to the eye or nervous system and depend on the location of infection. Other clinical signs of localised infection may include chronic weight loss or intestinal signs.

Diagnosis

Definitive diagnosis of the extra-intestinal (tissue) phase is difficult and is often made only at post mortem examination.

A presumptive diagnosis of clinical toxoplasmosis can be made on a combination of compatible clinical signs, high serum *Toxoplasma* IgM antibody titres, rising serum IgG antibody titres and response to treatment with an anti-*Toxoplasma* drug.

Treatment

Antibiotic treatment is only effective against active proliferating forms, and will not eliminate dormant cysts in the tissues. Clindamycin is currently the drug of choice and can also be used in the enteroepithelial cycle to stop oocyst shedding.

Prevention

Prevention of infection is an important public health issue, because toxoplasmosis is a zoonotic disease which has severe consequences for the foetus if the mother has her *first* exposure to infection during pregnancy. However, exposure to *Toxoplasma* is extremely common, with up to 90% of women of reproductive age having antibodies to the organism. Women who have previously been infected have enough immunity to prevent complications occurring during pregnancy. Humans are rarely infected by direct contact with cats, because the period of shedding is very short and it takes at least 24 hours for faecal oocysts to become infective. It is much more common for humans to become infected by eating undercooked meat.

A number of simple methods may be instituted to prevent infection:

- Both cats and humans should be fed only cooked meat or commercially processed food. The consumption of undercooked meat is by far the most common source of infection for humans.
- Litter trays should be cleaned daily, but handling of the tray should be avoided by pregnant women. It takes 1–2 days for oocysts to become infective. Gloves should be worn when gardening to avoid contact with cat faeces and infective oocysts, which can remain viable in soil for many months.
- Access to intermediate hosts (e.g. rodents) by cats should be controlled. Cockroaches and flies have also been known to act as mechanical vectors of faecal oocysts, and they may spread oocysts by carrying them on their bodies. Where possible, these insects should also be eliminated.

6.8 HAEMATOLOGICAL DISEASES

The most common haematological condition in cats is anaemia. Clinical signs include pale mucous membranes (sometimes with jaundice), weakness, and shortness of breath (dyspnoea) because of lack of oxygen carrying capacity in the blood. The signs of weakness, lethargy and dyspnoea are usually only seen if the anaemia is advanced, or rapid in onset. In chronic anaemia cats can adapt to the condition and become more sedentary, which enables them to cope with very low levels of red blood cells.

Management of anaemia is aimed at treating the primary cause, so correct diagnosis is vital. Initial investigation of anaemia involves identifying whether the bone marrow is able to produce new red cells to replace cells that are being lost (regenerative anaemia) or whether the anaemia has developed because of lack of production of new red cells (non-regenerative anaemia). Further tests can then be undertaken to identify the precise underlying cause.

Blood transfusion may be useful in the short term to support the cat while these investigations are undertaken, and is usually indicated if the packed cell volume (PCV) is <15%, especially if the PCV is falling rapidly. Close monitoring of the PCV is important, and is quick and straightforward to perform. It is important to use the minimum required volume of blood, as repeated blood sampling will contribute to further red cell loss and may make the anaemia considerably worse.

The main causes of anaemia in practice are:

1. Anaemia secondary to chronic disease.
2. Anaemia associated with chronic renal failure.
3. Anaemia associated with FeLV infection.
4. Anaemia associated with blood loss: This may be from acute loss following trauma, or chronic loss for instance in the gastrointestinal tract.
5. Feline infectious anaemia – *Mycoplasma haemofelis* infection.

Anaemia of chronic disease

This condition is multifactorial and partially due to sequestration of iron within macrophages, causing a non-regenerative anaemia (reticulocyte percentage <2.5%).

It is common in chronic inflammatory and neoplastic conditions and usually causes a progressive, relatively mild anaemia (PCV in the high teens to the low 20s). The main treatment is management of the primary cause. A blood transfusion may be indicated to support the cat while the treatment of the primary disease takes effect.

Haemolytic anaemia

Haemolysis in the cat causes a regenerative anaemia, and can be associated with infection by *Mycoplasma haemofelis* (see below). Certain drugs, toxins, metabolic conditions (hypophosphataemia in diabetes mellitus) and foods (e.g. onions) can cause oxidative injury to erythrocytes and subsequent haemolysis.

Immune-mediated haemolytic anaemia is less common in cats than in dogs.

Another form of haemolytic anaemia is neonatal isoerythrolysis. This can occur in newborn kittens when a queen with type B blood is mated to a stud cat with type A blood. The queen's milk will contain anti-A antibodies, which cause haemolysis if the kitten has type A blood.

Mycoplasma haemofelis (formerly Haemobartonella felis)

Pathogenesis

The organism that causes feline infectious anaemia has now been reclassified as a type of *Mycoplasma*, and it is recognised that there are at least two closely related organisms: *Mycoplasma haemofelis* is a pathogenic agent that causes anaemia, while *Mycoplasma haemominutum* appears to be less pathogenic in most circumstances. These organisms infect red cells and can be seen as small, dark staining inclusions on the surface of red cells (see Fig. 6.13). The number of organisms present fluctuates considerably during different phases of infection, and within the course of a single day. In the case of *M. haemofelis* infected red cells are recognised by the spleen and removed from the circulation, causing anaemia. The disease can exist in a carrier state, and the infected cat may suffer chronic intermittent relapses at times of stress or concurrent illness. Cats are probably infected via fleas and ticks, but vector transmission is unproven. Blood transfusions can also be a source of infection.

There are four phases of infection:

1. **Prepatent phase** – The organism is not detectable in the blood. This phase usually lasts for 1–3 weeks.
2. **Acute phase** – The number of organisms increases. Infected, damaged red blood cells are recognised as foreign and removed by the spleen causing anaemia. Without treatment, 33% of cats die during the acute phase of infection.
3. **Recovery phase** – The parasite burden reduces and the immune response to previously infected red blood cells gradually decreases. The PCV increases in this phase as new cells are produced by the bone marrow, and there are only low numbers of organisms in blood smears.

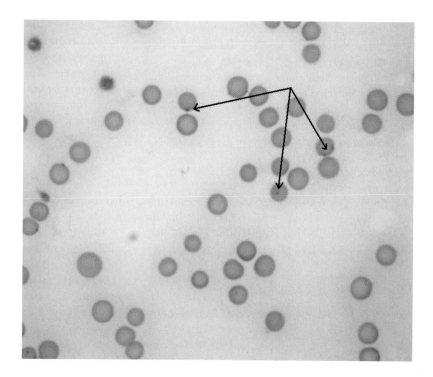

Figure 6.13 Diff-Quik stained blood smear from a *Mycoplasma haemofelis*-infected cat, showing organisms on the red blood cell membranes (arrows).

4. **Carrier phase** – A high proportion of recovered cats remain infected, but are clinically normal. Occasionally a few organisms are seen on blood smears, but infection is essentially silent in this phase. There may be a relapse of disease if the cat becomes stressed or ill.

Clinical signs

In the acute phase of infection cats may be presented with a history of depression, anorexia, weight loss and weakness. On physical examination there are pale mucous membranes, perhaps with jaundice, and there may be dyspnoea due to anaemia. Sometimes the spleen is enlarged on abdominal palpation, and about 50% of cats have a low-grade fever. Carrier cats may have milder episodes without showing marked clinical signs and the anaemia is less severe in these cases.

Diagnosis

On haematology there are usually signs of regeneration, i.e. increased numbers of circulating immature red cells (reticulocytes).

The most reliable diagnostic test is a PCR on a blood sample. This test has a high sensitivity and also differentiates between pathogenic and non-pathogenic strains of *Mycoplasma*.

The organism may also be seen on the surface of erythrocytes on blood smears forming chains, rods or rings (see Fig. 6.13). However, examination of blood smears is an unreliable means of diagnosis, partly because there are a number of other red cell inclusions and artefacts that may mimic *M. haemofelis*, and also because organisms are only detected around 50% of the time, depending on the stage of infection when blood is collected.

BOX 6.20   KEY POINT: *MYCOPLASMA HAEMOFELIS*

Mycoplasma haemofelis causes fluctuating haemolytic anaemia, and cats often become carriers. Relapses may occur during stress or concurrent disease.

Treatment

The main principles of treatment for *Mycoplasma haemofelis* infection are:

- To eliminate the organisms from the circulation: Doxycycline or tetracycline are the antibiotics of choice.

- To treat the anaemia: A blood transfusion may be required if the PCV is <15%, especially if it is decreasing rapidly.
- To suppress the immune reaction to infected and formerly infected red blood cells. In most cases, a secondary immune-mediated haemolytic anaemia contributes significantly to the severity of the clinical signs, so immunosuppressive doses of corticosteroids may be helpful.

It should be remembered that treatment of the acute phase of infection does not eliminate all organisms from the circulation, rather the infection moves from the acute phase into the carrier phase. Carrier cats often relapse, especially if they become ill for other reasons.

Anti-rodenticide coagulopathy

Most of the poisons that are commonly used to control rat and mouse infestations contain agents that act by prolonging blood clotting times, causing death from massive haemorrhage. These poisons stop the conversion of vitamin K to its active form, thereby halting the production of a number of key clotting factors by the liver.

Accidental ingestion of the toxin, or of a rodent that has eaten the toxin, can cause a significant coagulopathy. Younger cats are usually affected, and there is sometimes a history of access to rat poison, or of hunting affected rodents. First generation rodenticides (warfarin) do not cause a coagulopathy if ingested via a poisoned rodent, but second generation rodenticides (diphacinone, brodifacoum) may. Clinical signs of a coagulopathy generally occur 3–4 days after ingestion of the poison, and include pale mucous membranes, weakness and bruising. The underlying coagulopathy is treated with vitamin K and blood transfusion may be necessary to provide immediate support.

6.9   NEUROLOGICAL DISEASE

When considering the needs of a cat suffering from a neurological disorder it is helpful to categorise the condition according to which part(s) of the nervous system are affected. In broad terms the nervous system can be subdivided into three important regions:

1. **The peripheral nerves:** These are the sensory and motor nerves, which communicate between the organs and muscles of the body and the spinal cord and brain.

2. **The spinal cord:** The nervous tissue of the spinal cord provides the link between the peripheral nerves and the brain.

3. **The brain:** The brain receives and co-ordinates information from the sensory nerves, and initiates appropriate responses, which are activated via the motor nerves.

Disorders of the peripheral nerves

Disorders of the peripheral nervous system are relatively uncommon in cats. When they do occur, they may affect a single nerve or multiple nerves (polyneuropathy).

Disorders affecting a single peripheral nerve are most commonly a result of trauma, or loss of blood supply due to thromboembolism. Less common causes include pressure on the nerve from a neighbouring structure, e.g. a tumour or abscess, and tumours of the peripheral nerve itself.

The most commonly encountered polyneuropathy is the peripheral polyneuropathy that affects cats with long-standing poorly controlled diabetes mellitus. Other causes of peripheral polyneuropathy are rare, and include dysautonomia, metabolic disorders (e.g. hyperglycaemia and disorders of lipid metabolism), toxins (e.g. organophosphates, vincristine), some congenital disorders (storage diseases) and idiopathic peripheral polyneuropathy, which has some similarities to the human condition Guillain-Barré syndrome.

The nursing care requirements for cats affected by these conditions are similar to the requirements of cats with spinal disorders (see below). Management of the underlying disease, if any, is also important.

Disorders of the spinal column

Spinal cord damage in cats is usually traumatic in origin. Other potential causes include neoplasia, multifocal infections such as FIP and focal infections such as abscesses or discospondylitis. Paraparesis due to intervertebral disc disease is rare.

The spinal cord is arranged in segments. Neurological signs depend very much on which segment(s) of the spinal cord is affected as only the neurons at the level of and below the affected segment(s) are affected. Depending on the location of the lesion along the spinal column, clinical signs can be described as upper motor neuron or lower motor neuron.

Lower motor neuron signs (flaccid paralysis, muscle atrophy and loss of segmental reflexes) will occur in the muscles supplied by nerves of the spinal cord that are affected by the disease process.

Upper motor neuron signs will occur below the damaged segment, if the peripheral nerve is still working properly. The reduction of the normal inhibition of involuntary movement will result in exaggerated reflexes.

Affected cats may have deficits affecting their limbs, bladder or bowel. Limbs may be non-functional (paralysis) or partially functional (paresis); affected limbs may be on one side of the body (unilateral) or on both sides of the body (bilateral).

By doing a full neurological examination, which includes determining if there are abnormal upper or lower motor neuron signs, the veterinary surgeon can determine if the problem is unifocal or multifocal and where in the spinal cord the pathology is most likely to be.

Nursing care of the cat with peripheral or spinal neurological disease

Nursing care and physical rehabilitation are often just as important as specific medical or surgical treatments in the clinical outcome for a paralysed cat. This takes time, a gentle approach and patience. Given careful instructions, some owners may be able to provide this care at home once the initial acute nursing and treatment requirements have been supplied.

BLADDER CARE

Many peripheral nerve and spinal cord conditions cause loss of voluntary urination and the bladder must be kept decompressed to avoid overfilling and subsequent permanent damage to the bladder wall. The bladder must be emptied every 8 hours, using gentle bladder expression. Drugs which help relaxation of the bladder sphincter and stimulation of bladder contraction may be used. Bedding that draws moisture away from the cat, such as disposable diaper material, should be used to avoid urine scald. If increased urethral tone prevents manual expression, other methods such as cystocentesis, or placement of an indwelling catheter, will be required. Catheterisation should be avoided whenever possible because of the risk of bacterial urinary tract infection (see Home management of overflow incontinence, p. 149).

IN-HOSPITAL CARE

Paralysed cats should be turned frequently to prevent consolidation of the dependent lung lobe (hypostatic pneumonia), pressure sores or wound infections. Plenty of soft bedding covered in a surface material that draws moisture away from the skin should be provided. Heating pads may be necessary, but should be used with extreme care to prevent burns.

Regular grooming should be performed and perineal bathing with warm soapy water may be necessary if there is faecal incontinence. It is essential to keep the cage clean, comfortable and free of bacterial contamination. If there is faecal retention dietary manipulation or enemas as used in treatment for constipation, may help (see p. 139).

EXERCISE AND PHYSICAL THERAPY

Gentle assisted exercise is effective in maintaining joint mobility and stimulating circulation in weakened muscles. Limbs may be massaged vigorously to stimulate muscle tone and delay muscle contracture. A towel may be used as a sling to support the hindquarters in paraplegic cats, so that brief periods of walking can be encouraged.

PROGNOSIS

The long-term outlook for cats that have suffered spinal cord damage or have a peripheral neuropathy will depend on the underlying cause and severity of the problem. In some cases, if specific treatment can be started promptly after the incident, the prognosis for return to limb and bladder function is improved, e.g. orthopaedic repair of traumatic spinal injury. In the ideal scenario if the cat has been paraplegic for 48 hours or less and adequate surgical decompression and stabilisation of the spinal cord can be performed, voluntary urination and normal pain responses may return in 2–3 weeks. If the spinal cord injury is reversible, good voluntary limb movement should return within 4–5 weeks, and the cat should be able to stand unassisted within 6–8 weeks.

Central neurological disease

Some of the most common causes of central neurological disease in cats are infectious agents, such as feline infectious peritonitis virus, toxoplasmosis and fungal infections e.g. *Cryptococcus neoformans*. Other causes include trauma, non-suppurative meningoencephalitis, ischaemic encephalopathy, hepatic encephalopathy and thiamine deficiency.

Neoplastic disease of the central nervous system usually causes unifocal problems, where the neurological problems are referable to the specific location of the tumour in the brain. The most frequent intracranial neoplasm in cats is meningioma. These neoplasms are usually reported in older cats, and they cause chronic, progressive illness. Bone changes such as tumour mineralisation, and bone growth or lysis of the skull overlying the tumour are sometimes visible on skull radiographs. Advanced imaging with MRI/CT and stereotactic brain biopsy is the diagnostic method of choice for meningiomas. Meningiomas may be completely or partially removed surgically, and radiation is often used as adjunctive therapy.

Clinical signs of central neurological disease

Clinical signs are referable to the anatomical area of the brain that is affected (see Fig. 6.14).

- **Cerebral cortex** – Abnormal behaviour, depression, circling and seizures.
- **Thalamus and hypothalamus** – Abnormal behaviour, depression, possibly gait abnormalities.
- **Brainstem (midbrain, pons and medulla oblongata)** – Depression, stupor, coma.
- **Central vestibular system** – Depression, head tilt, incoordination, nystagmus. Involvement of surrounding tissues may result in paresis or paralysis.
- **Peripheral vestibular system** – Head tilt, incoordination, circling, nystagmus and sometimes vomiting.
- **Cerebellum** – Tremors, incoordination and sometimes nystagmus.

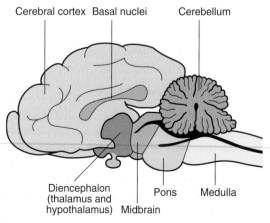

Figure 6.14 Anatomical areas of the brain.

Cerebral cortex Basal nuclei Cerebellum

Diencephalon (thalamus and hypothalamus) Pons Medulla Midbrain

- **Cranial nerves** – Disorders of the senses (e.g. smell, sight, and hearing) as well as paralysis or lack of sensation of the head, face or neck, depending on which nerve is affected.

BOX 6.21   KEY POINT: CNS DISEASE

A thorough diagnostic work-up should be performed in all cats with central neurological disease, including screening for common infectious agents such as FIPV, toxoplasmosis, FeLV, FIV and cryptococcosis.

Metabolic causes of CNS signs

These generally affect the cerebral cortex since the cortex is the area of the brain that receives the largest blood supply. Clinical signs are usually symmetric, and include depression, seizures, head pressing, and disorientation.

- **Hepatic encephalopathy** – This is caused by the build-up of metabolic by-products during liver failure. It is usually diagnosed in cats less than one year of age and is associated with a congenital portosystemic shunt but can also be diagnosed in older cats secondary to hepatic lipidosis or inflammatory liver disease.
- **Hypoglycaemia** – Hypoglycaemia is a common problem in neonatal kittens, as a result of immaturity of the liver enzymes involved in gluconeogenesis, coupled with inadequate food intake. Typical signs are of weakness, depression/lethargy and sometimes seizures. In adult cats, hypoglycaemia is most commonly seen with insulin overdose in diabetes mellitus. Affected cats can become lethargic, have tremors or twitching, dilated pupils and a 'drunken' staggering gait. Without treatment it may progress to semi-coma, seizures and/or coma. Insulinoma, an insulin-secreting pancreatic tumour, will cause hypoglycaemia, but is an extremely rare condition in cats.
- **Thiamine deficiency** – Thiamine plays an important role in energy metabolism, and cats require greater dietary amounts than dogs. A deficiency can occur if cats are fed meat that has been treated with thiamine-destroying preservatives; it can be secondary to anorexia or diuresis (urinary loss); and it can occur if the cat is fed an

all-fish diet (carp, herring), which contains high levels of thiaminase. On clinical examination there may be ventroflexion of the neck, and vestibular signs such as ataxia and nystagmus. There is often pupillary dilation with a poor pupillary light response in the absence of blindness. 'Convulsions' may occur. These are not thought to be true seizures, but rather an exacerbation of vestibular signs due to severe spatial disorientation. Thiamine deficiency may cause death within 24 hours of the convulsive stage if left untreated. Thiamine injections (100–250 mg b.i.d.) lead to a resolution of signs within 24–48 hours, although some residual signs may be present in severe cases.

Emergency treatment of central neurological disease

Treatment of the primary cause of central neurological disease, if possible, forms the basis of the therapeutic regime. If the cat has head injuries and has lost consciousness, the first priority should be to ensure that there is a patent airway. Supplemental oxygen should be provided, if necessary by an endotracheal tube, or tracheostomy tube if the airway is blocked. If the cat stops breathing, artificial respiration should be performed, using 12–15 breaths per minute. If the heart has stopped, cardiac massage should be commenced, using lateral compressions of the lower third of the chest at 80–120 compressions per minute.

If the cat has prolonged seizures (status epilepticus), control is essential to prevent further brain damage. An intravenous injection of diazepam (up to 0.5 mg/kg, given to effect) is usually the drug of first choice, as it is very safe, and is effective in the majority of cases. Further treatment with other anticonvulsant drugs may then be required to prevent future seizure activity.

Home care of the deaf or blind cat

Cats that have lost their hearing or sight may be kept as household pets, and often adapt remarkably well to their disability, especially if it is present from birth, or develops gradually. These cats are particularly vulnerable to road traffic accidents, or to attack by dogs or other cats. They should be kept indoors only, except perhaps for short periods outside supervised closely by the owner.

If the onset of blindness is slow, some cats cope so well with their disability that the owner is quite unaware of the loss of sight. Blind cats tend to spend their time in just a few rooms, where they can memorise the position of furniture. It is best to keep changes of furniture position to a minimum and have a constant position for food and water bowls and litter trays.

Deaf cats can be relatively independent, but should not be allowed outside unsupervised, as they are at serious risk of road accidents.

6.10   NEOPLASTIC DISEASES

Definition of neoplasia

A neoplasm (tumour) occurs when the cell division rate, which is normally well controlled by the cell, becomes uncontrollably fast. A tumour usually arises from one stem cell and is initially homogenous, but becomes more heterogenous with time as mutations occur. A tumour is considered highly malignant if it grows fast, is locally invasive and spreads easily to other organs (high metastatic rate).

Causes

Specific causes of feline tumours are poorly understood. Known associations are those between vaccination and vaccine-induced fibrosarcoma; feline sarcoma virus and fibrosarcoma; UV-light and squamous cell carcinoma; long-term progesterone therapy and mammary gland tumours; FeLV infection and lymphoma or other haematogenous tumours.

Undoubtedly there are genetic influences, but these are poorly understood in cats. There are some breed predispositions, such as mast cell tumours in Siamese cats.

Diagnosis

The veterinary surgeon may suspect a neoplastic process on the basis of the signalment, history, clinical signs and physical examination, but further diagnostic tests are necessary to confirm the diagnosis. The clinical signs are obviously very much influenced by the organ affected by the neoplasm.

Baseline biochemistry, haematology and survey radiography of chest and abdomen may give some clues as to the extent of the problem. In some cases a fine needle aspirate of the suspect organ may be sufficient to get a diagnosis, but in most cases histopathology of a biopsy sample from the organ is necessary to make a definitive diagnosis. It is essential to get a tissue diagnosis, as this will affect the treatment and prognosis. Additional tests may be required to stage the tumour, i.e. to evaluate the severity and degree of spread to other sites in the body, which again will affect the prognosis significantly.

Treatment options

Supportive treatment of neoplasia focuses on the specific organ system(s) involved. As well as pathological effects caused locally by the tumour, there are also more widespread effects, such as the release of substances by the tumour which cause the body to switch to a metabolic state where cells and tissues are broken down and used to help tumour growth (catabolism). Extra nutritional support is required to support healthy tissue and the diet should be high in protein, fat and calories, with relatively low proportions of carbohydrate, which may support tumour growth. Weight should be closely monitored in cats diagnosed with neoplasia.

A number of modalities can be used to treat feline neoplasia. For ethical reasons, the potential side effects of the treatment must be balanced against the possible benefit to the cat. The main treatments commonly used in general practice include chemotherapy using anti-cancer drugs, and surgery, while radiation therapy is available at some referral centres. Surgery alone usually provides a permanent cure for benign tumours, while surgery and/or chemotherapy and/or radiation therapy may be required to halt the spread of malignant tumours. In some cases, a combination of different kinds of therapy is considered optimal.

Anti-cancer regimes are potent therapies that often cause side effects in treated cats. Radiation therapy may cause local burns, which result in tissue sloughing and necrosis. The affected area needs to be kept clean and dry, preferably covered with a bandage that allows the wound to breathe.

Common side effects with chemotherapeutic drugs include vomiting and reduced counts of white blood cells. This is because chemotherapy is designed to attack rapidly dividing cells, and does not discriminate between tumour cells and normal tissues with a high rate of cell division, such as GI mucosa cells and white blood cells. It is therefore important to have baseline haematological values for comparison and to closely monitor haematological parameters in cats under treatment.

Correct handling of chemotherapeutic agents is essential (see p. 79).

Common tumours in the cat

Some of the more commonly diagnosed tumours in the cat include:

Lymphoma
This is a relatively common feline tumour of the lymphatic system, with peaks of prevalence in young and old cats. Tumours are classified according to their anatomical site: mediastinal (thymic), abdominal (GIT and associated lymph nodes, kidneys, or organs such as the liver or spleen without GIT or renal involvement), nodal (a single lymph node, a chain of adjacent lymph nodes in one area, or many/all peripheral lymph nodes) and atypical (includes lymphoma of non-lymphoid tissues such as the CNS, skin, larynx and nasal cavity). The tumours at each anatomical site have different characteristics in terms of the signalment of cats affected and the prognosis. Lymphocytic leukaemia is a related neoplasia. Other related conditions are myeloproliferative neoplasms such as myelogenous leukaemia. FeLV or FIV infection may predispose to the development of lymphoma or leukaemia, and serological tests for these viral agents should always be performed when a cat is diagnosed with lymphoma, as the predicted response to treatment and overall prognosis is affected by retroviral infection. Treatment of lymphoma usually involves a combination of chemotherapeutic agents, sometimes preceded by surgical resection of the tumour. As mentioned above, it is common for certain chemotherapeutic agents to have GI or haematological side effects, and cats undergoing chemotherapy should be closely monitored for these.

Squamous cell carcinoma
One of the sites for this tumour to develop is the skin. The cutaneous form of this tumour is commonly found on the ears and nasal planum of cats with white skin in these areas and is strongly associated with the amount of sunlight (UV radiation) that the cat has been exposed to. At first, non-healing sores or erosive lesions are seen on the nasal planum and ear tips, followed by progressive local tissue loss. It can be prevented in most areas by keeping the cat indoors, reducing exposure to direct sunlight. Effective treatment options include surgical resection, often followed by cryotherapy or radiation therapy.

Vaccine-associated sarcoma

This is a locally aggressive form of tumour that has been reported in recent years. It grows at the site of vaccination and sometimes other types of injections, and its exact cause is as yet poorly understood. Aggressive surgical resection, ideally combined with radiation therapy, is required to slow the growth of this tumour, and the prognosis is guarded at best.

EMERGENCY CARE AND FIRST AID

CHAPTER 7

Myra Forster-van Hijfte, DVM CertVR CertSAM DipECVIM MRCVS
Annette Litster, BVSc PhD FACVSc(Feline Medicine)

When an owner finds that their cat is in need of emergency care they may contact their veterinary practice by telephone, or they may arrive in the practice requiring immediate attention. In either situation a veterinary nurse is often the owner's first point of contact, so it is essential that they are able to make a rapid assessment of the patient's requirements, are competent to provide veterinary first aid, and are able to offer sound telephone advice to an owner to ensure that a cat's emergency care requirements are met with minimum delay.

7.1 EMERGENCY SET-UP

First of all it is important to develop certain protocols within your practice in order to be able to deal with an emergency in the best possible way. Some practices may have a referral institution or emergency clinic nearby and it is advisable to have an internal agreement whether certain emergencies are not better referred immediately. Most veterinary practices will however not have these options and will have to deal with an emergency to the best of their ability.

Staff

Especially in a larger group practice it may be worth dedicating a few veterinary surgeons and nurses to deal with emergencies. This should ideally be a team that is especially interested in emergency care and has received further training in this field. There may also be several veterinary surgeons within the practice that have an increased knowledge in certain areas, such as internal medicine, surgery, ophthalmology etc. who potentially could deal with emergencies within their field of expertise.

Tasks need to be assigned, such as placing of an intravenous catheter, taking of blood and urine samples, and maintaining airway patency and oxygenation.

Equipment

You have to determine *where* within the practice you are going to deal with an emergency so that staff know where to bring/find the patient and also where all the equipment will be available.

The level of equipment will dictate the level of emergency care that is available. The following list is a minimum requirement for all practices:

- Oxygen (including masks, endotracheal tubes, tracheostomy tubes).
- Laryngoscope.
- Intravenous-catheters (including butterfly catheters).
- Clippers.
- Stethoscope.
- Thermometer.
- Surgical pack and blades.
- Urinary catheters.
- Surgical spirit, chlorhexidine scrub.
- Syringes/needles.
- Heating pad.
- Blood and urine tubes.
- Mini laboratory (urinary dipsticks, refractometer, microhaematocrit tubes, centrifuge, blood glucose sticks, blood urea sticks, microscope).
- Intravenous fluids (including saline, Hartmann's solution, mannitol, hypertonic saline).
- Drugs: atropine, adrenaline 1:10 000, calcium gluconate, methylprednisolone, frusemide, dobutamine, dopamine, dextrose, euthanasia solution, pentobarbital, sodium bicarbonate (if blood gas analysis available), propofol, diazepam, pethidine, glyceryl trinitrate ointment.

It is essential that staff are familiar with the use of all this equipment, including the drugs. Dosage charts (see Box 7.1) should be readily available for rapid reference. It is no use stocking any of these drugs if the staff are not familiar with the use and side effects of the drugs.

Further more advanced equipment includes:

- Fluid pumps, ECG, pulse oximetry, blood pressure monitor, inhalation chamber, face mask and metred dose inhaler (MDI), blood gas analyser, coagulation analyser, suction pump, full laboratory including electrolyte monitoring, central venous pressure monitoring.

165

This more advanced equipment is very useful in the right hands and will provide a higher level of emergency care.

BOX 7.1   EXAMPLE DOSAGE CHART

Adrenaline (1:10 000 = 100 µg/ml):

Cardiac arrest:

10–20 µg/kg i.v.

200 µg/kg intratracheal

Anaphylactic shock:

2.5–5 µg/kg i.v.

50 µg/kg intratracheal

Atropine: 0.02–0.04 mg/kg i.v.

Calcium gluconate (100 mg/ml): 0.5–1.5 ml/kg i.v. slowly

Dextrose 50% (dilute 1:1saline): 1–2 ml/kg i.v. slowly to effect

Diazepam: 0.5 mg/kg i.v.

Dobutamine: 0.5–2 µg/kg/minute i.v. infusion

Dopamine: 1–5 µg/kg/minute i.v. infusion

Frusemide: 1–2 mg/kg i.v. b.i.d.or t.i.d.

Mannitol: 0.25-2 g/kg i.v. slowly over 30–60 minutes

Methylprednisolone sodium succinate: 30 mg/kg i.v.

Nitroglycerine ointment: 1/4 inch ointment topically

Pentobarbital: 25–30 mg/kg i.v.

Propofol: 6.6 mg/kg i.v.

Pethidine: 5–10 mg/kg i.m.

b.i.d. or t.i.d., twice or three times daily; i.v., intravenously, i.m., intramuscularly.

7.2   INITIAL ASSESSMENT: TRIAGE

On arrival at the practice the emergency care patient must be rapidly but systematically assessed in order to identify the severity of the situation, and the immediate requirements for treatment. This process is known as 'triage' and it is an essential first step in the care of any injured or collapsed cat. The aim is to perform a quick but thorough examination of the major body systems in order to identify and reverse any life-threatening problem. Once the cat has been stabilised a more detailed examination will be required, and attention can then be paid to any non life-threatening injuries.

All veterinary nurses should be familiar with the aims and priorities of triage, and be able to undertake basic life saving first aid measures while awaiting veterinary assistance. Always remember the 'ABC' of emergency care – 'A' is for airway; 'B' is for breathing; 'C' is for circulation.

When making your assessment do not get drawn into obvious injuries and overlook less obvious major problems. For instance a cat that has suffered a road traffic accident may have a very obvious degloving injury and fractures, but a life threatening pneumothorax may not be immediately apparent. A cat will not die from a lack of immediate treatment to a degloving injury or fracture, but will almost certainly die from a neglected pneumothorax.

Respiratory system

Apnoea

The absence of breathing (apnoea) is an emergency and an airway needs to be established as soon as possible. A veterinary surgeon needs to be contacted immediately but the veterinary nurse should not delay in establishing an airway. CPR should be started immediately (see later). Failure to maintain a supply of oxygen to the lungs will rapidly cause permanent brain damage, or death.

Dyspnoea

Increased breathing effort (dyspnoea) may be seen as more pronounced movements of the chest wall, open-mouthed breathing or marked abdominal effort during the breathing cycle. If this is the case a veterinary surgeon should be consulted immediately and the cat should be handled as little as possible. It is important to realise that a cat with increased breathing effort is already oxygen deficient, and any increase in oxygen requirement due to stress or struggling may tip the balance and cause life-threatening hypoxia. These cats must be handled with as little stress as possible and it is often prudent to supply additional oxygen at this stage (see Section 7.4).

Some cats suffering from respiratory distress may also have increased upper respiratory noise (stertor or stridor), which indicates an obstruction along the respiratory pathway.

When faced with a severely dyspnoeic cat the following needs to be taken into account:

1. **Do not stress the cat.** The first priority is to sustain life, so the cat should be handled as little as possible.

Observing the cat may give clues to the location of the problem (upper airway versus lower airway).

2. **Place the cat in an oxygen-rich environment,** e.g. an oxygen tent, incubator or oxygenated cage. Light sedation may be beneficial to calm a panicking cat.

3. **Use symptomatic therapy** based on the history and clinical examination.
   - For emergency treatment of lower airway disease use steroids and bronchodilators, via an inhaler if available
   - For cardiac failure, use intravenous diuretics and nitroglycerine cream applied to the inside of the pinna, or a shaved patch in the groin or axilla.
   - For pleural effusion, emergency drainage is required.

4. **Delay further investigations,** e.g. radiography, ultrasonography and blood sampling, until the clinical condition is more stable.

Pulse

The pulse rate in the cat is normally between 120–180/minute: the rhythm should be regular, without pulse deficits. Any irregularity in rhythm should be noted. Abnormal heart rates, whether too slow (bradycardia) or too fast (tachycardia) should be reported to a veterinary surgeon immediately.

An absence of femoral pulses is always an emergency. It may mean that the heart has stopped contracting, the blood pressure is too low, or there is a blockage in the circulation preventing blood entering the femoral artery, e.g. a blood clot (thrombus). If femoral pulses are not palpable, the heart beat needs to be palpated through the chest wall, or auscultated with a stethoscope. If the heart beat is absent cardiopulmonary resuscitation (CPR) should be started immediately (see later).

Neurological system

In an emergency triage situation the most common neurological emergency is the cat that has ongoing seizure activity. Anti-seizure medication is usually indicated to prevent further seizure activity and 'status epilepticus'. A veterinary surgeon should be contacted immediately.

Body temperature

Many cats that require emergency care will have a subnormal body temperature (hypothermia) and gentle re-warming, using blankets, heat pads and/or hot water bottles is required. This will improve mental state, circulation and metabolism, as well as making the cat more comfortable.

Less commonly the body temperature will be significantly elevated due to heat stroke, or due to massive muscle activity during a prolonged seizure (hyperthermia). Affected cats require cooling to prevent permanent damage to the nervous system. This is best done using a fan, or by applying cool water to the coat, paws or ears. Ice packs and very cold water are best avoided as they may cause peripheral vasoconstriction, which will reduce heat loss. Cooling is not appropriate, and may be harmful, if the raised temperature is due to fever: if in doubt seek advice from a veterinary surgeon before applying cooling methods.

On the basis of the initial assessment the cat can be classed as:

- Class I – Catastrophic/dying: needs to be dealt with immediately. A patient suffering cardiac arrest, respiratory arrest or continued seizure activity is in class I.
- Class II – Critical: needs to be dealt with as soon as possible. Patients with toxic ingestion, shock, haemorrhage or breathing difficulties belong in this category.
- Class III – Urgent: needs to be dealt with within a few hours. Patients with open fractures, severe dehydration, urethral obstruction etc.
- Class IV – Less seriously ill, but requires attention within 24 hours. Patients that are anorexic or lame fall into this category.

Having assessed these vital signs and provided immediate treatment as required, a brief history can

BOX 7.2   KEY POINTS: EMERGENCY TRIAGE

- Contact a veterinary surgeon as soon as practically possible.
- Gain consent, verbal or written.
- Aim is to prevent suffering.
- Be aware of your limitations.
- Be methodical.
- Do not overlook the life-threatening to treat the obvious.

be taken and consent for further treatment can be obtained from the owner.

7.3 CARDIOPULMONARY RESUSCITATION (CPR)

When the triage examination reveals lack of respiratory or cardiac function, immediate cardiopulmonary resuscitation is required.

Airway

The first priority is to check for, and clear, any obvious obstruction to breathing. Extending the cat's neck to straighten the trachea, and pulling the tongue forward to clear the back of the mouth may be enough to re-establish an airway. Take care not to get bitten if the cat is conscious or semi-conscious.

Breathing

If the cat remains apnoeic assisted breathing will be required. In unconscious patients it is most appropriate to place an endotracheal tube, which will allow effective intermittent positive pressure ventilation (IPPV) to be provided. In cases of laryngeal or tracheal obstruction, it may prove difficult or impossible to place an endotracheal tube and a tracheotomy will be necessary to deliver oxygen. Around 10–15 breaths/minute need to be delivered.

If oxygen is not immediately available then mouth to nose resuscitation can be administered to force air into the lungs. This requires the first aid provider to place their mouth over the cat's nose and mouth and to blow firmly to introduce air into the cat's lungs, watching the chest wall to check that the lungs are being inflated. The first aid provider then removes their mouth from the cat's face to allow exhalation by elastic recoil of the thoracic wall, before repeating the process a few seconds later. Watch carefully for recovery of spontaneous breathing efforts. This is a short-term measure and is only appropriate if no equipment is available to provide more effective help, or until such help is available. It should not be performed unless it can be done without risk of the cat biting the first aid provider.

A tight-fitting mask connected to an oxygen supply can also be used for assisted breathing and is preferable to mouth to nose resuscitation. The mask is fitted over the cat's mouth and nose and the re-breathing bag on the anaesthetic circuit is squeezed to provide IPPV.

A pulse/oxygen monitor should be placed on the patient to ensure that he/she is maintaining good oxygen saturation levels of the haemoglobin.

Circulation

When faced with cardiac standstill it is important to start cardiac compressions immediately. The rate of compressions should be between 80–120/minute and palpating the femoral pulse at the same time can assess the effectiveness of the compressions. If compressions are not effective there is the option of open chest cardiac massage.

The circulation needs to be restored and at the earliest possible moment an i.v. catheter needs to be placed to have intravenous access and also to provide fluid therapy to maintain circulation.

Drugs can be used to try and start the heart or to deal with dysrhythmias, but in the latter case an ECG is necessary to document the type of dysrhythmia.

Shock

Shock is defined as 'a condition associated with circulatory collapse, during which the blood pressure is too low to maintain adequate perfusion to the tissues' (see Box 7.3).

The clinical signs are tachycardia, weak peripheral pulses, hypothermia, delayed capillary refill time and pale mucous membranes. The cat will also appear generally quiet, even depressed.

The aims of treatment are to reverse the symptoms of shock before there is irreparable damage to the underperfused tissues, and to prevent further deterioration and death. Appropriate fluid therapy is the key to treatment of shock. The use of intravenous fluids, plasma expanders or blood transfusions is the choice and decision of the veterinary surgeon.

Patients should be gradually warmed in cases of hypothermia using indirect heat, blankets and 'space blankets'. Cooking foil can be used to wrap around extremities to retain and reflect heat. If a pre-warmed incubator is available the cat can be placed in it.

BOX 7.3 THE MAIN CAUSES OF SHOCK

- Haemorrhage – internal or external.
- Dehydration – burns, vomiting, diarrhoea.
- Sepsis and anaphylaxis.
- Heart failure.
- Drug overdosage.

Warming should be started while other treatments are being prepared or administered. The aim for re-warming is to raise the core body temperature by around 1°C per hour.

Once the patient is stable a full physical examination can take place. A detailed history should be taken. Baseline urine evaluation, blood tests (biochemical panel and haematology) and routine survey radiographs are essential to establish the full extent of the problems. A problem list can be drawn up and further diagnostic tests started.

This is another point in time where it is important to determine if the practice can deal with the further diagnostic tests, treatment and monitoring or if referral would benefit the patient.

It is important to continue intensive monitoring to pick up subtle changes. Intensive monitoring is known to reduce the number of complications and the time spent in intensive care and reduces the ultimate cost to the client.

7.4 OXYGEN THERAPY

Dyspnoeic patients can be difficult to nurse, as they are often extremely distressed. It is important to know how to recognise signs of dyspnoea at the earliest possible stage in order to allow early intervention.

Signs of dyspnoea can vary from a slightly increased respiration rate to a patient that is extremely distressed and desperately struggling for every breath, often involving open-mouth breathing (cats do not normally pant, unlike dogs). Once a cat becomes obviously dyspnoeic the situation is critical and action needs to be taken to improve the cat's oxygen exchange.

The colour of the mucous membranes varies depending on the cause and severity of the dyspnoea. Mucous membrane colour ranges from pale pink to a deep shade of purple/blue (cyanosis) or brick red if carbon monoxide is the cause of the dyspnoea.

Reducing oxygen demand

When dealing with dyspnoeic patients, it is important to try and reduce their demand for oxygen as much as possible. When a cat becomes distressed or anxious, or is struggling, its demand for oxygen increases. Reducing oxygen demand is easily achieved by trying to keep the patient as calm and quiet as possible. Most

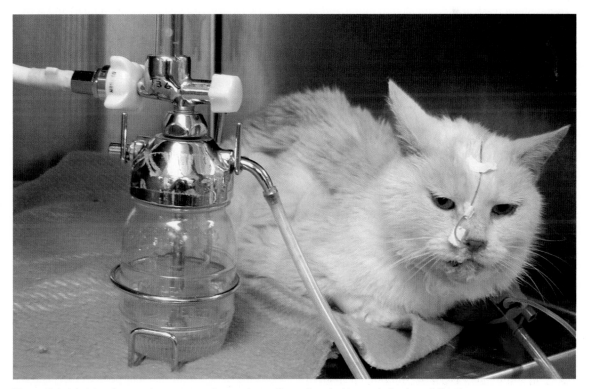

Figure 7.1 Administering nasal oxygen to a dyspnoeic cat. Reproduced with permission from J. Beatty.

cats prefer to be left in a quiet kennel with as little interference as possible. They often find a comfortable position to settle in, which is most suitable for their condition. Vigilant monitoring is often still required and it is important to strike the right balance between not disturbing the cat and monitoring progress.

Many cats will not tolerate handling and restraint when dyspnoeic and repeated attempts to restrain them could lead to excessive struggling which will often result in a respiratory crisis or death.

Oxygen supplementation

While the cause of the respiratory distress is being diagnosed or treated, it is often useful to provide increased levels of inspired oxygen. An increased oxygen supply can be delivered to the patient by various methods. The most suitable method will depend on the temperament of the patient as well as the reason for oxygen therapy.

Facemask delivery of oxygen

Most cats poorly tolerate this method of supplying oxygen, especially when they are compromised to such an extent that they begin to mouth breathe. Facemasks can often increase a patient's stress levels causing an increase in the rate of respiration and an increased demand for oxygen. However some patients, particularly patients that are very collapsed, or patients in need of short-term oxygen therapy may tolerate it adequately. Transparent plastic facemasks are often more acceptable to patients than the solid rubber type.

An advantage of this method of delivery is that the patient can be closely observed and monitored. Disadvantages include the need for relatively high flow rates, as most patients will not tolerate a close fitting facemask. This can be both costly and can have a drying effect on the respiratory mucosa, which will further distress the patient.

Oxygen face tent

This involves fitting an Elizabethan type collar with clear plastic or cling film covering across the front of the collar, in order to form a seal, leaving only a very small gap to allow expired air to exit.

Oxygen can then be delivered via a tube, which can be secured in place under the patient's collar. This allows a reasonable concentration of oxygen to build up within the face tent, without the patient feeling overly restricted. The patient is free to move

and can be allowed to make itself comfortable in a cage. Occasionally the tube may become dislodged.

Some patients will become distressed with the Elizabethan collar and if this is the case then an alternative method should be used.

Oxygen tent/cage

Covering a normal cage with clear plastic, leaving a small hole for expired gas, will make a suitable oxygen tent. An incubator can also be used as they are often fitted with an oxygen inlet. This method of providing a patient with oxygen is well tolerated as the patient can be left to settle without disturbance but can still be closely observed.

A disadvantage is that every time the patient has to be examined or the cage door opened, the oxygen rich atmosphere disperses into the room. When the patient is returned to the cage it will take a while for the oxygen to build up again, unless high flow rates are used, so this method of oxygen supplementation can prove more costly. Care should also be taken to ensure that the patient does not overheat in this enclosed environment.

Intra-nasal oxygen therapy

This technique is not always well-tolerated by cats, but it allows a patient to be closely monitored and it only requires minimum equipment. Of all the techniques for providing oxygen therapy this one requires the lowest oxygen flow rate as the oxygen is delivered straight to the naso-pharyngeal area.

The placement of the tube is as for a naso-oesophageal tube (see p. 112), but the tube is only placed as far as the naso-pharynx, which means that the tip of the tube should not be placed further than the medial canthus of the eye. This can be measured beforehand and the tube can be marked at the appropriate place.

This method is most suitable for long-term oxygen therapy, in which case it is advisable to bubble to the oxygen through a bottle of sterile water, to help provide some moisture to the respiratory tract mucosa (see Fig. 7.1).

The nasal catheter should be changed every 48 hours, and when changing the catheter it is advisable to alternate between both nostrils.

7.5 FIRST AID

First aid can be administered by people other than veterinary surgeons according to the Veterinary Nurses and the Veterinary Surgeons Act 1966. Schedule 3 of the Act allows anyone to administer first aid in an emergency for the purpose of saving life and relieving suffering.

Veterinary nurses must be familiar with first aid techniques themselves, and be able to advise owners on how to apply them at home as an interim measure while transporting their cat to the veterinary practice.

Haemorrhage

Bleeding (haemorrhage) may occur from an external wound, or due to internal injuries.

External haemorrhage

Most external haemorrhage is a combination of arterial, venous and capillary haemorrhage.

- Arterial haemorrhage usually has a definite bleeding point and pumps out with the rhythm of the heart. The blood is a vibrant oxygenated red. The volume of blood and the rate of loss depends on the size of the artery severed.
- Venous haemorrhage has a definite bleeding point and occurs in a steady stream. The blood is darker in colour and bleeding is easier to control, although a large severed vein can cause rapid blood loss and even death.
- Capillary haemorrhage will be present in all external wounds, causing general ooze with no definitive bleeding point.

The easiest first aid measure is to apply direct digital pressure either around the wound edges if small enough, or directly over the wound with a clean lint free cloth.

First ensure your hands are clean. When applying pressure to a wound, take care to check you are not making the condition worse or more painful by pushing a foreign body further into the wound, or putting pressure on fractures below the wound. If a foreign body is present, do not be tempted to remove it as this could cause pain, further bleeding or damage to deeper structures. A doughnut bandage can be put around the foreign body, raising the point of pressure above it (see later). When continuous pressure is applied most haemorrhage will cease after 5 minutes, as a clot will form. Do not be tempted to remove the pad to check progress until at least 5 minutes (timed by the clock) has elapsed, as this will dislodge the clot causing bleeding to re-start.

Another method is to use pressure points (Box 7.4) but this is only useful for life threatening arterial bleeds, and is not always practical to apply, especially if the cat is conscious. Effective application requires good knowledge of anatomy, and practise at locating the pressure points quickly and effectively.

A tourniquet can be used for short-term control of haemorrhage from the distal limbs or tail. This approach is only recommended if other attempts have failed to stem the haemorrhage, or if the wound is such that amputation of the affected region is likely to be needed. A suitable piece of pliable rubber tubing, latex (for instance a Penrose drain) or commercially available rubber bandaging is used to make the tourniquet. String or rope should not be used as it will crush the soft tissues and cut into the skin. Once the tourniquet is in place a stop clock or watch should be set, as it should not be left in place any longer than 15 minutes. The tourniquet should be released gradually to allow the blood pressure to increase slowly and if bleeding re-starts the tourniquet must be reapplied, or the wound must be explored and managed surgically. If a tourniquet is required for longer than 15 minutes, it should be reapplied distal to the original application site in order to allow the vessels to recover. Patients should always be monitored and never left in the cattery whilst a tourniquet is in place.

Once the bleeding has stopped a temporary dressing needs to be applied, as the patient's blood pressure will rise on recovering from shock or loss of consciousness and this may cause bleeding to start again. If the wound is on a limb or the tail, a pressure bandage, e.g. a 'Robert Jones' type, should be applied; elsewhere pressure dressings should be used. Pressure dressings require a sterile dressing on the wound itself. Pressure bandages require a lot of padding under the conforming bandage layer to ensure that even pressure is applied. If haemorrhage persists and shows through the dressing do not attempt to remove the primary dressing, but place further layers of

BOX 7.4   ARTERIAL PRESSURE POINTS

Pressure point	Location	Site of bleed
Brachial artery (humerus)	Medial shaft	Below elbow
Femoral artery	Medial thigh	Below stifle
Coccygeal artery	Ventral tail base	Length of tail

padding and a new conforming layer to apply more pressure to the wound.

Internal haemorrhage

Signs of significant internal haemorrhage include pallor of the mucous membranes, tachycardia and weak pulse pressure. Minor internal bleeding is very difficult to detect.

Internal bleeding is treated by providing fluid replacement or plasma expanders (see p. 82), and by identifying and surgically managing the site of haemorrhage. For abdominal haemorrhage application of a pressure wrap around the abdomen may partially reduce the rate of haemorrhage until more effective treatment can be instigated.

Burns

Burns can be classified for this purpose as severe, moderate and mild. Burns are classified as severe when a substantial proportion of the total skin area is affected or when the burns are very deep. These patients will be in a great deal of pain and require analgesia (administered under veterinary instruction), and supportive care for shock (see p. 168). Burns are exudative wounds and cause heat loss through evaporation. Affected cats should be covered in foil blankets to retain heat. Do not use direct heat as this will increase pain and cause peripheral vasodilation, which will draw circulating volume to the periphery and away from vital organs.

Moderate burns or scalds should be flushed with copious amounts of cooled water or saline to stop further burning of the tissues. If the patient has been burnt by contact with hot fat, other greasy substances or caustic chemicals, the addition of a detergent to the fluid will help to remove it and prevent continued burning. The choice of fluid initially is not important, and the easiest and cheapest method is to use tap water; this is useful to remember when giving advice to owners over the phone.

For chemical burns it is helpful to find out, when possible, the exact nature of the chemical: acid burns can be ameliorated by application of an alkaline solution (e.g. bicarbonate of soda or washing soda), while alkaline burns will be neutralised by application of a mildly acidic solution (e.g. dilute vinegar).

Once all debris and contaminates have been removed the area should be covered with a sterile dressing protected by a layer of plastic, e.g. a small carrier bag or cling film, to help retain moisture in the wound and prevent further contamination.

Electrical burns are often found in or around the mouth of a patient (the cat may have chewed through an electrical cable) and also on the paws as the point of exit. **Remember to turn off the electrical supply if the patient is in situ.**

Fractures

Fractures should be stabilised at the earliest opportunity to prevent movement of the fractured ends of the bones, which causes pain and further soft tissue damage. The application of a splint or a strong support bandage such as a Robert Jones dressing should achieve this, and application of a bandage has the added advantage of reducing and preventing further swelling, thereby minimising further pain. However, most conscious, injured feline patients will not tolerate the amount of handling and limb manipulation that is required to apply an effective support bandage, and in attempting to restrain the cat you may achieve the complete opposite of your goals! Most injured cats will require good analgesia and/or sedation to enable initial effective stabilisation of a fracture.

7.6 TOXINS

Cats are fastidious eaters and rarely ingest unsuitable food, or eat poisonous plants. However their natural grooming behaviour does mean that any toxins that get onto their coat, or that they walk through, will be cleaned from their fur and swallowed. Cats hunt and may occasionally catch and eat a prey animal that has previously ingested a toxin, e.g. a rodenticide or slug bait.

Cats have very limited capacity to detoxify compounds using the glucuronidation pathway in the liver. This pathway converts a wide range of toxic compounds into less toxic, water-soluble, easily excreted compounds. Many common drugs and chemicals such as insecticides are metabolised by this route, so cats are more susceptible to their toxic effects. Owners must be made aware that drugs that are safe for humans may be highly toxic to cats (e.g. aspirin and paracetamol). Also, some flea control products that are marketed for dogs (e.g. permethrin) may cause fatal toxicity in cats. When contacted by an owner who suspects that their cat has come into contact with a toxin, it is of the utmost importance to find out which toxin is involved, how long ago the incident occurred and approximately how much of the toxic substance was involved.

Many veterinary practices will have access to the Veterinary Poisons Information Service (UK) or National Poisons Bureau (Australia), or similar services, which will provide detailed advice on specific treatments for different poisons.

Basic principles of toxin removal

There are a number of methods that can be employed for removal of toxins and prevention of further absorption. The most appropriate method will depend on whether the toxin is on the skin or has been ingested, and how long ago contact occurred.

- **Bathing** – When the toxin is on the skin, it can be removed by bathing the cat in lukewarm water using a mild detergent (e.g. baby shampoo, or washing up liquid). Hot water should not be used as it may cause peripheral capillary dilation and encourage increased toxin absorption. Solvents e.g. white spirit or paint stripper must never be used, as they are themselves toxic to cats. If the cat resents bathing it may be safest to avoid complete immersion or to tranquillise the cat before bathing. A number of changes of water may be required and care should be taken to avoid contact with the eyes. The cat must be kept warm, and out of all drafts, until its coat is completely dry. The cat should also be prevented from licking its coat and an Elizabethan collar may be necessary.

- **Emesis** – Inducing vomiting may purge recently ingested toxins. This will only be effective if it can be done within 4 hours of toxin ingestion, and should only be undertaken in cats that have an adequate cough reflex. If the substance that was swallowed is caustic or corrosive, then inducing vomiting may cause further severe damage to the oesophagus. If induction of vomiting is considered appropriate, it can be achieved by dosing the cat with washing soda crystals (sodium carbonate), or by an injection of apomorphine.

- **Gastric lavage** – This is performed using a stomach tube passed under general anaesthesia and is suitable for treating recently ingested toxins. A cuffed endotracheal tube should be placed first, to prevent aspiration of the lavage fluid into the lungs. Substances that may absorb the toxin, such as activated charcoal or kaolin, may be added to the lavage fluid and left to bathe the GI-tract in the final lavage.

- **Fluid therapy** – While diuresis induced by fluid therapy is of little use in removing toxins, the fluid and electrolyte needs of the cat should be attended to. Some toxins such as ethylene glycol, aspirin and barbiturates cause metabolic acidosis, which is treated by i.v. administration of sodium bicarbonate. The acid–base balance should be monitored by blood gas analysis.

Specific poisons

Aspirin

Well-meaning owners may administer aspirin to cats, but cats are sensitive to its toxic effects, and the therapeutic dose range is relatively close to the toxic dose range.

Aspirin has a range of toxic effects:

- It inhibits platelet aggregation, causing prolonged bleeding times.
- It causes accumulation of the metabolic by-product lactic acid, resulting in metabolic acidosis.
- It causes changes to glucose metabolism resulting in high blood glucose concentrations and glucose in the urine.
- It severely restricts blood flow to the gastric mucosa, causing ulceration and bleeding of the stomach.

Cats are usually presented with a history of vomiting, depression, anorexia, fever and hyperventilation. There may be signs of liver failure, jaundice and anaemia.

If exposure to aspirin is recent (within 4 hours), emesis should be induced and gastric lavage may be performed. Activated charcoal and Glauber's salts (Na_2SO_4 – 3 g p.o. as a 6% solution) can then be instilled into the stomach, if they are available. Intravenous fluid therapy should be commenced using fluids containing sodium bicarbonate to treat the metabolic acidosis. Close monitoring is necessary

BOX 7.5 KEY POINTS: MANAGING POISONING

Supportive care, such as supplemental oxygen, artificial ventilation, fluid therapy for cardiovascular support, warming mats, pain relief and control of seizures are vital nursing measures used in caring for poisoned, critically ill cats.

to prevent over-perfusion. Blood transfusion may be indicated if there is severe anaemia. Gastric mucosal damage should be treated using gastric protectants such as sucralfate and gastric acid inhibitors such as cimetidine or ranitidine.

Paracetamol (acetaminophen)

Cats have a very poor ability to metabolise paracetamol because of their limited capacity for hepatic glucuronidation, so relatively low doses of paracetamol (e.g. a single 325 mg tablet) may be fatal. A common cause of intoxication results from owners dosing their sick cat, mistakenly believing that it will be helpful.

There are three main toxic effects:

- Methaemoglobinaemia – Normal haemoglobin is converted to methaemoglobin causing hypoxia and resulting in chocolate brown or blue mucous membranes.
- Heinz body formation – Heinz bodies are particles of denatured haemoglobin which attach themselves to the red blood cell surface. Cats are particularly prone to the formation of Heinz bodies, and affected cells are removed by the spleen (haemolysis) resulting in acute anaemia.
- Toxic effects on the liver – occur only if the cat survives the initial toxic insult.

Early clinical signs of paracetamol toxicity include cyanosis or chocolate brown mucus membranes; swelling of the face and paws; excessive tear production; and acute itchiness. Anorexia and depression gradually increase in severity and haemolysis and jaundice become apparent within 2–7 days, if the cat survives the initial crisis.

Prompt and aggressive treatment of paracetamol toxicity is extremely important if there is to be any chance of saving the cat. If the cat is presented within 4 hours of exposure, emesis should be induced, or gastric lavage performed. Addition of activated charcoal and sodium sulphate to the lavage fluid markedly improves the survival rate. Oral acetylcysteine (140 mg/kg as a loading dose, followed by 70 mg/kg every 4–6 hours for up to 3 days) can be administered as an antidote, as it supplies glutathione, which can aid in metabolising paracetamol. S-adenosyl methionine (SAME) may be helpful for similar reasons. Methylene blue (in 10% sterile saline, given intravenously at 1.5 mg/kg) and ascorbic acid (500–1000 mg daily p.o.) may be used to treat the methaemoglobinaemia.

Supportive therapy such as supplemental oxygen, warming mats and intravenous fluids are also critical to successful treatment.

Ethylene glycol (antifreeze)

Ethylene glycol is a widely used as antifreeze in car radiators and windscreen cleaning solutions and accidental intoxication is relatively common in areas where it is used. It is highly toxic to cats (a dose of just 1 to 2 ml/kg can cause clinical signs and death), so for example, a cat walking through a pool of spilt antifreeze may ingest a potentially fatal dose when it subsequently washes its paws.

Ethylene glycol is rapidly absorbed from the GI tract and subsequently metabolised to glycol, which has euphoric effects similar to alcohol. Metabolism of glycol to acidic compounds causes severe metabolic acidosis within 3 to 4 hours of ingestion and acute renal failure, which becomes clinically apparent within 1–3 days.

There are three clinical phases:

1. **First phase** – Early signs (1 to 4 hours after ingestion) include incoordination, increased heart rate and respiratory rate, and dehydration.
2. **Second phase** – Four to six hours after ingestion, a second more serious phase begins. This is characterised by gradually worsening anorexia, depression, vomiting, reduced body temperature and constricted pupils. This may be followed by severe depression, increased respiratory rate, coma and death.
3. **Third phase** – The cat that survives the acute metabolic acidosis of the second phase will develop acute renal failure. This phase has a very poor prognosis because of the very limited capacity of the kidneys to recover from a toxic insult.

Early diagnosis and treatment of ethylene glycol toxicity are essential for a successful outcome, and nonetheless many cats will not survive. If the cat is presented within four hours of ingestion, gastric lavage with activated charcoal should be performed. An intravenous infusion of ethanol (20%; 5 ml/kg every 6 hours for five treatments, then every 8 hours for four treatments) is the only specific antidote to ethylene glycol that is suitable for use in cats. Intravenous fluid therapy is also essential in successful treatment and 4.5% NaCl with 2.5% dextrose may be used initially to establish urine flow. Potassium containing fluids should not be used until urine flow is established.

Sodium bicarbonate may be administered to correct the metabolic acidosis, and plasma bicarbonate should be monitored serially every 2–4 hours if possible during the initial period. Glucocorticoids may be used to treat shock and pulmonary oedema.

Pyrethrins

Pyrethrins are natural insecticides produced from extracts of pyrethrum flowers, whereas pyrethroids are synthetic insecticides that resemble pyrethrins in their chemistry and actions. Pyrethroids are often considered to be 'safe' natural compounds and may be used inappropriately by some owners. These compounds are used in a wide range of flea control products and excessive use may cause intoxication. In particular, permethrin is a synthetic pyrethroid insecticide and neurotoxicant which is safe and effective for use in dogs, but is not suitable for use in cats.

Pyrethroids can be absorbed orally, via the skin or inhaled. This causes the generation of repetitive nerve impulses, resulting in both neurological and GI signs such as heightened response to stimulation, muscle tremors, seizures (Fig. 7.2), paralysis, salivation and vomiting. Clinical signs generally resolve in 24–72 hours if the animal survives.

Diagnosis is based on history of exposure and presence of appropriate clinical signs.

Treatment is based on removing the toxin and supportive therapy:

- If there has been skin exposure, the cat should be bathed in warm soapy water, preferably using a number of rinses. Care should be taken not to stress the cat and sponge bathing may be safer for cats that become distressed by immersion bathing. Clipping the hair from the affected region is also effective, but affected cats may be hypersensitive to noise, so care is required when restraining them.
- If there has been ingestion of the toxin, gastric lavage should be performed, preferably adding activated charcoal to the lavage fluid to reduce absorption and aid elimination.
- Seizures should be controlled using diazepam, but it is often not possible to completely control tremors without producing an unacceptable level of sedation. Body temperature should be monitored closely and managed appropriately. Hyperthermia may occur as a result of excessive muscle activity, but hypothermia may occur once seizures and tremors

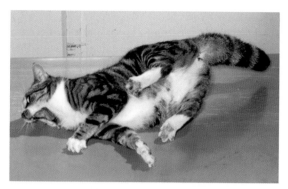

Figure 7.2 Cats poisoned by pyrethrin or pyrethroid flea control products may present with seizures.*

are controlled. Atropine can be used sparingly to treat excessive salivation and vomiting.

Caustic chemicals

There are numerous caustic chemicals that are frequently used around the house, which may cause acute burns if the cat comes into contact with them. Common examples include bleach and cleaning fluids for ovens, bathrooms, drains or swimming pools.

If these are spilled on the coat or if the cat walks in them, they can cause oral burns and subsequent necrosis when the cat grooms itself. More severe burns and ulceration of the pharynx, oesophagus and stomach may occur if the caustic compound is ingested, for example if the cat drinks water from a recently cleaned bath or shower tray. Clinical signs such as drooling may commence within 24 hours of exposure and tongue ulcers usually develop 24–48 hours later.

If the cat is presented within the first 2 days after exposure, it should be washed to remove the caustic agent. In the initial stages drooling may cause dehydration, and subcutaneous or intravenous fluids may be required. Analgesics may be administered for pain relief. Oral ulceration may be treated with anti-inflammatory agents and antibiotics may be necessary to treat secondary infections. Nutritional support may also be required if the cat is unwilling to eat.

*Every effort has been made to obtain permission to reproduce Fig. 7.2 (Photographer G. Wilkinson). Any concerns should be addressed in writing to Elsevier Ltd, The Boulevard, Kidlington, Oxford, OX5 1GB. UK.

Lily toxicity

Hemerocallus (day lily) and *Lillium* species (lilies) are common garden and indoor ornamental plants that can cause severe acute renal failure if cats ingest any part of the plant. The specific toxic compound is unknown.

Early clinical signs include depression and vomiting, followed in 2–4 days by signs of acute renal failure, i.e. anorexia, depression and lack of urine production.

Since no antidote or effective treatment is available, preventing exposure is imperative. If the cat is presented within 24 hours of ingestion, emesis should be induced, followed by gastric lavage with activated charcoal added to the lavage fluid. Intravenous fluid diuresis should be commenced, whilst avoiding volume overload as the kidneys are often unable to eliminate excess fluid. If not treated aggressively within 24 hours of ingestion, lily toxicity is uniformly fatal to cats.

ANAESTHESIA AND ANALGESIA

CHAPTER **8**

Graham Bilbrough, MA VetMB CertVA MRCVS

Safe feline anaesthesia can present a challenge. Cats have a unique physiology, anatomy and temperament, which means that anaesthetic drugs, techniques and equipment must be chosen carefully to suit their needs.

As with all species, safety is improved by a thorough clinical examination prior to administration of any drugs. However, with some aggressive cats this will not be possible.

The cat should be fasted for a period of at least six hours prior to sedation or anaesthesia (except in an emergency) to ensure that the stomach is empty. This reduces the risk of regurgitation and aspiration of stomach contents. Pregnant queens for caesarian section or young kittens should only be starved for one to two hours. All cats should be allowed free access to water until the sedative or premedication is given.

8.1 SEDATION

Sedative drugs are given to cats with the intention of calming them either prior to inducing anaesthesia or performing diagnostic procedures. It is in the interests of both the patient and the staff that the cat remains calm at all times. Aggressive cats may be impossible to work with without adequate sedation and even an apparently friendly cat can become difficult to restrain, risking injury to the cat or the handler.

As a cat becomes frightened, release of adrenaline will increase the likelihood of cardiac arrhythmias and also elevate its oxygen requirement. Any cat with a decreased ability to transport and deliver oxygen to the tissues (e.g. due to anaemia, cardiac or pulmonary disease, or hypovolaemia) is at grave risk of death during these episodes.

The effect produced by a particular dose of a sedative agent will vary considerably between individual animals. The doses suggested in this chapter should not result in excessive cardiovascular or respiratory depression but every patient should be carefully observed following the administration of a sedative drug. Some patients will vomit and staff must be avail-

able to ensure this cannot result in respiratory obstruction or aspiration. Prolonged sedation, such as that induced by high doses of alpha-2 adrenoceptor agonists, may result in hypothermia.

While it is vital to observe every patient after giving a sedative, the cat should be left in as quiet an environment as possible, where it will feel safe, for sufficient time for the drugs to take effect.

Most sedative drugs are given by intramuscular injection, however when handling an aggressive cat some of the drugs (e.g. ketamine and buprenorphine) may be squirted directly into the mouth.

Sedative drugs

Acepromazine
Acepromazine is a sedative that is commonly used as an anaesthetic pre-medication (see Section 8.3) but it provides only mild sedation. It is unlikely to provide sufficient sedation for most procedures, especially when used alone.

Ketamine
Ketamine can be used in combination with other drugs, to provide sedation or anaesthesia. Sedation protocols use lower doses than anaesthetic protocols. Sedative combinations that include ketamine are particularly useful when the cat is fractious or in pain. However, its sedative effect is relatively short-lived, around thirty minutes, and during the recovery phase the cat may be harder to handle, rather than easier.

This drug should only ever be used in combination with other sedative drugs as when used alone it can result in excitement. After giving this drug, particular care should be taken not to stimulate the cat with either light or sound. Respiratory arrest may occur and cats should be observed closely until signs of sedation are no longer apparent. Excretion of this drug is dependent on renal function, and so it should be used with caution when dealing with urinary obstruction or kidney failure.

177

In the UK, ketamine must now be treated as if it is a Schedule 2 Controlled Drug, in that it must be stored within a locked metal cabinet, secured to the wall, and each dose used must be recorded within a bound register.

Alpha-2 adrenoceptor agonists

There are two alpha-2 adrenoceptor agonists licensed for use in the cat: medetomidine (Domitor™, Pfizer) and romifidine (Romidys™, Virbac). The use of xylazine (Rompun™, Bayer and others) can no longer be justified, as it has no advantages over the alternatives but causes more pronounced side effects.

The alpha-2 adrenoceptor agonists have profound and complex cardiovascular effects and should only be used with due consideration of the patient's health. After initial administration, the cat will develop significant peripheral vasoconstriction, producing very pale mucous membranes and an elevation in the arterial blood pressure. The physiological response to this rise in blood pressure causes slowing of the heart rate. Overall there is a dramatic fall in the volume of blood that the heart will pump over a given period of time, however, the blood flow to the essential organs seems to be relatively well-preserved. Later, the vasoconstriction will abate while the heart rate remains low and this may result in mild hypotension.

Collective experience with the use of medetomidine in cats seems to suggest that it is associated with fewer untoward events in cats than dogs. When given by intramuscular injection, it is an extremely reliable sedative making it particularly useful in fractious cats. It is popular for short procedures as its sedative effects are readily reversed by the antagonist drug atipamezole (Antisedan™, Pfizer). If it is used in a premedication combination, there is a marked reduction in the dose of anaesthetic agents required for induction and maintenance.

Romifidine has only recently been licensed for use in the cat. Given the similar modes of action of this and medetomidine it likely that there will prove to be few clinically significant differences between these two drugs. Romifidine can also be antagonised by atipamezole.

Benzodiazepines

A benzodiazepine is frequently given in combination with ketamine to provide good sedation for minor and diagnostic procedures. Midazolam is preferable to diazepam as it produces less pain on injection. When given alone, diazepam and midazolam seem to result in no apparent sedation, except in very sick cats. The combination of midazolam and butorphanol (Torbugesic™, Forte Dodge) is useful in very young kittens.

Opioids

Opioids have little sedative effect when given alone but they have a synergistic effect when given with other sedatives. They are a useful element in sedative combinations to reduce the required dose of the other drugs and to provide analgesia. While sedative combinations do not have to include an analgesic component, sedation will only be successful in the patient in pain if they are included. The analgesic properties of the opioid drugs are discussed further in Section 8.2.

8.2 ANALGESIA

Providing adequate analgesia is essential for the well-being and care of cats, but in the past they have tended to be under treated for pain. Many practitioners have incorrectly believed analgesics to be unnecessary for cats, partly because they have an innate ability to mask pain so that the behavioural clues they do give may only be obvious with experience (see p. 69). Cats also have limited capability to metabolise many analgesic drugs and few of these agents have undergone extensive trials in the cat. This has resulted in the use of inappropriate drugs or excessive doses in feline patients and as a consequence widespread misunderstandings have evolved as to what is safe and what is not.

In the vast majority of cases, the benefits of managing pain outweigh the risks associated with drug administration. Analgesia should not be denied to cats simply because the species is not fully understood. In addition to the use of analgesic drugs, other important aspects of care in the clinical setting should be considered. Provision of warmth, appetising food and general attention will make the cat 'feel much better'. Good nursing, with particular attention to careful bandaging and grooming, is equally important. This time spent with the patient will enable better observation of the subtle changes in a cat's behaviour, which will indicate the patient's level of pain.

When administering analgesics to cats, it is important to consider that an individual's response to a given agent can be extremely variable both in terms of analgesia and side effects. For this reason, each agent should be carefully titrated to effect rather than rigidly supplied at a standard dose rate. By using a combination of drugs from different analgesic classes, a good overall effect can be achieved using relatively low doses of each one.

Pre-emptive analgesia

Any analgesic drug will produce a much more potent effect if it is given before a painful event rather than being used after the pain has already developed. That is to say that if analgesic drugs are given before an operation, the requirements for further postoperative doses will be dramatically reduced. Premedication (see Section 8.3) provides an ideal opportunity to take

advantage of this by including an opioid and a non-steroidal anti-inflammatory agent (NSAID) whenever appropriate.

Opioid analgesics

In the past veterinary surgeons have avoided using opioids in cats because they were believed to cause excitement and profound respiratory depression. Doses many times higher than those suggested here (Table 8.1) are required to produce such problems. Cats have a limited ability to metabolise some opioids,

Table 8.1 Suggested dose rates for analgesics in cats

Drug	Suggested dose	Duration of analgesic effect	Comments
Buprenorphine (Vetergesic™)	0.01 mg/kg s.c.[a], i.m[b]. or sublingually t.i.d[f].	6–8 h	If analgesia is insufficient, the dose may be increased to 0.02 mg/kg
Morphine or methadone	0.1–0.2 mg/kg s.c. or i.m. q.i.d.[g]	4–6 h	If analgesia is insufficient, the dose may be increased up to 0.5 mg/kg
Meloxicam (Metacam™)	**Day 1**: 0.3 mg/kg s.c. or p.o[c]. s.i.d.[e] **Days 2–5**: 0.1 mg/kg p.o. s.i.d.	18–24 h	Then decrease to lowest effective dose, usually 0.1 mg/cat s.i.d.
Carprofen (Rimadyl™)	Single injection of 4 mg/kg s.c. or i.v.[d]	Extremely variable; up to two days	Do not repeat within seven days. This drug should not be used for multiple administrations, even at a reduced dose
Ketamine	0.5 mg/kg i.v.	30–60 min	This is usually given in the postoperative period to a cat that appears to be in severe pain. It should not be given to a patient undergoing an excitable recovery unless a sedative drug is to be given concurrently
Lidocaine	Up to 4.0 mg/kg by perineural injection	1–2 h	
Bupivacaine	Up to 1.0 mg/kg by perineural injection	2–8 h	

NB: All analgesics have the potential for causing side effects and the appropriate data sheet should be consulted for full details. Few of these products are licensed for use in the cat. The duration of analgesic effect can be extremely variable in the cat.
[a] s.c., subcutaneous injection; [e] s.i.d., once per day; [b] i.m., intramuscular injection; [f] t.i.d., three times daily; [c] p.o., given by mouth; [g] q.i.d., four times daily; [d] i.v., intravenous injection.

so they often require relatively low doses and some have a longer duration of action in feline patients than in other species.

An alternative to periodic dosing with opioids is to use a continuous rate infusion (CRI). These have been described for both morphine and fentanyl and can be a very effective way of managing severe pain. An infusion pump or syringe driver makes this a more practical option.

Morphine and methadone

Morphine and methadone are very effective analgesic agents, which can be safely used in cats as long as an appropriate dose is used. Morphine has a relatively slow onset of effect in cats, which may be in part because it needs to be metabolised (by glucuronidation) after administration to produce the active components and cats have limited ability to do this. Sufficient time (up to one hour after intramuscular injection) must be given for the drug to take full effect before considering giving a second dose.

Buprenorphine

Some recent work with cats suggests that in this species buprenorphine is superior to morphine in providing analgesia, possibly because it does not require glucuronidation after administration. Buprenorphine (Vetergesic™, Alstoe) is not licensed for use in cats but it has widespread use in the UK as a safe and effective analgesic. It is usually chosen for long-term opioid use as it provides good analgesia and requires less frequent dosing than morphine. It is also more convenient than morphine or methadone as its use does not need to be recorded in a controlled drug register. In cats that resent injections, buprenorphine can be given via the buccal route (placing it under the tongue with a syringe). The alkaline nature of cat saliva means that it has good bioavailability via this route.

Butorphanol

Butorphanol (Torbugesic™, Forte Dodge) is an extremely useful sedative when combined with other drugs like acepromazine or medetomidine (see Table 8.2), but it is a poor choice of opioid for analgesia. Its duration of effect is too short (about one hour) and there are real concerns that repeat dosing, or combination with other opioids, could actually result in a reduction in analgesia.

Fentanyl

Fentanyl is a highly potent opioid that is usually administered by bolus intravenous injection (typically $2 \mu g/kg$). It has a very short onset time so an effect will be noticed almost immediately but it also has a short duration of action (usually less than thirty minutes). This drug can be used intra-operatively in advance of an acute, intensely painful part of the procedure, such as just prior to reducing a fracture, providing potent analgesia without the need to deepen the plane of anaesthesia. It is a potent respiratory depressant, which means it should only be used intravenously when the cat can be ventilated.

Recently, fentanyl has also been used in cats by the transdermal route. Skin patches designed for humans are applied to an area of clipped skin. This technique

Table 8.2 Suggested anaesthetic premedication combinations for cats			
Suitable for:	Drug combination	Route	Dose (mg/kg)
Friendly healthy cat	Acepromazine	i.m.[a] or s.c.[b]	0.05 mg/kg
	Buprenorphine	i.m. or s.c.	0.005–0.01 mg/kg
Friendly unwell cat	Acepromazine	i.m. or s.c.	0.02 mg/kg
	Buprenorphine	i.m. or s.c.	0.01–0.02 mg/kg
Fractious healthy cat	Medetomidine	i.m. or s.c.	0.04 mg/kg
	Buprenorphine	i.m. or s.c.	0.01–0.02 mg/kg
Fractious unwell cat	Ketamine	i.m. or s.c.	3 mg/kg
	Buprenorphine	i.m. or s.c.	0.01–0.02 mg/kg
Alternative opioid doses (substitute for buprenorphine)	Morphine	i.m. or s.c.	0.10–0.15 mg/kg
	Methadone	i.m. or s.c.	0.1–0.2 mg/kg
	Pethidine	i.m. only	3.3 mg/kg
	Butorphanol	i.m. or s.c.	0.25 mg/kg

[a] i.m., intramuscular injection; [b] s.c., subcutaneous injection.

is useful for controlling chronic pain, but in cats it can be difficult to keep the patch in place. The analgesic effect is slow in onset (usually about six hours in the cat) but lasts for a long time. Plasma levels of the drug do not fall rapidly after the patch is removed and it may take 12 to 18 hours to drop below the therapeutic level. There are a variety of patch sizes available, which deliver different doses of the drug; the patch that releases 25 µg/hour is used in domestic cats. This dose may be too high for some individuals (small cats, geriatrics and the systemically ill) so these cats should be dosed with a half patch. The patch should not be cut in half; rather only half of the backing material should be removed so that only half of the surface area of the patch is in contact with the skin. Each patch should be removed, or replaced, after four days.

Non-steroidal anti-inflammatory drugs (NSAIDs)

NSAIDs act by inhibiting the production of some inflammatory mediators. Many of the older NSAIDs are very toxic to cats (e.g. paracetamol, aspirin) because they are unable to eliminate them effectively. However new generations of these drugs (e.g. carprofen and meloxicam) can be used safely if they are reserved for well-hydrated cats with normal arterial blood pressure, normal renal and hepatic function, and no clotting abnormalities. The newer agents have proven to be very effective, even when treating severe pain.

Care must be taken to avoid concurrent treatment with NSAIDs and corticosteroids.

Meloxicam

Meloxicam (Metacam™, Boehringer Ingelheim) is currently only licensed for use as a single perioperative dose (0.3 mg/kg s.c.) but it has been successfully used to provide longer-term analgesia by the oral route (see Table 8.1). The drug's honey syrup presentation is particularly well-received by many cats. The lowest possible dose should be used while strictly monitoring the patient for the potential side effects of any NSAID. The benefits of this drug to a cat's welfare often outweigh any concerns regarding adverse effects.

Carprofen

Carprofen (Rimadyl™, Pfizer) has a similar licence (one perioperative injection, 4 mg/kg s.c. or i.v.) and has been widely use for this purpose with very few

reports of toxicity. However, the speed at which this drug is eliminated by a cat seems to vary greatly, so particular caution is required for repeat dosing, even if a reduced dose is used. Recently, some authors have recommended 2 mg/kg twice per week; however, until further data is available it is prudent to not use carprofen more than once per week (see Table 8.1).

Local anaesthetics, e.g. lidocaine and bupivacaine

Cats are considered to be more susceptible than dogs to the toxic effects of local anaesthetics but problems are very rare if appropriate doses are used (see Table 8.1). Accidental intravenous injection should be avoided. Perineural injection is the most common route of administration. They are particularly useful in dental nerve blocks, which are quick and easy to perform and will help to achieve a rapid return to eating, even following several tooth extractions. Local anaesthetics are also used for epidural analgesia/anaesthesia.

EMLA™ cream (Astra Zeneca) is a combination of lidocaine and prilocaine, which can be applied to the skin prior to inserting a venous cannula. It can provide effective skin anaesthesia if it is applied in a sufficiently thick layer and then covered with an occlusive dressing, which must be left in place for about 45 minutes to achieve a complete effect. This is particularly useful when training an inexperienced member of staff or for cats that will not be given any sedation prior to placing an intravenous catheter.

Ketamine

Ketamine (see p. 177) is very useful as a post-operative analgesic when used at subanaesthetic doses and given in combination with opioids. It acts on the central nervous system to help to prevent central sensitisation ('wind up'). It can either be given as a single dose approximately every hour (see Table 8.1) or as a continuous rate infusion.

8.3 GENERAL ANAESTHESIA

Anaesthetic pre-medication

Pre-medication is an important part of anaesthesia, giving sedation to the patient prior to induction.

It aims to:

- Calm the patient.
- Facilitate placement of intravenous catheters.
- Give a smooth induction and recovery.
- Reduce the required doses of anaesthetic agents.
- Start pre-emptive analgesia.

Inducing anaesthesia in a stressed cat is dangerous and must be avoided whenever possible. Prior to induction of anaesthesia, the feline patient should have a stoical indifference to its environment. This will be achieved through an appropriate degree of sedation from the premedication and by careful, sympathetic handling (see Chapter 3). If the cat does become distressed it is almost always safer to give further sedative drugs and/or try again later when the patient has become calm, rather than to risk inducing anaesthesia in a stressed cat.

Commonly used pre-medication combinations are listed in Table 8.2. Many of the drugs have been described elsewhere in this chapter; other commonly used pre-medicants are described below.

Acepromazine

Acepromazine is commonly included in combinations of drugs given for premedication as it helps to calm nervous patients. It has a very variable effect in cats, but usually only produces a mild sedative effect.

Typical doses for cats are around 0.05 mg/kg; doses above this do not seem to result in greater sedation, just more pronounced side effects.

Its use is contraindicated in hypovolaemic patients and it should be used at much lower doses in sick patients.

Anticholinergic agents

Atropine used to have widespread use in cat premedication combinations to reduce the volume of respiratory secretions and saliva that could potentially block small tracheas. It is no longer recommended as it has a number of undesirable effects including eliciting an excessively fast heart rate. Atropine causes dilation of the pupils, making bright light uncomfortable, potentially resulting in panic. If an anticholinergic drug is to be included in the premedication, glycopyrrolate (0.01 to 0.02 mg/kg i.m.) is preferred as it does not cause pupillary dilation and, during pregnancy, does not cross the placenta.

An anticholinergic drug (typically atropine at 0.02 mg/kg i.v.) should always be available for use in an emergency, such as during cardiopulmonary cerebral

resuscitation or when the patient has a sufficiently low heart rate to result in a low arterial blood pressure.

Induction of anaesthesia

Using inhaled anaesthetic agents

Inhaled anaesthetic agents can be used to induce anaesthesia using either a facemask (see Fig. 8.1) or an induction chamber (see Fig. 8.2). This is unlikely to be the technique of choice in all but a few patients as it results in significant pollution of the working environment and it does not allow the cat's airway to be rapidly secured by intubation. However, some 'needle-shy' cats are surprisingly tolerant of a facemask, while extremely aggressive cats can be quickly transferred to an induction chamber and appear to become more relaxed as they inhale the agent. Halothane, isoflurane and sevoflurane have all been successfully used in this way, but sevoflurane is the agent of choice, as it has the fastest onset time and it is also less irritant to the respiratory tract than isoflurane.

Using injectable anaesthetic agents

Most patients will be induced into anaesthesia using an injectable agent. The dose of the agent that is required will depend on the degree of patient sedation that has been achieved by the pre-medication. All agents must be given to effect rather than according to a dose rate. In particular, if an alpha-2 adrenoceptor agonist, such as medetomidine, was included in the premedication, the dose of induction agent should be significantly reduced.

Excitement at induction will result in far higher doses being required, risking overdose. For all the agents described below, an intravenous bolus of a benzodiazepine (e.g. diazepam 0.5 mg/kg or midazolam 0.2 mg/kg) given just before the induction agent will further reduce the required dose. For this purpose, a lipid emulsion of diazepam (Diazemuls™, Dumex) is superior to the preparation containing propylene glycol, as it will cause less irritation to the vein.

PROPOFOL

Propofol is widely used in the cat and is generally safe and well-tolerated if used appropriately; however its use is associated with a number of problems. A period of apnoea is very common following induction with propofol although this effect can be reduced by very slow administration. Cardiovascular depression is also evident after induction.

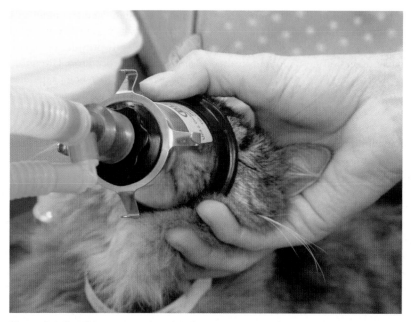

Figure 8.1 Supplying oxygen via a tight fitting mask.

Propofol should not be used to repeatedly anaesthetise cats, as they are rather poor at metabolising this drug and repeated exposure results in damage to feline red blood cells and haemoglobin. These cats will also be seen to have delayed recoveries from the anaesthetics and develop general signs of illness such as malaise and poor appetite. This effect has been seen if propofol is used for induction more frequently than once in every four days; however, as is common with feline drug metabolism it is likely that individuals will vary greatly in their susceptibility. For the same reason, propofol is unlikely to be the agent of choice in the cat for maintaining anaesthesia using intravenous 'top ups' or constant rate infusion.

THIOPENTAL

Thiopental is regarded by many practitioners to be an old-fashioned induction agent; however, for general feline practice no alternative drug has been shown to have demonstrable benefits over it.

Thiopental must only be given by intravenous injection, and it is very irritant if it is accidentally given extravascularly (i.e. if it leaks from the vein during the injection). It is therefore recommended that a very dilute solution (1.25%) be used in cats. This dilution also makes for more practical volumes of injection in small patients, making overdose less likely. Generally, in small animal practice, 100 ml of sterile water will be added to a 2.5 g bottle of thiopental to give a 2.5% solution. To produce a 1.25% solution for use in a cat, a 5 ml syringe is filled with 2.5 ml of 0.9% saline and then 2.5 ml of conventional 2.5% thiopental. Typically, when this solution is given to effect, the volume in the syringe will be more than sufficient to induce anaesthesia. Thiopental should not be diluted to concentrations of less than 2% using sterile water as this may cause haemolysis.

If extravascular administration does occur, the area should be infiltrated with 1 ml of 2% lidocaine diluted with 4 ml of 0.9% saline, providing analgesia and helping to correct the pH. If the extravascular injection

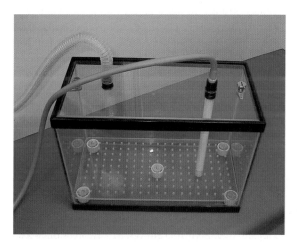

Figure 8.2 An anaesthetic induction chamber

183

occurred as a result of an incorrectly placed intravenous catheter, this catheter should be used to inject the lidocaine solution, prior to removal from the leg, so that the local anaesthetic will be deposited in the area required.

ALPHAXALONE-ALPHADOLONE (SAFFAN™, SCHERING-PLOUGH ANIMAL HEALTH)

Saffan™ is a combination of two steroid anaesthetics. It is usually given by intravenous injection so that it can be given in incremental amounts until sufficient anaesthesia is achieved. If intravenous injection is not possible it can also be given by intramuscular injection, but large volumes are required. It usually produces less respiratory and cardiovascular depression than either propofol or thiopental.

The problems associated with this product are attributed to the solubilising agent, cremophor EL. This produces histamine release in the cat, potentially causing hyperaemia and oedema of the pinnae, face and paws. Generally these effects are transient and not problematic. However, occasionally either bronchospasm or laryngeal oedema occurs which will have more serious consequences. In these cases endotracheal intubation and ventilation with oxygen is usually sufficient to support the cat until the problem resolves. A tracheostomy tube may be required if there is severe laryngeal oedema. Acepromazine has some antihistamine properties that may reduce these effects, so it is recommended to include this in the premedication for cats that will be induced using Saffan™. The sedative effects of acepromazine will also reduce the incidence of restlessness or excitement in recovery.

KETAMINE

Ketamine (see p. 177) is rarely used alone as an induction agent as it causes profound muscle rigidity and will result in profound excitement in the recovery phase. In man its use without sedatives or tranquillisers is associated with extremely unpleasant hallucinations and mood alterations; from the behaviour of cats it is likely they experience similar events. Ketamine often induces profuse salivation so precautions must be taken to ensure the airway is patent (see later).

The alpha-2 adrenoceptor agonists are potent sedatives and extremely useful as adjuncts to ketamine based anaesthesia. As well as providing muscle relaxation, the additional analgesia provided by these drugs significantly reduces the dose of ketamine that is required for surgery. The combination of medetomidine, ketamine and an opioid, given by intramuscular injection, is extremely popular in general practice as it conveniently provides satisfactory anaesthesia for short surgical procedures. Given the profound physiological changes that both ketamine and the alpha-2 adrenoceptor agonists are capable of producing, this 'triple combination' has proven to be surprisingly safe if it reserved for healthy patients and as long as the patient is adequately monitored until full recovery. The recovery can be hastened by the use of atipamezole (see earlier) to 'reverse' the alpha-2 adrenoceptor agonist. The atipamezole should not be given until the ketamine has been largely eliminated (45 minutes is usually sufficient) or the patient will become excitable.

Endotracheal intubation

Intubation is particularly difficult in cats due to their small size and the highly reactive nature of their larynx. Cats have a powerful laryngeal reflex; they are very prone to laryngeal spasm (see p. 186) and both their larynx and trachea are particularly delicate and easily damaged. If poorly executed, endotracheal intubation can cause more harm than good so great care and good training are required.

Cats are rather better at maintaining an airway under general anaesthesia than dogs and for some short procedures providing oxygen via a facemask (see Fig. 8.1) may be quite acceptable. Generally, intubation is preferred for procedures lasting longer than about ten minutes. It is essential if intermittent positive pressure ventilation (IPPV) will be required or if there is an increased risk of aspiration.

Choice of endotracheal tube

Prior to induction a range of endotracheal tube sizes suitable for the patient should be prepared. Most domestic cats require a tube with an internal diameter of between 3 and 5 mm; each practice should hold a range of widths, including half sizes, of both uncuffed and cuffed endotracheal tubes. Modern endotracheal tubes are more flexible to minimise damage to the trachea; the use of a stylet may provide more rigidity while intubating. Care should be taken that the stylet does not extend beyond the end of the tube and that it is removed as soon as the tube is placed.

For feline practice, uncuffed endotracheal tubes are generally favoured, as a cuffed tube has a larger external diameter for any given internal diameter. Also, if the deflated cuff itself does not lie flat against the tube it may cause irritation to the vocal folds as it is placed. More modern cuffed endotracheal tubes have a smooth profile and do not greatly increase the external diameter. If the cuff is inflated, great care should be taken to fill it with only just enough air to prevent a leak around the endotracheal tube. Cats have complete tracheal rings and so the trachea will not increase in size if stretched by the cuff. This makes cats particularly susceptible to tracheal necrosis if the pressure in the cuff is high enough to impede blood flow.

With dental procedures there is an increased risk of material trickling down the trachea, so a cuffed tube may be preferred, taking care not to over-inflate the cuff. Alternatively an uncuffed tube can be used and the pharynx can be packed with a damp gauze bandage. Usually the end of this bandage is left to trail from the mouth, so that it cannot be forgotten at the end of the procedure.

Commercially available endotracheal tubes of a suitable diameter are always too long for feline practice, and need to be cut to an appropriate length – the distance from the point of the cat's shoulder to the dental arcade. Using an over-long tube must be avoided because:

- Excessive dead space in the breathing system or endotracheal tube will lead to re-breathing of the expired gases, resulting in hypercapnia. Even a few extra millilitres can present a hazard to the domestic cat.
- An over-long tube may extend into one of the main bronchi resulting in one of the lungs not being ventilated.

If a capnograph is being used to monitor ventilatory function, its adaptor will fit between the endotracheal tube and the breathing system. The smallest possible adaptor, usually intended for human neonatal use, should be used to avoid creating excessive dead space.

INTUBATION TECHNIQUE

The cat has powerful laryngeal reflexes that must be overcome prior to placing an endotracheal tube in order to avoid laryngeal spasm. Typically, this is achieved by applying a few drops of local anaesthetic by aerosol. Care should be taken to follow the manufacturer's recommendations regarding the maximum dose in order to avoid local anaesthetic toxicity. The local anaesthetic spray should only be applied when the laryngeal area is well-exposed; and must be given

twenty seconds to take effect before endotracheal intubation is attempted.

Intubation is greatly facilitated by positioning the cat correctly and by the use of a laryngoscope with a short, flat blade such as a Miller size zero blade.

The cat is positioned in such a way that the mouth and neck are straight (see Figs 8.3 and 8.4) in order that the tube can be passed with ease. The tongue is gently pulled out of the mouth to hold the mouth open while the tube is placed. The weight of the head is supported from just behind the upper canine teeth: a length of gauze tape may be used so that the head can be held without obscuring the view of the larynx.

The best exposure of the larynx is provided by using the laryngoscope blade to gently press down at the base of the tongue, taking great care not to touch the sensitive epiglottis. If a suitable laryngoscope is not available an alternative technique for intubation of the cat may be useful (see Fig. 8.4). The intubator stands behind the cat and supports its head, such that

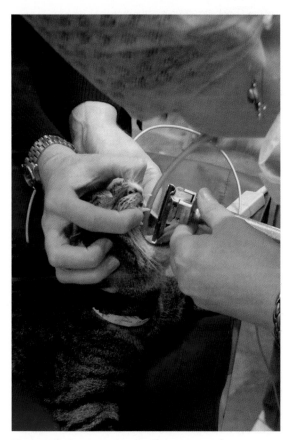

Figure 8.3 Correct positioning for endotracheal intubation.

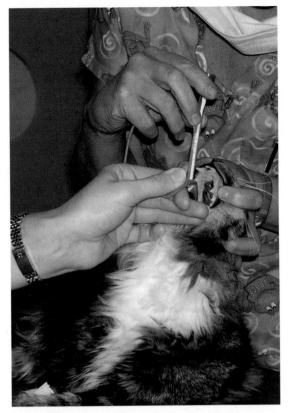

Figure 8.4 An alternative technique for intubation of the cat if a suitable laryngoscope is not available.

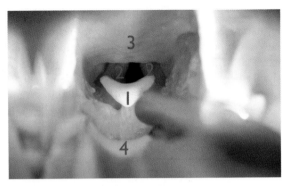

Figure 8.5 Exposure of the larynx with a laryngoscope. (1) Epiglottis; (2) vocal folds; (3) soft palate; (4) laryngoscope blade.

the head and neck are extended. The tongue is then gently pulled out of the mouth by an assistant allowing the intubator to visualise the larynx. This method becomes rather more awkward if a very flexible endotracheal tube is used and the use of a stylet is then recommended.

With the cat correctly positioned, the larynx well exposed and local anaesthetic applied, it is relatively simple to pass a suitably large endotracheal tube between the vocal folds (see Fig. 8.5). Occasionally, the soft palate may be caught on the epiglottis; if so, the soft palate should be carefully pushed out of the way with the end of the endotracheal tube. It is tempting to use a smaller tube to facilitate intubation but this should be avoided, as it will increase the resistance to breathing. If the diameter is too large it will result in trauma to the larynx.

Placement of the tube can be facilitated by passing a narrower tube (e.g. a dog urinary catheter) through the endotracheal tube prior to placement (see Fig. 8.6). The narrow tube can be passed through the larynx more easily than the larger endotracheal tube,

then when the narrower tube is in place the endotracheal tube can be smoothly passed along the narrower tube into the trachea, and the narrower tube can then be removed, leaving the endotracheal tube in place.

Once the tube is in place it should be secured with a length of gauze bandage; care must then be taken to ensure that the endotracheal does not become occluded by kinking or become dislodged from the larynx when the cat is moved or re-positioned. When re-positioning the cat it is also prudent to disconnect the breathing system from the endotracheal tube, so that it does not scrape against the internal surface of the trachea.

Laryngeal spasm

Laryngeal spasm can occur in all species, but is particularly likely in the cat due to the highly sensitive nature of their larynx. It is more likely to occur with poor intubation technique or if extubation is delayed until after the return of the gag reflex.

If laryngeal spasm occurs, do not continue trying to intubate as this will prolong the spasm. Provide oxygen via a facemask and wait for the spasm to wane, which will usually take less than twenty seconds. After this time, examine the larynx with a laryngoscope and only try to intubate if the larynx is open. If the larynx remains closed it may be necessary to give more anaesthetic agent (beware of overdose) or a neuromuscular blocking drugs such as suxamethonium.

In an emergency, it may be possible to pass a dog urinary catheter between the vocal cords. The luer fitting at the end of the catheter will accept a 3.5 mm endotracheal tube adaptor (see Fig. 8.6) that can then be joined to an anaesthetic breathing system. If the expiratory limb of the breathing system is closed and the oxygen set to about 3 litres per minute a small jet of oxygen will be created to provide temporary

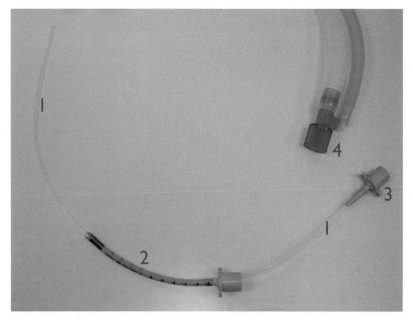

Figure 8.6 A dog urinary catheter can be used to supplement oxygen during laryngeal spasm. (1) Dog urinary catheter; (2) endotracheal tube; (3) 3.5 mm endotracheal tube adaptor; (4) anaesthetic breathing system.

oxygen support until the laryngeal spasm wanes. Passing the urinary catheter through a suitable endotracheal tube prior to placing it may facilitate intubation once the spasm has relaxed, as previously described.

Extubation

Laryngeal spasm can be initiated at the end of an anaesthetic if the endotracheal tube is not removed early enough. The tube should be removed at a rather deeper plane of anaesthesia in the cat than in the dog, and since cats are rather better at maintaining an airway, this does not seem to be problematic. The tube should be removed before the cat starts to swallow and cough as this will irritate the larynx.

Maintenance of anaesthesia

It is prudent to always supply supplemental oxygen during anaesthesia and have the facility to be able to ventilate the patient. Usually, placing an endotracheal tube facilitates this; however, in an emergency, cats may be ventilated for short periods of time with a tight fitting facemask and a suitable anaesthetic breathing system.

Maintenance of anaesthesia using inhaled anaesthetic agents

BREATHING SYSTEMS

Breathing systems for cats must have minimal dead space to reduce the potential for rebreathing of exhaled gases, and any valves must be of suitably low resistance. Table 8.3 lists the breathing systems commonly used for cats in the UK; they are all non-rebreathing systems but the more efficient systems reduce the requirements for fresh gas flow and inhaled anaesthetic agent. These breathing systems will maintain a better body temperature as well as reducing pollution and cost. The anaesthetic equipment commonly used in veterinary practice is often not sufficiently accurate at very low fresh gas flows, so it is recommended that unless capnography and a well-calibrated vaporiser is available, the total fresh gas flow should not be less than one litre per minute.

Any breathing system where the scavenging outlet is connected directly to the reservoir bag should be avoided, as it is common for the scavenging pipe to twist, occluding the expiratory limb. This prevents the cat from exhaling and can overinflate the lungs with potentially fatal consequences. Modifications of the Ayre's T-piece are available which incorporate a low resistance

Table 8.3 Breathing systems for use in the domestic cat and suggested fresh gas flows

Breathing system	Total Fresh Gas Flow	Suitable for IPPV	Picture
Modifications of Ayre's T-piece (including Intersurgical's Mapelson F)	400 ml/kg	Yes	
Mini-Lack (Burtons Medical Equipment Ltd.)	200 ml/kg	No	
Humphrey's ADE (Arnold's Veterinary Products Ltd.)	200 ml/kg	Yes	

NB: Total fresh gas flow should not be less than one litre per minute unless a capnograph and an accurately calibrated vaporiser is available.

adjustable pressure limiting (APL) valve before the reservoir bag allowing more convenient scavenging and greater safety (e.g. Intersurgical's Mapelson F, which is a T-piece with a paediatric APL valve).

INHALATION AGENTS

There are three inhaled anaesthetic agents which are currently in common use in feline clinical practice in the UK: halothane, isoflurane and sevoflurane. Despite sevoflurane (Sevoflo™, Abbott Animal Health) not being licensed for use in the cat it is rapidly gaining popularity. All of these anaesthetic drugs depress cardiovascular and respiratory function in a dose dependent manner. Halothane produces more cardiovascular depression than isoflurane, but isoflurane is a more

potent respiratory depressant and is more irritant to the respiratory mucosa. Overall there is no evidence to suggest that one agent is safer for the patient than another.

The agents vary in their potency and this is demonstrated by their different MAC values (see Table 8.4). A higher MAC value implies that more of the agent will be required to achieve the same effect, so the vaporiser will need to be set to a higher percentage. In general these agents appear to be less potent in cats than dogs.

When a premedication including acepromazine and an opioid has been used, the choice of inhaled anaesthetic agent will have little impact on the recovery time. However, the speed at which anaesthetic depth can be varied is different between the agents; sevoflurane gives the most rapid changes, and halothane the

Table 8.4 Minimum alveolar concentrations (MACs) of commonly used inhaled anaesthetic agents		
	MAC in cats (%)	MAC in dogs (%)
Halothane	0.8–1.2	0.9
Isoflurane	1.6	1.3
Sevoflurane	2.6–3.4	2.4
Nitrous oxide (N$_2$O)	255	188–222

NB: There is significant individual variation, so all of these drugs must be titrated to effect.

slowest. This potential advantage of sevoflurane is only useful if someone is able to pay close attention to the patient's depth of anaesthesia at all times.

Nitrous oxide is not suitable as a sole anaesthetic agent as it is impossible to achieve a high enough alveolar concentration. Its analgesic efficacy in cats varies between individuals, but will be non-existent when it forms less than 70% of the fresh gas flow.

Maintenance of anaesthesia using injectable anaesthetic agents

In cats there are limited safe options for prolonging anaesthesia using injectable agents. Saffan™ may be given as either 'top up' doses or as an infusion to prolong anaesthesia. Propofol is less than ideal for use in incremental doses or as a continuous rate infusion in

cats (see p. 182) and administration of incremental doses of thiopental results in a prolonged recovery.

Monitoring anaesthesia

The small size of the domestic cat can present a number of difficulties with regard to monitoring the patient during anaesthesia. The cat is frequently 'lost' under the surgical drapes, making it hard to assess the patient. An oesophageal stethoscope can be used to help monitor the heart rate from a distance; however, it will give no indication of how effectively the heart is pumping. The nurse should be constantly vigilant to ensure that surgical instruments are not being rested on the thorax, potentially impeding respiratory movement. As with all species, it is essential to constantly monitor the ABC of anaesthesia (see Table 8.5).

Repeated studies have shown that having an individual dedicated to caring for the patient during anaesthesia significantly reduces mortality. Use of a simple anaesthetic monitoring chart (see Fig. 8.7) can be very helpful in ensuring that all aspects of the anaesthetic are closely followed, as well as providing a permanent record for the clinical notes.

DEPTH OF ANAESTHESIA
The depth of anaesthesia should be monitored particularly carefully as the small size of the domestic cat means overdose of inhaled anaesthetic agent can

Table 8.5 The ABC of anaesthesia	
A = Airway	Endotracheal intubation does not guarantee an airway. The small diameter tubes frequently kink or occlude with respiratory secretions.
B = Breathing	The cat's small thoracic excursion and the surgical drapes make it difficult to observe respiratory movements. It is imperative to watch the reservoir bag carefully.
	Heat probe monitors can be placed between the endotracheal tube and the breathing system to detect ventilation. These typically emit a beep with each breath and indicate the respiratory rate. However, a near normal respiratory rate does not ensure that ventilation is adequate. Hypoventilation during inhaled anaesthesia typically results in the patient taking a normal number of breaths per minute, but each of a small volume. Capnography is superior, as it will indicate if the cat is hypoventilating.
C = Circulation	The heart rate should be constantly monitored. Changes in the pulse volume can indicate a great deal about the circulation but these differences can be relatively difficult to detect in a patient as small as a cat. Clinically, the best way of assessing the circulation is to measure the arterial blood pressure. Generally, aim to keep the systolic arterial blood pressure above 100 mmHg (see p. 105).
	An electrocardiogram (ECG) can be used to assess the electrical activity of the heart.

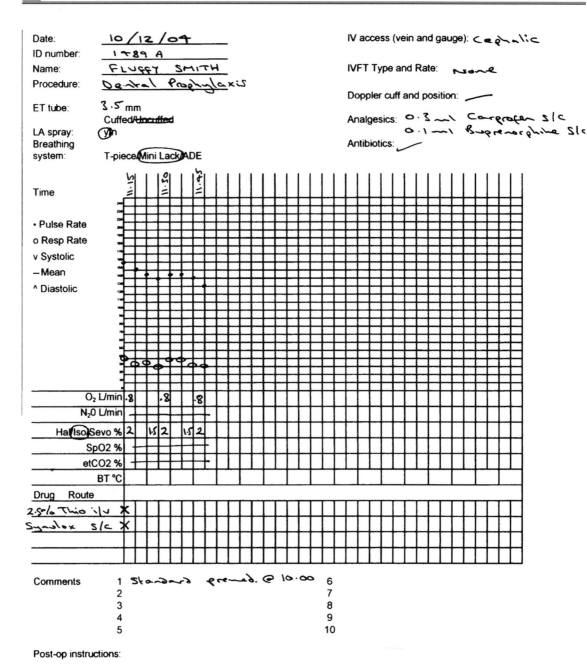

Figure 8.7 Anaesthetic monitoring chart.

develop very quickly. Furthermore, changes in the depth of anaesthesia can occur rapidly when a non-rebreathing system is used, as is typical in cats. As body temperature falls, the requirement for inhaled anaesthetic agent will also fall: if the vaporiser is not changed accordingly, then the anaesthetic plane will progressively become deeper, heading towards overdose.

Most assessments of the depth of anaesthesia are based around the degree of muscle relaxation, the presence or strength of certain reflexes and the side effects of anaesthetic drugs on the respiratory and cardiovascular system. For example, a low heart rate, respiratory rate and arterial blood pressure are usually associated with excessive anaesthetic depth, while the reverse would imply an inadequate depth. An absent palpebral (blink) reflex and relaxed jaw muscles suggest deep anaesthesia while the reflex will be brisk and the jaw tone stronger during light anaesthesia. However, none of these features are specific for anaesthetic depth and these responses vary with individuals and the anaesthetic agents used. As many features as possible must be examined before drawing any conclusions. The position of the eye is particularly useful (except when using ketamine): as anaesthesia deepens the eye will rotate downwards from a central position such that it will be hard to see the iris. The anaesthetist should be aware that at an excessive 'depth' the eye may return to a central position and so other assessments are required to clarify the situation.

FLUID BALANCE

Cats are considered to be particularly intolerant of either circulating volume excess or depletion. Ideally, any perturbation should be corrected prior to induction as fluid homeostasis will be further disturbed by anaesthesia and surgery. Upsetting this balance will have more serious consequences for old, very young and diseased patients. The use of appropriate fluid therapy can improve the outcome following anaesthesia and surgery. Of particular concern are cats with chronic renal failure; these patients will often compensate for their disease by consuming large quantities of water. As cats will often refuse food and water while hospitalised there is a major risk of further deterioration if intravenous fluid therapy is not used.

The effects of anaesthetic drugs and fluid loss on the circulation during anaesthesia and surgery can be minimised by the use of intravenous isotonic crystalloid solutions (see p. 82). The rate of administration is often arbitrarily set as 10 ml/kg/hour during the period of anaesthesia. This rate may be excessive for patients with severe cardiac disease or insufficient if significant haemorrhage occurs during surgery. The cat has a small circulating blood volume (approximately 60 ml per kilogram body weight) and even apparently minor losses can result in a significant fall in circulating volume. Blood loss during surgery should be followed meticulously; this volume should be returned to the circulation by giving additional crystalloids. If the haemorrhage is severe then the use of artificial colloid solutions or blood products should be considered.

BODY TEMPERATURE

As cats are so small they have a high surface area to volume ratio making hypothermia a common problem.

Temperature probes can be placed into either the oesophagus or rectum so that the temperature can be conveniently and continuously monitored without disturbing the surgeon by repeatedly placing a thermometer in the rectum.

Methods that can be used to conserve body temperature during anaesthesia include:

- Anaesthetising the patient in a warm environment.
- Keep clipping and the use of alcohol-containing cleaning products to a minimum.
- Place insulating material between the cat and the operating table. Positioning the cat on a warm water heating pad is considered to be ineffective, other than in providing insulation.
- Wrap any part of the cat away from the surgical site in an insulating material such as plastic bubble packing sheets ('Bubblewrap'), or a heat reflecting material, such as aluminium foil. This particularly applies to the extremities, namely the tail and legs.
- Use breathing systems that have a minimal requirement for fresh gas flow; the use of capnography may allow further reductions.
- Heat exchangers (e.g. Thermovent™, Portex) can be used between the endotracheal tube and the breathing system to reduce the loss from the respiratory tract. These must be intended for use in small patients (typically human neonates), as they will contribute to the equipment dead space.
- The air around the cat can be warmed. Ideally this should be with a forced air warmer (e.g. Bair Hugger™, Augustine Medical); examination gloves filled with hot water ('hot hands') or heated gel packs can be effective but care must be taken to ensure these do not burn the skin. When a forced air warmer is used it is not uncommon to over-heat small patients and body temperature must be continually monitored.
- The use of intravenous fluids at room temperature will have a minimal effect on body temperature (even when given at 10 ml/kg/h) compared with other losses. Nevertheless, when giving fluids rapidly it may be helpful to administer them at body temperature, using an incubator or electrical fluid warmer to pre-heat the fluid.

ARTERIAL BLOOD PRESSURE

The small size of a cat's peripheral arteries places a practical limit on which techniques can be used to monitor arterial blood pressure. The most appropriate choice is to use a non-invasive Doppler ultrasound technique (see p. 105). The ultrasound probe can be taped onto the limb, over an artery allowing repeated measurements to be conveniently taken. It is important to ensure that the occlusion cuff is empty between measurements, otherwise it will act as a tourniquet. Doppler techniques tend to underestimate the true systolic arterial blood pressure in such small patients by about 15 mmHg. Non-invasive oscillometric techniques, for example with Critikon's DINAMAP, offer a more convenient way to follow trends in arterial blood pressure; however, these machines frequently struggle to get readings on small patients such as cats. The invasive techniques of monitoring arterial blood pressure involve placing a catheter into an artery, so that the blood pressure can be measured directly. It takes great technical skill to achieve this in the domestic cat and it is usually unduly time consuming to place the catheter.

Whatever technique is used, the trend in values is more important than any one reading. In the majority of cases, hypotension results either from an overdose of anaesthetic agent or from a loss of circulating blood volume. Aim to keep the systolic blood pressure over 100 mmHg throughout anaesthesia.

Anaesthetising kittens

Kittens are at particular risk of developing anaesthetic complications due to their small size and, in very young kittens, their reduced ability to metabolise some anaesthetic and sedative drugs.

When anaesthesising kittens:

- Do not withhold food for more than 1–2 hours prior to anaesthesia as hypoglycaemia can easily develop in a short period of time.
- Ensure access to fluids until the time of anaesthesia.
- For very small kittens (less than 1 kg body weight) induce and maintain anaesthesia with an inhaled anaesthetic agent.
- Endotracheal intubation should be undertaken with great care, as it is very easy to damage the trachea and larynx. It is best avoided unless the kitten's airway is large enough to accommodate an endotracheal tube with an internal diameter of at least 2 mm.
- Always have suction ready (cut down dog urinary catheter and 5 ml syringe) to clear respiratory obstruction.
- Ensure meticulous attention to maintaining body temperature.
- Take particular care to ensure a normal circulating volume.

- Ensure that all the drugs are safe for use in such young animals.

8.4 POSTANAESTHETIC CARE AND MONITORING

Surveys reviewing anaesthetic deaths in veterinary practice have indicated that the postoperative period is associated with a high death rate in feline patients, especially when cats are left unobserved during recovery. This suggests that if a trained member of staff had been present, the problem could have been solved and the patient might have survived. The ABC of anaesthesia (see Table 8.5) should be monitored until full recovery.

Excitement

All efforts should be made to avoid an excited recovery, as this will often result in injury and produces a dramatically increased requirement for oxygen. Some patients lack the ability to increase their supply of oxygen (e.g. due to anaemia, lung or cardiac disease) and this may result in an oxygen deficit, potentially causing cardiac arrhythmias and death. While it is essential to be able to observe the patient, the recovery is more likely to be smooth if the cat is left undisturbed in a quiet environment.

The quality of the recovery will in large part be determined by what agents have been used to provide anaesthesia. Ketamine and Saffan™ based anaesthetics are particularly likely to produce 'stormy recoveries'; however, excitement can occur with any agent and someone must be available to calm the cat or provide further sedation as necessary. Postoperative pain and the application of bulky bandages will also contribute to the problem.

Hypothermia

As the cat is a small patient, it is very likely to have a low body temperature during recovery. A prolonged period of hypothermia is likely to be associated with an increased morbidity and mortality. The cat should have its body temperature monitored and be warmed if necessary, until it is able to support its own body temperature. Warming can be achieved with a forced air warmer, such as a Bair Hugger™, a warmed cage or a modified human neonatal incubator. Patients will often shiver in recovery, as they raise their temperature. This will result in a dramatically increased requirement for oxygen. Generally, preventing hypothermia is better than treating it, so steps should be taken from the time of induction to prevent heat loss.

Encouraging the cat to eat as soon as it has regained full consciousness will help to return the body temperature to normal. Local anaesthetic spray used prior to intubation has a very short duration of action and does not cause any increased risk of aspiration of food or fluid once the patient has recovered from anaesthesia.

Laryngeal oedema

Laryngeal oedema may develop some hours after a difficult intubation or extubation. It is not uncommon for a cat to appear to be recovering well from anaesthesia, and to be returned to its cage, only to be discovered dead some time later. These patients must be monitored closely, for a long period of time, paying particular attention to respiratory effort. Some authors advocate the use of short-acting corticosteroids to reduce oedema and swelling if any difficulty was experienced during intubation or extubation.

Further reading

Hall LW, Taylor PM (eds) 1994 Anaesthesia of the cat. Balliere Tindall, London.

Lamont LA 2002 Feline perioperative pain management. The Veterinary Clinics of North America. Small Animal Practice 32:747–763.

OWNER COMMUNICATION

CHAPTER 9

Paul Manning, MA VetMB MSc(VetGP) MRCVS

Communication is a vital part of the delivery of excellent veterinary care. In surveys of vets in the UK, carried out by the SPVS Masters Group and by the author, communication was strongly endorsed as being very important to both veterinary surgeons and their clients. Clients felt strongly that they judged the service they received from their vet on their ability to communicate and care, and this was rated more important than their clinical ability.

Many clients have very strong relationships with their pets and most, if not all of them, consider their pets to be members of their family. Some concerns clients have may seem unimportant to those with clinical knowledge, but finding out what those concerns are, and dealing with them in a sympathetic way is the key to gaining an excellent reputation as a caring veterinary nurse within a caring veterinary practice.

A key factor in successful communication within a veterinary practice is the enthusiasm and commitment of the entire team: nurses, vets, receptionists and administrators. It is important to remember that the nurse is one part of the whole practice team. There are many ways in which clients will receive information from the practice, but the nurse can help in reassuring the client and answering their questions or redirecting the questions back to the vet concerned with the case, or perhaps to another colleague. Ensuring that a practice has team members with good people skills is a prime requirement for the delivery of excellent care, and it seems likely that in the future more practices will select and train their team members with this in mind.

First impressions count

The communication process starts with that all important first impression: the initial telephone contact with the receptionist, the moment that the client walks into the waiting room, or even their immediate impression of the car park. Failure to make a good start can make handling both the client and the patient more difficult during a consultation, and this can impede the whole process of trying to deliver best practice. Success in making a good introduction can make all the difference to producing a successful outcome and greater job satisfaction for the dedicated nurse.

Making a good first impression involves attention to a number of 'hard issues', involving the building structure and layout of the practice, but this chapter will focus mostly on the 'soft skills' that you can develop and offer to the practices in which you work.

There is no substitute for a good bedside manner and a positive and proactive attitude to client and patient care. Good teamwork, time management and good interpersonal skills are all vitally important. Sometimes you feel that a consultation hasn't gone well, even though you have done everything 'right'. It can be difficult to understand what went wrong, until you discover that the client was already upset before they actually got into your consulting room.

The nursing team can make a very big difference to the success of any practice by ensuring that clients have already received an excellent level of service before they ever step into a consulting room. They can have an important influence on those caring actions such as discussing the client's concerns on the phone, making sure they are comfortable with their appointment time, ensuring high standards of cleanliness and tidiness in the surgery, and making sure that all clients are greeted in an appropriate manner at the reception desk.

A friendly warm greeting, using the names of the client and their cat when they arrive at the practice and when you call them in to see you are so important in getting off to a good start.

There is also a need for nurses to help with prioritising appointments where possible, and keeping nurse rotas organised to ensure that the varying needs of clients and their pets are met as far as possible within the normal constraints of time, cost and efficiency.

9.1 COMMUNICATION SKILLS

The significance of good communication in veterinary practice has been recognised in veterinary practices for many years, but its importance to the delivery of clinical excellence has only recently become widely accepted by the academic community. Previously it had largely been assumed to be a skill that must be learned by experience, not taught or measured. However the medical profession have been investigating communication skills for some time now, with vastly more resources than are available to the veterinary profession. As a result of this research the 'Calgary–Cambridge' guide to consultation technique has been developed. This detailed analysis of all aspects of a consultation includes some 70 individual 'competencies' within the medical consultation process. These competencies illustrate many aspects of the continuous stream of communication that is needed in order for the patient to receive the best treatment and for the client to have understood and appreciated what is involved. It is a very detailed analysis, but it does provide an excellent basis for the nurse or vet who is dedicated to improving their medical communication skills in order to provide the best care for their patients and clients.

The many aspects of the medical communication process are broadly divided into five key areas:

- **Initiating the session:** greeting the client and listening to their concerns.
- **Gathering information:** exploring and discussing the concerns.
- **Building the relationship:** developing support for the client. Involving them in the thought processes arising from the findings in the history and clinical examination.
- **Explanation and planning:** Involving the client in developing a plan, which is mutually acceptable to the nurse or vet and to the client.
- **Closing the session:** Summarising the main points for the client. Checking that they understand, agree with and are comfortable with the recommendations and finishing with a question such as 'Is there anything you feel you do not understand, or anything else that I can help you with?'

In all these key areas asking questions, and listening to the answers form vital components of the communication process. Learning to ask appropriate 'open' and 'closed' questions as part of the art of conversation can make a big difference to the outcome of a conversation with a client:

- An 'open' question invites the client to discuss the answer. 'How much is your cat drinking?' is an example of an open question, and it usually generates a response along the lines of 'definitely more than usual', or 'Well, actually, I hardly ever see him drinking, except from the fish pond, and I'm worried that he isn't drinking enough'.
- A 'closed' question invites a specific answer. Is your pet drinking more than normal?' is an example of a closed question, which is likely to elicit a simple 'yes' or 'no'.

Open questions allow the client to answer the question in their own way, and to add information that they feel may be helpful. However they will not always produce a definite answer, or the answer given may not be the answer to the question that was asked! A closed question gives the client less opportunity to discuss the answer, but by 'forcing' a yes/no response can sometimes produce misleading information.

It is often most useful to start by asking an open question, and then if necessary to follow it up by asking a closed question to elicit more detailed information. For example, you might start by asking 'How much is your cat drinking?' then when the client answers 'Definitely a bit more than usual' you can follow up by asking 'Do you think it is nearer quarter or half a pint of water each day?'

Closed questions may also elicit an answer that brings the conversation to a premature close. For example, if you ask 'Have you wormed your cat recently?' the client is likely to respond with either 'yes' or 'no'. That can effectively close the discussion and prevent the nurse obtaining more useful information about whether the cat is actually being wormed in accordance with the practice's recommended protocols. Asking 'How have you been worming your cat in the past 12 months?' encourages the client to tell the nurse how many times, with what product, and whether or not they would like to find a more convenient and effective solution.

The important point is that during a consultation different types and styles of questions are needed to explore each issue in a way that both the nurse and the client feel comfortable with.

Training sessions

Not everyone is a natural communicator, and nurses will need to develop their skills by observing their more experienced colleagues, and by discussing and comparing their consultations with their colleagues. This may be done in one to one sessions, in group meetings, or in any other way that the nurses find they are comfortable with. 'Role play' sessions tend to fill nurses (and vets) with horror and are not always useful if the people involved are nervous and self-conscious about acting a part.

'Semi-structured interviews' may be more useful. Here an interviewer, who can be another nurse, stands in to observe a consultation, and afterwards separately interviews the client and the nurse who did the consultation, asking each of them similar questions. This can help nurses to develop their consultation skills in ways that are user friendly, non-threatening, constructive and directly relevant to their consultations. They can also provide very useful feedback from the interviewer and the nurse and client involved. Many clients are happy to be involved in this process because there is a real perception that the practice is taking that extra bit of trouble to ensure that their clients get the best service from their practice. By participating in the training the client appreciates that they are helping to improve the service for their next visit to the practice.

The interviews will work best if plenty of planning is done. Everyone in the practice has some impact on every consultation, so the planning stages should involve nurses, vets and in fact all of the practice team. The client must also be aware of the process and be asked before their consultation if they would mind answering a few questions afterwards. Some explanation is needed to reassure all involved that the exercise is intended to be a positive learning experience. In the author's experience clients are generally kind in their comments and very supportive, so there is little to fear. If there is criticism from the client, it is normally well meant and constructive. Addressing these comments creates an opportunity for the interviewer to discuss any queries that the client may have, and to promote more of the practice products and services to provide the best care for the pet.

Some questions that might be used to open up constructive feedback and discussion are shown in Table 9.1. The questions will need to be adapted to suit the particular nature of the consultation that took place. For example, in supporting and evaluating a nurse

Table 9.1 Analysing the outcome of a 'semi-structured interview'	
Question for the client	**Question for the nurse**
Did the nurse tell you the name of the condition your pet is suffering from, or did the vet tell you this before you saw the nurse?	What was the diagnosis you understood the practice gave the client?
What treatment did the nurse say was needed?	What treatment, in detail, was recommended? e.g. Diets for obesity or oral hygiene, explanation of postoperation instructions, care of bandages, application of worming and flea products, grooming equipment and advice.
Did the nurse supply everything that you need to carry out the recommended treatment? If not why not?	Did you supply everything that the client will need to carry out the recommended treatment? If not why not?
What did the nurse say the outcome is likely to be in terms of your pet getting better?	What is the prognosis for this cat?
When does your cat need to be re-examined? Did the nurse schedule the appointment?	When does the cat need to be re-examined? Did you schedule a re-visit appointment?
How did you rate the care that the nurse and the practice gave to you and your pet? Use a scale of 1 to 5, where 1 is 'Not very helpful or supportive' and 5 is 'Excellent, really supported me and cared for my cat'.	How do you think the client would rate you on a scale of 1 to 5, where 1 is 'Not very helpful or supportive' and 5 is 'Excellent, really supported me and cared for my cat'.

weight clinic, the interviewer could ask both nurse and client how likely it is that the client will feed the recommended diet, offering options such as 'Every day without fail because the cat will eat anything', 'Will try hard but might be tempted to feed the cat's usual food if he/she does not like the diet' and 'Will try offering the diet but will not know what to do if he/she refuses to eat it the first time'.

Getting feedback

Further information can be obtained by using questionnaires for clients to complete after they have finished their visit to the surgery. The questionnaires, such as the one illustrated in Fig. 9.1, can be left in the waiting room, on the reception desk, sent out with booster reminders, or handed to clients individually by vets, nurses or receptionists. Provide a box in the waiting room for the completed replies, which may make interesting reading.

9.2   NURSING CONSULTATIONS

Every practice has a cost base which influences the number of nurses they can employ, but nurses who demonstrate their value to the practice help to reinforce the investment that the practice is making in them and simultaneously help to improve the standards of care that are being delivered.

Nurses have a very important role to play in caring for distressed owners and their pets in emergencies and bereavement situations. Efficiency in organising time and readiness to help are vitally important for the practice working hard to provide the best of care.

Veterinary nurses and their employers often make subconscious judgements about their worth, and often tend to undervalue the contributions that the VNs can make if they are given the chance. Practices can and should make the best use of the veterinary nurses, and they should be valued team members. Some enlightened doctors are of the opinion that, while the doctors make the diagnoses it is the nurses that get the patients better.

Some veterinary nurses are much more confident and happy to do consultations than others, and that does not always depend on age or experience. Some love talking to clients about their pets, and only need some honing of their skills. Some are very shy or lack confidence and have plenty of knowledge but need encouragement to talk. A trainee VN once told me she had no confidence in her knowledge or ability and this

was preventing her from taking on basic nursing consultations. I shared a thought that she could compare what she had learned in her two years of training with what a checkout assistant who had worked in a pet superstore for the same period of time would know about pet health. My trainee had no hesitation in replying that she knew 'a LOT more', and this was the start of her realisation of what she had to offer and what she could be contributing in her role as a student veterinary nurse.

Covering all the issues

It is not always possible, and indeed it is highly unlikely, that every nurse in a practice will be skilled in all types of consultation, and even the most experienced nurses can occasionally slip up. So it can be helpful to have a 'crib sheet' of the subjects that need to be covered in each of the main types of nursing consultation, including lists or sequences of general questions to suit the different types of consultation.

Questionnaires can also be used effectively to prompt clients and nurses to ask the questions that will get the best out of the consultation. Table 9.2 lists some of the questions that might be included for different nursing consultations. The receptionists can ask the client to fill in these questionnaires while they are waiting to be seen, so they are valuable both in the content of the answers and in saving the nurse time that can be better spent in the consultation, explaining the issues and the importance of the obesity diet, the dental care or the postoperative care etc.

9.3   ADMISSION PROCEDURE

Owners of animals being admitted to the practice are likely to be feeling very anxious indeed and they will often find it difficult to take in everything that is happening, or being said to them. From the point of view of the veterinary practice it is essential that clients have understood the procedures that are to be performed, the risks involved and the likely cost of those procedures. However the key question for the client at this critical time is often 'is my cat going to die?' and this one point may preoccupy their mind so much that they cannot take in anything other than the advice that relates to the safety and high standard of care that the nurse is offering to them.

It is therefore very important that good preparation is done in the time leading up to the admission and that as much as possible is discussed and explained ahead of time. The consultation at which

At XYZ veterinary practice our aim is to provide you with an excellent level of service and support. To help us to continue to improve our service to you we would be grateful if you could take a few moments to complete this questionnaire.

To show our appreciation we will be happy to donate 20p to your chosen animal charity. Please circle the charity of your choice:

RSPCA / Cats Protection / PDSA/ Animal Ambulance / Local Wildlife Rescue Centre

QUESTIONNAIRE
Please write your answers in the space provided, or circle the appropriate choice

Background Information

1) How long have you been a client of ours?
_____

2) Where did you hear about us?
_____

3) Which animal did we treat on this visit?
_____

4) What day of the week was this visit?
_____

On this visit, was the surgery: VERY BUSY / BUSY / STEADY / QUIET

Hospitality

1) When making the appointment did you find the service:
        EXCELLENT / GOOD / SATISFACTORY / POOR

2) When you arrived for your appointment did you find the greeting
        EXCELLENT / GOOD / SATISFACTORY / POOR

3) How long did you have to wait before your appointment?
        Less than 5 mins / 5-10 mins / 10-20 mins/ 20-30 mins / More than 30 mins

4) If you were kept waiting for longer than 30 minutes were you given progress reports via reception?   YES / NO

Any further comments ?_____
_____

Consultation

1) Was the quality of care for your pet:
        EXCELLENT / GOOD / SATISFACTORY / POOR

2)Was the understanding of your pet's problem
        EXCELLENT / GOOD / SATISFACTORY / POOR

3) Was the transfer of information about treatment of your pet
        EXCELLENT / GOOD / SATISFACTORY / POOR

Any further comments ?_____
_____

How would you rate our staff for
1) Appearance: EXCELLENT / GOOD / SATISFACTORY / POOR
2) Friendliness: EXCELLENT / GOOD / SATISFACTORY / POOR
3) Knowledge: EXCELLENT / GOOD / SATISFACTORY / POOR
4) Compassion: EXCELLENT / GOOD / SATISFACTORY / POOR
5) Helpfulness: EXCELLENT / GOOD / SATISFACTORY / POOR
6) Clarity of explanation: EXCELLENT / GOOD / SATISFACTORY / POOR

Taking into account all of the above how would you rate the service you received?
        EXCELLENT / GOOD / SATISFACTORY / POOR

Would you be happy to introduce a friend?   YES / NO
How could we improve our service?
_____

_____

_____

Thank you for your help
This is a confidential questionnaire, but if you would like further information about any of the following; please circle the appropriate item(s) and fill out your name and address below.
Flea control / Diets / Worming / Dental Care / Vaccinations / Other Services we offer

Name _____

Address _____

Figure 9.1 Client feedback questionnaire.

Table 9.2 Example of a pre-consultation questionnaire

Consultation	Question	Answer
Dental health check	How often are you feeding the special diet we recommended to help care for the teeth?	(a) All of the time (b) A few days a week (c) Once a week (d) Less than once a week (e) Never
	How often have you been brushing the teeth with the toothpaste we recommended?	(a) Twice every day (b) Once every day (c) Twice a week (d) Once a week (e) Other combination (please specify)
Obesity clinic	How often does your cat eat the food we recommended for his weight problem?	(a) Every day (b) Most days (c) Once a week we manage to persuade him to eat it (d) Never
	How does he like the food?	(a) He loves it (b) He absolutely refuses to eat it (c) He quite likes it but also eats the other cat's food (d) He only eats it if we mix it with normal cat food
	How often does your cat get fed extra treats?	(a) Never (b) He sometimes pinches some of the other cat's/dog's food (c) The children feed him scraps from their plate (d) The neighbours feed him whenever he visits them
	How often does your cat spend all day indoors?	(a) Every day (b) Once a week (c) If it's raining (d) He goes out hunting every day

the inpatient procedure was first recommended is the ideal time to issue any literature about the procedure, to offer advice about preoperative procedures such as pre-anaesthetic blood tests and to inform the owner what to expect after the procedures have finished.

Estimate of costs

The owner needs to be made aware of the costs before the animal is admitted to the hospital. This is best done in the form of a written estimate of the cost of the procedure (see Fig. 9.2).

Informed consent

When the client brings their pet in on the morning of the hospital admission, it is very important to ensure that the client understands what procedures are to be done that day, whether they will involve sedation or anaesthesia, and whether there are any specific risks associated with procedure. Sometimes the client will not have fully understood the procedure that was being recommended when the vet explained it to them, so great care is needed to ensure that there is no misunderstanding at this point in time. This is what is commonly known as 'obtaining informed consent', in simple and practical terms it means that the client understands what they are signing for when they complete the consent form. It is good practice to ask the client to confirm what they think will be happening that day and to ask if they have any other requests for the day. If there is any doubt, or if the client's expectation is different to the clinical notes, the nurse should check with a vet and ensure that the correct

DESCRIPTION OF WORK PROPOSED: _____

ESTIMATED COST
This Estimate is given on the strict understanding that it is only an approximation, and that any unforeseen complications that might occur will be charged for as an additional cost.

1.	Consult Fee	£15 to £16.00
2.	Hospitalisation / Nursing Care (per day)	£11 to £35.00 × 3days
3.	Cost of operation	£50 to £350
4.	Anaesthetic costs	£20 to £60
5.	X-rays (1st / 2nd /3rd)	£30 to £60
6.	Drips	£25
7.	Injections	£6 to £50
8.	Tablets	£10
9.	Dressings	£3 to £15
10.	Blood tests	£20 to £70
	TOTAL	£200 to £800

I accept the terms and conditions as outlined above and agree that I will pay for any unforeseen charges which may occur in the treatment of my animal.

Pet's Name:
Client Name:
Address:
Signed: Date:

Figure 9.2 Example of an estimate form for non-routine operations.

procedure has been agreed upon before the client leaves the practice.

In order to ensure that the client has fully understood what is being done it can be helpful to include a checklist of questions on the consent form (see Fig. 9.3), and to offer the client time in the waiting room to read through the consent form before the consultation for the hospital admission. This gives the anxious client some quiet time to think a little about what is happening, and to prepare for that tense moment when they will leave their pet in the hospital. It also provides a head start on filling out the consent form because the basic information will already have been supplied such as:

- Have you been provided with an estimate of costs?
- How are you planning to pay?
- Where/how can we contact you through the day?

This makes more time available to ask the really important clinical questions such as 'which lumps/ teeth are you expecting us to remove?' and 'do you understand the potential risks?'

Contact details

When admitting an animal into the hospital it is important to make sure that arrangements are made to contact the owner at appropriate times. This allows the

practice to discuss any unexpected findings or complications, but it is also extremely important for the anxious client to be kept informed about what is happening to their pet through the day. Important points include:

- Contact details for the day – take down as many numbers as possible, including home, work and mobile numbers as appropriate.
- Times during the day that the client will be available on each number, and any periods during which the owner will be unavailable to speak.
- Anticipated time that the outcome of the procedure can be discussed or that the results of any tests will be available.
- Suggested time at which the client can call the practice to find out how things are going and/or to arrange a time to collect their pet.

Remember that for even the most routine procedure the concerned client will want to know how soon they can find out how everything went. Some clients are so worried that they would like to be telephoned at each stage, especially at the completion of an operation, to let them know that their pet has made it through that important stage. If this is the case, make sure that it has been clearly agreed with the client when they will be contacted and make sure that the vet in charge of the case knows that this agreement has been reached. It is

Client name:
Client address:

Animal name:
Animal breed:

Operation / Procedure _____

I hereby give permission for the administration of an anaesthetic to the above animal and to the surgical operation detailed on this form, together with any other procedures, which might prove necessary.

I understand that all the anaesthetic techniques and surgical procedures involve some risk to the animal.

I request that the practice will telephone me, on the number(s) shown below (delete as appropriate):

- After any investigations but before any surgery is carried out.
- If the original estimate does not include a procedure which is found to be necessary after further diagnostic work has been carried out.
- Only in the event of a decision as to whether or not the animal should be euthanased.

I confirm that (delete where applicable):

- I have received enough information for me to understand the likely costs involved. YES/NO
- I undertake to pay all fees incurred in the treatment of the above animal at the normal practice rates / I am paying for the operation with a CPL/RSPCA voucher.
- I do/do not wish a pre-anaesthetic blood test to be performed
- I do/do not wish to have my pet identichipped whilst under the anaesthetic, for the price of £XX

PAYMENT METHOD (please tick)
Cash . . .   Debit Card . . .   Credit Card . . .   heque . . .

Contact number(s) and availability

Home . . . .

Work . . . .

Mobile Phone . . . .

Name (please print clearly) . . . .

Signature . . . .

Date . . . .

Verified by . . . .

PLEASE NOTE THAT PAYMENT MUST BE MADE AT THE TIME OF COLLECTION A charge of 3% per month will be payable on any outstanding amounts. This is in no way to be taken as an offer of credit. It is an additional charge to cover our administration costs.

Figure 9.3 Example of a consent form.

good practice to try to exceed clients' expectations in this regard, for example by telephoning them to let them know that all is well, or by calling them to let them know there has been an unavoidable delay and that their cat's procedure will be happening later than predicted. Try to avoid clients telephoning at times when there is uncertainty as to the timetable or the outcome for their pet by establishing ahead of time when will be a good time to call. The real point here is that the practice needs to retain the initiative and aim to keep clients closely informed of progress. Sometimes this is impossi-

ble; the client may not be contactable by telephone at certain times or they may have 'just popped out shopping' when you make the telephone call. At the time of the admission, these points need to be borne in mind and arrangements made for telephone calls to be made at suitable times. It is very important to the client to know that at a certain time they will know the outcome of the day's procedure, and it is essential that once contact times have been agreed they are kept, even if only to report that there is no news yet and to make a new arrangement for contact.

9.4 COMMUNICATION WHILE THE CAT IS HOSPITALISED

As we have seen, arrangements should have been made at the time of the admission as to when and how contact telephone calls will be made or suitable hospital visiting times arranged. Once made, these arrangements must be observed, to protect the client from unnecessary anxiety. A telephone call or hospital visit that happens at the prearranged time is very reassuring to an owner, and is an essential part of the care being provided. These aspects of customer service offer many opportunities for the nurse and the practice to excel and to bond with the client.

Good nursing requires proactive communication, which includes a great deal of tact and empathy, and there are considerable opportunities for VNs to achieve personal success and satisfaction through taking up this challenge.

Consistency in communication

It is important for VNs to appreciate that they are part of a team which must communicate as a whole, as well as through the individuals involved in each case. Breakdowns in communication can easily arise if a client is given the wrong information, or even the right information in the wrong way. Clients often think, perhaps subconsciously, that the person they are speaking to has a seamless consistency of knowledge, qualifications and skills to be able to communicate the same message, whenever they choose to telephone or visit the practice. To avoid confusion it is essential that all members of the practice give clear information to the client about who is speaking to them and in what capacity. Compare the client's experience with a visit to a medical hospital: they would expect to see their consultant surgeon infrequently but would expect to see the nurses quite regularly every day. The human patient's needs are met, but they would not expect their nurses to know as much as their consultant and nor would they expect to receive detailed information from their consultant every time they pick up the telephone. In veterinary practice, we have some work to do in explaining the roles of the different members of the healthcare team to ensure that the clients understand us. Where possible the potential for this sort of confusion can be reduced by having a named vet and a named nurse responsible for each hospitalised case, especially those that will be in the hospital for some time. This approach minimises

the risk of confusion, and is popular with clients who like to be able to talk to the same person each time they ring, and who then build up a relationship with the person in charge of the care of their pet. This is a real aspect of personal client care that is greatly valued and appreciated by clients.

Breakdowns in communication

Breakdowns in communication can happen at any stage along the way from preparation to admission or during the hospitalisation stage, and it is the responsibility of every member of the practice team to play their part. This can be hard work and it can be frustrating, but it is an essential element of modern veterinary practice, and success in this area can make a major contribution to the feeling of satisfaction at a job well done.

Sometimes, despite all your efforts, it is not possible to make contact with the client because they are unavailable, or the wrong telephone number has been given to the nurse on admission. In this case it is good practice to record all attempted telephone calls on the clinical records so that when subsequent calls are made or received, other members of the practice can see that attempts were made to keep the client informed. Clients really appreciate these efforts, but some will tend to assume that the practice 'didn't bother' unless there is a record, which proves the practice team tried to keep in touch.

The delivery of nursing care during a patient's stay in hospital is an aspect of care that nurses take great pride in. To their credit, veterinary nurses often take this role extremely seriously and do this job very well indeed, and yet it is often undervalued by the vets, the practice as a business and even the clients. Recognition by these 'stakeholders' of the level of nursing care provided, can only be gained through excellence in communication. The term 'stakeholders' seems particularly appropriate here, because:

- For the client it is their pet's life that is at stake.
- For the vets it is their clinical success that depends on the nursing care and delivery of the prescribed treatment.
- For the practice as a business it is the recovery of the costs of treatment and of running the practice and making a return on the investment that is important.

For the nurse involved, it is often the satisfaction of knowing that they did a good job that really matters, but hard-working nurses can feel very frustrated and let down when they work through the day and sometimes during the night to care for a patient without getting any apparent appreciation from the stakeholders, whether the pet dies or the pet survives. It is difficult for a practice, or a client, to praise and thank the nursing team if they have not communicated the good job they have done or are doing for the patients in their care, and the really important point is that doing that good job depends on how well the nurse communicates with the clients, the vets and the practice team. It could be that the nurse faces all sorts of difficulties in feeling that the stakeholders have not communicated well themselves, but part of the job of a veterinary nurse involves being responsible for initiating some of the communication rather than relying on being told everything by someone else.

9.5 DISCHARGING THE PATIENT

In many practices veterinary nurses play an important role in the discharging of patients to their owners; the vet in charge of the case communicates essential information to the nursing team and relies on them to convey the message to the client.

Discharging a patient from the hospital involves the communication of a considerable amount of important information, and often involves coordinating information from different nursing and vet shifts, which can be fraught with pitfalls. Nurses cannot, and should not, be expected to give detailed clinical information about the case, because it is so easy for those messages to be misunderstood, but the nurse can provide an important caring service including:

- Gentle handling of the cat when returning it back to the relieved owners.
- Listening to, and sharing with the owners their concerns and anxieties.
- Explaining basic information about any medication, feeding, dressings and special care.

If the client has been kept well-informed during their cat's stay, with daily discussions or visits it may be assumed that there is little to add at the time of discharge. However in many cases the client will still need reassurance that they have understood everything, and duplication of the information they have already received. The client will expect this detailed information to be available, and may not anticipate that the nurse who discharges the cat only has basic

discharge notes from the vet involved. The nurse cannot reasonably be expected to know every detail of the case, or all aspects of the telephone conversation between the client and the vet earlier in the day. In this case it is reasonable for the nurse to pass on what information they do have and to offer the client the option of finding out more at the next visit to see the vet. However, conveying this message requires care and tact, to avoid giving the client a poor impression of the practice, and to ensure that the nurse does not feel inadequate.

Discharge notes and advice sheets are extremely valuable. They can contribute greatly to the practice team's efforts to deliver all of the correct information, in the correct way, to each and every individual client and for patients with a whole range of different medical or surgical problems. A discharge note from the vet in charge of the case (see Fig. 9.4) can serve as a useful check-list to the nurse responsible for discharging the patient, to ensure that all important areas are discussed. In addition a discharge advice sheet can be prepared for the client to take away with them, with a set of relevant instructions to read when they get home, and to act as a reminder of all the verbal information that has been given but which the client can too easily forget.

There is no doubt that at the moment that the cat is handed back to them, what the client needs most is reassurance and good clear instructions as to how they should be caring for their pet. At this time it is often the 'soft' skills of the nurse that are most important to the anxious client rather than the detailed diagnostic analysis from the vet. Compare the situation with the support that we hope to get from a good nurse when we, or one of our relatives are recovering from a stay in hospital. The 'care' that was taken home from the conversation with the nursing staff, feels just as valuable as the pills and advice from the consultant.

It is also important to establish when is the most appropriate time for the client to bring the pet back to the surgery for a re-check and whether this should be at an appointment with a vet or with a nurse. This will vary from case to case and is another essential piece of information that must be communicated from the vet in charge of the case to the nurse who discharges the animal, and on to the owner. Try to ensure that an appropriate appointment is made before the client leaves the surgery, as it is all too easy for the owner to forget to ring back to schedule the re-visit once they are away from the surgery.

Discharge Note for Mrs Whisker's cat Felix of 'The Cat's House', Feline Road, Moggietown.

Vet in Charge: _____

Problem: _____

Procedures Performed: _____

Working Diagnosis: _____

Likely Prognosis: _____

Vet has/has not spoken to the client after the procedures were carried out and given explanations via telephone (delete whichever applicable)

Points arising from the vet's telephone call _____

_____

_____

Client instructions:

a) care of the wound / teeth / dressings _____

_____

b) feeding instructions / prescription diets. _____

_____

c) Medications:

    Drug Name: _____

    What it's for: _____

    Dose rate: _____

d) Keep indoors / allow out until next visit (delete whichever applicable)

e) Any other instructions: _____

_____

f) Appointment for the next check-up with the vet / nurse (delete whichever applicable) _____

g) 'Is there anything I can help you with at this stage Mrs Whisker?' (LISTEN CAREFULLY and respond appropriately.)

h) Thank you for trusting us with your precious 'Felix'. We look forward to seeing you again soon. Please call at our reception desk to make your appointment for the post op check up.

i) I see that you said you would pay by credit card/cash/cheque (delete as applicable from the notes on the consent form). Reception will be happy to supply your medicines from our pharmacy as you settle your account.

Figure 9.4 An example of a discharge note for communication between the vet and the nurse.

It is very easy for important information to become confused or lost in the system of a practice, whether or not it is busy or quiet. The large number of interpersonal interactions that are required produce many opportunities for messages to be missed, or to be misunderstood. Recording information centrally, on computerised clinical records, in addition to pinning a written copy to the cat's hospitalisation cage means that whatever happens to the hard copy of the form, the nurse discharging the patient can re-print it when she needs it.

9.6 FOLLOW-UP CALLS

A valuable contribution to the care given to owners from a member of the practice can be made by picking up the telephone and calling an owner whose cat is under treatment, to check that all is well and that the owner has no new concerns. This is particularly valuable if it is scheduled for the day after any surgery or major diagnostic procedure.

A follow-up telephone call can send a powerful caring message that clients really appreciate. They may be worried about an aspect of the home-care that they would like to talk about, but which they did not feel was important enough to disturb the vet or the nurse before their next appointment. The follow-up call gives them an opportunity to ask any questions and discuss their cat's behaviour, and an unsolicited call exceeds their expectations and can encourage them to pursue the practice's home care recommendations. This leads to greater owner compliance and better care for the patient.

A little preparation is needed to ensure that the veterinary nurse making the call has an up-to-date understanding of the case notes and the plan for the care of the cat. A simple reminder system needs to be established, listing which owners are to be called, on what day, and by which nurse. Some drug companies are already starting to offer the support of a nurse to telephone owners on behalf of the practice, and this can be helpful when a practice is very busy, but it is no substitute for the individual attention that a personal phone call from the practice provides. A little time spent setting up a practical system can pay dividends; be encouraged, and get involved because that is the true hallmark of both a caring nurse and a caring practice.

9.7   CARING FOR BEREAVED OWNERS

Bereaved owners need to be offered a support system to help them through what can be an extremely traumatic and emotional time for them. When euthanasia is the final step, the care of the owner starts before their final visit to the surgery, or the home visit, and extends beyond it. Some important considerations include:

- Comfort and reassurance in the telephone call from the receptionists can help enormously.
- Schedule the appointment to allow plenty of time to reassure the owner that this is the right decision and to allow them time to express their grief. Some clients will spend up to 1 hour in the surgery during the whole process, and most owners will spend at least 20–30 minutes, so they need some space.
- Try to find out the owner's requirements for disposal of the body before they come on the day. Make sure they are aware of the costs involved when they make the decision.

- Adopt a calm and friendly but professional manner when they arrive at the practice, and ask if they would like to settle their account ahead of time, so there is no delay after the event.
- If possible use a room with easy, unobtrusive access, at a quiet time of day, so that the bereaved owner does not have to walk through a waiting room full of people. This can be distressing for the owner concerned, but also for the other people who witness their distress.
- Once the client is in a quiet consulting room, or another suitable room if these rooms are all occupied, a quiet, reassuring but competent manner is essential. Be prepared to give clear, but firm instructions in an emergency or if the cat is in pain or distressed.
- Offer the client some quiet time alone with their pet before administration of the final injection.
- Offer them the opportunity to stay with their cat, and if appropriate to hold their cat while the injection is being given.
- Many clients value some time alone with their cat after the event. It is always a good idea to offer this to them at this point when they often become emotionally overcome.

After the event a personal expression of sympathy from the practice, through a phone call or by sending a sympathy card will provide many clients with the extra reassurance that they have done the right thing. This is a distressing time for all concerned, but if handled well it can make a lasting good impression. Many clients produce thank you letters in appreciation of the care they and their cats receive at this difficult time and it reinforces all of the care that has been given.

Communication can be very hard work, and it can be under-estimated and under-appreciated within a practice, but within it lies the real heart of the matter. Above all else, clients want to know how much you care, because the vast majority of them care enormously themselves.

References

Silverman J, Kurtz S, Draper J 1998 Skills for communicating with patients. Radcliffe Medical Press, Abingdon.
Kurtz S, Silverman J, Draper J 1998 Teaching and learning communication skills in medicine. Radcliffe Medical Press, Abingdon.

INDEX